Clinical Decision Making for the
Physical Therapist Assistant
ACROSS THE CONTINUUM OF CARE

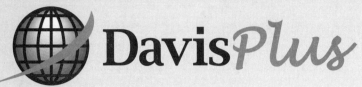 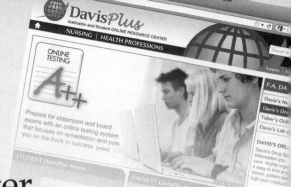

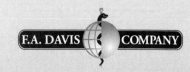

Clinical Decision Making for the Physical Therapist Assistant

ACROSS THE CONTINUUM OF CARE

REBECCA A. GRAVES, MSPT
Physical Therapist
Signature Home Health
Bellingham, WA

F.A. Davis Company • Philadelphia

F. A. Davis Company
1915 Arch Street
Philadelphia, PA 19103
www.fadavis.com

Printed in the United States of America

Last digit indicates print number: 10 9 8 7 6 5 4 3 2 1

Acquisitions Editor: Melissa Duffield
Manager of Content Development: George W. Lang
Developmental Editor: David Payne
Design and Illustration Manager: Carolyn O'Brien

As new scientific information becomes available through basic and clinical research, recommended treatments and drug therapies undergo changes. The author(s) and publisher have done everything possible to make this book accurate, up to date, and in accord with accepted standards at the time of publication. The author(s), editors, and publisher are not responsible for errors or omissions or for consequences from application of the book, and make no warranty, expressed or implied, in regard to the contents of the book. Any practice described in this book should be applied by the reader in accordance with professional standards of care used in regard to the unique circumstances that may apply in each situation. The reader is advised always to check product information (package inserts) for changes and new information regarding dose and contraindications before administering any drug. Caution is especially urged when using new or infrequently ordered 'drugs.

Library of Congress Cataloging-in-Publication Data

Graves, Rebecca A.
  Clinical decision making for the physical therapist assistant : across the continuum of care/Rebecca A. Graves.
    p. ; cm.
  Includes bibliographical references and index.
  ISBN 978-0-8036-2591-4
  I. Title.
  [DNLM: 1. Physical Therapy Modalities—Case Reports. 2. Physical Therapy Modalities—Problems and Exercises. 3. Allied Health Personnel—Case Reports. 4. Allied Health Personnel—Problems and Exercises. 5. Clinical Medicine—methods—Case Reports. 6. Clinical Medicine—methods—Problems and Exercises. 7. Decision Making—Case Reports. 8. Decision Making—Problems and Exercises. 9. Decision Support Techniques—Case Reports. 10. Decision Support Techniques—Problems and Exercises. WB 460]

  615.8´2076—dc23

2012012289

To my husband Greg for the constant support
and encouragement in so many ways
and to William and Joseph for helping me
learn more in the past 12 years as a mom
than I ever thought possible.

PREFACE

Purpose

This text was written specifically for the physical therapist assistant (PTA) student and is designed to be used across the curriculum of a PTA program and especially to complement courses in pathology. It could also be used by new graduates or PTAs who have worked in the field for some time who are looking to change practice setting or just improve their critical thinking skills. The purpose of the text is to help students learn to think critically in order to make sound clinical decisions as PTAs. These skills can be difficult to teach and difficult to learn. Using simulated real-life cases and giving students an opportunity to work through them enable students to learn these skills and apply their "head knowledge" in the clinical situations they will encounter. It is my hope that students will be able to use the tools they already have along with this textbook to help them gain confidence in making clinical decisions as a PTA.

Approach

The text uses hypothetical but probable case studies that include information typically found in a patient chart in a hospital setting, such as the physician's history and physical, physical therapy evaluation, summaries of occupational therapy and speech therapy evaluations, and nursing and social work notes. Each chapter is based on a different patient with a specific diagnosis. The cases vary in complexity depending on the number of comorbidities; any additional psychosocial, socioeconomic, cultural, or other contextual factors; and the number of settings in which the patient receives physical therapy. A table in Appendix B summarizes some of these factors to help the student see the details of a patient case quickly in order to choose appropriate cases to study. In each additional setting after the acute setting, applicable documentation that the PTA would use is included. To maintain simplicity, the term *patient* is used when referring to the patient/client, rather than *client*. With the use of the word patient rather than client, the student is reminded that the person is vulnerable and in a situation in which he or she needs the professional help of the health-care team. On the other hand, the term client can imply someone who is looking for a consultation for a problem, but is not in quite the vulnerable situation that many patients are in the hospital setting and truly can be considered a client. This use of terminology is certainly my choice and does not necessarily reflect how all physical therapy professionals view it.

Students will also note abbreviations throughout the text, many of which may be unfamiliar. Although the trend across disciplines is to use fewer abbreviations in order to facilitate improved understanding between and among disciplines, the student will still see many used in the medical chart. Perhaps in the future, abbreviations will be used less frequently. In order for students to understand the abbreviations used throughout this text, I have provided a list of abbreviations and their definitions in Appendix C. Students should remember that when using abbreviations in their documentation, they should always consult the approved abbreviations list of the facility in which they work.

Terms describing the functional levels of assistance (e.g., minimal assist, moderate assist) are used throughout this text and will be familiar to students who have started their technical portion of a PTA program. Some terms that may not be familiar include *modified independent* and *total assistance*. These terms are used primarily in the inpatient rehabilitation setting and other places where the Functional Independence Measure (FIM) is used. Modified independence generally means that a patient is independent but must use equipment such as an assistive gait device or shower bench. Total assistance means that a patient performs less than 25% of the task. In other places, the student will see the term *dependent*, which means the patient is unable to perform any of the task. As is the case in all matters of terminology, the PTA must understand the rating scale used in the facility where he or she works in order to understand how to progress the patient in functional mobility tasks.

Critical thinking questions are included in each chapter. Although they are very similar from chapter to chapter, they are included in each chapter to encourage students to think through each case individually. Space is included to write down thoughts as the student reviews each case to further facilitate learning. Students are encouraged to first think through the questions themselves, write down their thoughts, and then compare their own responses with those of their classmates, academic teachers, and/or clinical instructors. Appendix A includes my comments on Chapter 2 and comments of experienced PTAs on selected cases that can also be used to compare responses. The intention of these inclusions is to help the student see a variety of responses to selected cases, not to say that this is the only way to approach a patient. After such comparisons, students are encouraged to reflect on their own responses and modify them as necessary; then, they can consider different scenarios that might change the outcome or approach toward the patient.

Some students, especially early in the technical program, will find some questions very challenging. These will require a higher level of critical thinking. Particularly, the questions regarding the expectation of patient progression over time will be difficult considering the lack of experience that students have with patients. It will be helpful for the student to remember that he or she does not need to have all the answers and that beginning to think about these things now as a student will help them to think in more detail later. And, of course, with more experience, students and graduates will find these questions easier to think about.

Throughout the cases, students are asked to consider what they already know about a particular pathology and then find additional information presented about the case that will help them make sound clinical decisions. The text does not provide information on the pathologies themselves or physical therapy techniques; but, instead, it encourages students to learn how to use a variety of resources to help them decide how to implement the physical therapy plan of care written by the PT. Specific texts that are recommended and are referred to throughout this text are the *Guide to Physical Therapist Practice*, published by the American Physical Therapy Association in 2001; and *Pathology: Implications for the Physical Therapist, Second Edition*, written by Goodman, Boissonnault, and Fuller and published by Saunders in 2003.

Key Features of the Text

The following is a summary of key features of the text:

1. Chapter outlines that organize the information presented in each chapter
2. Learning objectives to clarify topics covered in each chapter
3. Introductions of the patient as a whole person in each chapter
4. Realistic patient case scenarios
5. Simulated medical chart information
6. Medical terminology use consistent with the APTA's *Guide to Physical Therapist Practice*
7. Cases representative of various ages, each gender, and a variety of practice settings and socioeconomic or cultural challenges
8. Questions leading the student to further develop critical thinking skills
9. Significant focus on pathology and the implications for treatment interventions
10. Photos of patients participating in a variety of physical therapy settings
11. Opportunities to practice documentation skills
12. Relevant information regarding other health-care team members and their roles as well as how they affect physical therapy interventions
13. Information on selected physical therapy specialty areas
14. Current websites that provide further information on selected topics
15. Information on protocols that are referred to in some chapters
16. Comments by an experienced PTA on selected cases
17. References that will support the students' learning, such as the APTA's *Guide to Physical Therapist Practice*

Learning Objectives for Chapters 2 through 14

The following learning objectives apply to each chapter following Chapter 1, so they are included here rather than repeated throughout.

After working through each case study, you will be able to:

1. Locate pertinent information in a simulated patient chart
2. Discuss information from a variety of health-care professionals' notes
3. Consult references to gain further information about particular pathological processes
4. Explain the relationship between physical therapy and the disease process
5. Explain the relationship of short- and long-term goals in the physical therapy POC
6. Identify appropriate interventions within the POC to use with specific patients
7. Explain when and how to modify interventions within a POC

8. Identify when and what kinds of information to communicate to the primary PT or other health-care team members to ensure safety of the patient and effectiveness of the therapy interventions

9. Practice documentation of interventions and progress notes for simulated patients

Study Tips

Some keys to getting the most out of this text are highlighted here. Feel free to be creative in your use of the text to facilitate your learning and to fit your own learning style.

- Have references available, such as a pathology text, a medical terminology reference, a drug handbook, and a laboratory and diagnostic test handbook along with other physical therapy textbooks. Two specific texts that will be referenced throughout the chapters are the *Guide to Physical Therapist Practice,* published by the APTA, and *Pathology: Implications for the Physical Therapist* by Goodman, Boissonnault, and Fuller, published by Saunders.
- Look up terms you don't know.
- Use the Internet with a critical eye for valid websites to enhance your learning.
- Make use of school and public libraries for additional information.
- Try not to get overwhelmed by the vast amount of information; focus on a single part of the case or chapter before trying to put it all together.
- Take time to review individual cases in the order given. You probably will not complete a whole case in a single study session or lab, but try to maintain the order from session to session. Perhaps you will take several weeks to finish reviewing a case. That's OK. The purpose is to strengthen your critical thinking skills, not rush through the cases. (There will come a time, though, when productivity and time management will be more important!)
- As you learn new treatment interventions and more about the implications that various pathologies have on the patients whom you work with throughout your technical program and clinical experiences, feel free to review what you have done and see if there is anything else you would add to your responses to the cases.
- Take time to review the cases on your own before you do so with others.
- Try to remember that there are a variety of ways to approach a patient.
- Challenge yourself beyond what is required and you will gain more. Make learning your own responsibility and use your instructors as resources to help you reach your goals.
- Find a mentor who can help encourage you in your professional growth and decide to become a mentor for new graduates yourself one day.
- Try to get beyond the many details and see the patient as a person, as someone you might meet one day. After all, it could be your own parent or child or yourself that needs physical therapy care.
- Ask a lot of questions and listen to the answers; try to answer some of your own questions first before you ask them.
- Learn from your mistakes.
- Focus on what you need to know and finding that information quickly from the patient's chart.
- Enjoy your chosen profession. You have the opportunity to change the life of someone else. Have fun!

As you delve into the case studies and begin practicing clinical decision-making skills, please remember that this text was written to be somewhat broad in scope in that it includes a variety of patient ages, both genders, common diagnoses seen across the continuum, and a sprinkling of cultural, socioeconomic, and ethical considerations. It cannot include everything. For example, some very common pathologies are not included. Students are reminded of some of these at the end of the pathology implication questions in each chapter. Also, not all health-care team members are highlighted. Please use the cases as tools to learn critical thinking and clinical decision-making skills that can then be transferred to real cases in the clinical setting.

CONTRIBUTORS

Mariisa Bonsen, PTA
Signature Home Health
Bellingham, Washington

Jennifer Koivisto, PTA
Signature Home Health
Bellingham, Washington

Susan Schofield, BS, PTA
Whatcom Community College
Bellingham, Washington

REVIEWERS

Denise M. Abrams, PT, DPT, MA
Chairperson/Professor
Physical Therapist Assistant Program
Broome Community College
Binghamton, New York

Marja P. Beaufait, MA, BS
Associate Professor
Physical Therapist Assistant Program
St. Petersburg College
St. Petersburg, Florida

Barbara J. Behrens, PTA, MS
Program Coordinator
Physical Therapist Assistant Program
Mercer County Community College
Trenton, New Jersey

Leigh-Anne Boggs, PTA, MAEd
Instructor
Health Sciences Department
Caldwell Community College and Technical Institute
Hudson, North Carolina

Kyndall L. Boyle, PT, PhD, OCS, PRC
Associate Professor
Physical Therapy Program
Northern Arizona University
Flagstaff, Arizona

Ann L. Charrette, PT, DPT, MS, PCS
Associate Professor
Physical Therapy Program
Massachusetts College of Pharmacy and Health
    Sciences
Worcester, Massachusetts

Karon Coupo, PT, DPT, MSEd
Faculty
Physical Therapist Assistant Program
Keiser University
Orlando, Florida

Maria Holodak, PTA, MEd
Associate Professor
Physical Therapist Assistant Program
Broward College
Coconut Creek, Florida

Adrienne R. Parry, PT, DPT
Teaching Assistant
Physical Therapy Program
AT Still University
Tucson, Arizona

Carrie Perkins, PTA
Physical Therapist Assistant Program
Mohave Community College
Lake Havasu City, Arizona

Julie A. Plake, MS, CCC-SLP
Speech Language Pathologist
Rehabilitation Department
San Juan Rehab
Anacortes, Washington

Maureen Raffensperger, PT, DPT, OCS, MS
Director
Physical Therapist Assistant Program
Missouri Western State University
St. Joseph, Missouri

Donnalee Shain, PT, MS, DPT
Chair
Physical Therapist Assistant Program
Bay State College
Boston, Massachusetts

Jackie Underwood, PTA, MS
Online Instructor
Physical Therapist Assistant Program
San Juan College
Farmington, New Mexico

Debbie Van Dover, PT, MEd
Program Director, Instructor
Physical Therapist Assistant Program
Mt. Hood Community College
Gresham, Oregon

Krista M. Wolfe, DPT
Director
Physical Therapist Assistant Program
Central Pennsylvania College
Summerdale, Pennsylvania

ACKNOWLEDGMENTS

This textbook has been a dream of mine since directing and teaching in the PTA program at Whatcom Community College. I am indebted to the students, faculty, and staff there who helped me realize the need for such a text.

I am grateful to my patients over the years who continue to teach me more than I can ever teach them.

My husband, Greg, provided much support in the way of helping with so many things from housework to caring for two rambunctious boys, allowing me to spend the time I needed on the book along the way. Working with him to obtain photos of real patients doing real therapy for the textbook was a fun part of the project, and I appreciate his willingness to help in that way.

My sons William and Joseph helped, too, by being patient and finding things to occupy their time while "Mom" was working on the book. Thanks, boys.

I thank my mother Suzanne Boyer, sisters Debby White and Lori Bridges, and my father- and mother-in-law Ken and Irene Spady also for their continued support and interest in my project along the way. My father-in-law, Dr. Spady, a retired family practice physician, put in many hours reviewing the medical aspects of the text, and for this I am deeply appreciative.

For her technical help in learning how to use my new version of Word and my new laptop, I thank Della Wisdom, my kids' computer teacher at school.

To those who helped arrange many patient encounters to be photographed at different facilities, I especially thank Daisy Garvey, PT, the staff of the cardiac rehab department, physical therapy and other rehab staff, and Linda Wright at Skagit Valley Hospital in Mt. Vernon, WA; Susan Brownrigg and the physical therapy staff at Peacehealth St. Joseph Medical Center in Bellingham, WA; Alice Stride at Cornerstone Prosthetics and Orthotics in Mt. Vernon, WA; Sheila Von Bergen, PT, Becky Rice, PT, and the physical therapy staff at Northsound Physical Therapy in Stanwood, WA; John McWilliams, owner of Bellingham Physical Therapy in Bellingham, WA; Rick Schafer, owner of Cascade Physical Therapy in Sedro Woolley, WA, along with the many patients who were willing to be photographed during a vulnerable and often painful time in their lives.

For general advice and suggestions for the case studies themselves, I wish to thank Linda Thomson, OT; Jennifer Sakamoto, PT; Margaret Anderson, PT; Connie Rockstad, RN, MSN; Kathy Kraynack, PT; Loni Carambot, OT; Julie Plake, SLP; James Walsh, Special Education Teacher; and Dr. Tracy Ouellette, MD.

The physical therapist assistants who took time to put into writing their own thoughts about several of the cases to include in Appendix A are Susan Schofield, PTA; Mariisa Bonsen, PTA; and Jennifer Koivisto, PTA. Their contributions were invaluable.

I thank my friend Alma Sasser, PT for showing me that physical therapy might be a good choice of careers back when I was in high school.

I owe a big thanks to my friend Katie Walker, PT for encouraging me and mentoring me when I was a new grad and as I transitioned into teaching in the PTA program. Before she lost her battle with breast cancer, she taught me so much about how to be a mother to two growing boys and how to provide for my family's needs while growing in my chosen career.

I thank the editors at F. A. Davis for their help and encouragement in the long process of writing and revising this textbook, especially Melissa Duffield for her constant encouragement and David Payne who helped to revise many parts and make them more understandable to the readers, as well as those who will be helping to finish this book.

Lastly, I wish to thank God, the Creator of life and the human machine, for such a magnificent topic of study. Through the years I have become amazed at the way the human body is able to function and heal itself despite the many stresses we place on it. I could not have completed this textbook without God's help and direction in all aspects of my life all along the way.

CONTENTS

Essentials of Clinical Decision Making

CHAPTER OUTLINE

Introduction

To be a successful PTA, you must know more than just muscle attachment sites, how to perform different kinds of transfers, and how to perform an electrical stimulation intervention. You must know how to apply your book knowledge to the clinical world of patients and their problems, a process we call clinical problem solving. This chapter helps you prepare for this role of clinical problem solver by providing an overview of some foundational concepts that you will use throughout the book in making clinical decisions related to specific patients. We first consider the role of the PTA in the plan of care. Next, we cover what documentation you must complete as part of this role. Evidence-based practice and its relevance to you will be explained, as well as the purpose and content of the *Guide to Physical Therapist Practice*. Finally, you will be introduced to the concept of clinical problem solving and how it relates to the role of PTA.

The Role of the PTA in the Plan of Care

One critical aspect of your education as a PTA is an understanding of how your role fits in to the overall POC for a patient. Central to this role is the relationship between the PTA and PT. The APTA describes the ideal PT/PTA relationship as one that is "characterized by trust, mutual respect, adaptability, cooperation, and an appreciation of individual and cultural differences."[1] Furthermore, it involves "effective communication," as the PT directs and supervises the PTA, who is helping to provide the physical therapy services.

This communication is two-way and requires not only effective speaking and delegating by the PT but also active listening skills. At the same time, the PTA must be able to speak out when necessary, especially when patient safety is at risk, but also listen closely and follow directions given.

The responsibilities associated with the role of the PTA are recommended by the APTA in its documents, including the *Guide to Physical Therapy Practice* (the *Guide*) and the Standards for Ethical Conduct of the Physical Therapist Assistant, which this text reinforces. The APTA describes in the *Guide* the preferred patient/client management process as one that includes the following components of care:

- Examination
- Evaluation
- Diagnosis
- Prognosis
- Intervention
- Outcome

The only portion of the process that may be delegated to a qualified PTA is that of intervention. The *Guide* describes intervention as the "purposeful and skilled interaction of the PT with the patient/client and, if appropriate, with other individuals involved in care of the patient/client, using various physical therapy methods and techniques to produce changes in the condition that are consistent with the diagnosis and prognosis."[2]

So, as a PTA, your job is to provide the interventions and data collection as delegated by the supervising PT to help the patient achieve the goals set forth in the

POC. What does this mean and what does it look like in the clinical setting? In all settings across the spectrum, the PT first collects data from the history and examines the patient. He or she then evaluates the patient, determines the diagnosis and prognosis, and then writes goals and a plan for meeting those goals. This information is generally found in the initial documentation, sometimes (and also in this text) referred to as the initial "evaluation." Different facilities use different formats. In addition to short- and long-term goals, the POC should have a list of interventions to be used as well as the planned frequency and duration for the physical therapy "episode of care." The PTA must review the initial documentation, including the POC, and decide which interventions to use during the first and subsequent sessions, how best to sequence those interventions within a session, and the appropriate tests and measurements to use to measure progress toward the goals as well as patient response to the interventions used. The session must then be documented according to facility policy. The PTA may modify the approach and the sequencing of specific interventions as long as they are within the POC written by the supervising PT. Modifications within the POC are generally for the purpose of ensuring patient safety and comfort or to progress the patient toward the goals.

What if you, as the PTA, find something within the POC that you question? What if you are asked to do something you are not trained in? What if you observe a change in the patient's status that might indicate a need for the supervising PT to reassess the patient? After communicating your concerns with the PT, he or she will decide whether to reassess the patient and modify the POC if needed. Although it is the responsibility of the PT to modify or change the POC, input from you is vital to the process. Although the PT expects that you will closely follow the POC, making modifications in approach as needed and communicating to him or her any changes in patient status, remember that it is your responsibility to provide only care that is within your scope as a PTA and for which you are trained.

Beyond legal and ethical considerations, there are likely as many ways that PTAs are utilized in the clinical setting as there are clinical settings. Each individual PT and PTA, who work together and within a group of other therapists and health-care team members, brings a unique set of background and experiences that make the relationship unique. In all, one of the most important aspects of the PT/PTA team and relationship is that of communication. Effective written and verbal communication will not only enhance your working environment but will also allow you to provide the safest, most effective interventions for the patient. Besides one on one direct communication, much of the communication between PT and PTA occurs within the documentation of patient care.

Documentation

After providing a physical therapy intervention, how will you document it? In this text, you will be given opportunities to practice documenting your physical therapy interventions and the patient's response to those interventions. Sometimes it seems to take more time and effort to document your interventions accurately than to provide them in the first place. You are probably learning about the basics of documentation and, in particular, the SOAP format. In addition, some therapists and clinical settings are now using a format that more closely follows the patient client management model described in the *Guide*. In addition, the APTA also has published guidelines for documentation that can be helpful as you put into practice what you are learning in your technical PTA program. Please refer to your documentation textbook for detailed instructions on how to document in your classes; it is recommended that you use these same guidelines when using this text. During your clinical classes, you should also follow each facility's guidelines. Usually, these different formats are designed to meet requirements of third-party payers such as Medicare.

Other differences you will see in documentation involve whether and how much technology is used. You must be able not only to use the technology to write your notes but also to access, read, and understand the information provided. Many facilities still use handwritten notes, although often the PT's initial documentation will be transcribed and provided in a typed format. You may also be asked to dictate your daily or progress notes so that they can be transcribed and signed later before being placed in the patient chart. More and more facilities, both inpatient and outpatient, are now using computerized documentation software. Hospital settings may have all disciplines computerized; this allows easier access by the therapy staff to notes written by physicians, nurses, occupational and speech therapists, and other health-care providers. Some even provide access to digital imaging pictures as well as the imaging summary results, latest laboratory results, and other important information used in planning a physical therapy session. As you practice documentation for the case studies in this text, remember that often you will need to modify any format used to fit the requirements of the facility in which you work. Also remember that documentation in the real-world clinical setting can be more challenging than it is in the classroom. However, maintaining high standards in documentation is critical not only for legal reasons and limiting liability but also, more importantly, to ensure a high-quality service to our clients and patients.

What kinds of notes will you write? Primarily, you will document the daily notes, recording each physical therapy session. In addition, in some settings, PTAs document interim progress notes addressing the patient's progress toward the goals set forth in the POC. The need for various kinds of notes to be cosigned by the supervising PT varies from state to state.

Documentation can also promote problem solving. Using the format of the patient progress note can help organize your thinking and help you to make sound decisions as you provide the interventions for your patients.

Evidence-Based Practice

One important role of documentation is that of demonstrating the patient's progress or lack of progress toward the goals. Your documentation is crucial in helping the PT understand where the patient is in relation to the goals. Another term used for measuring this progress through the use of tests and measures is outcome measurement. Third-party payer requirements over recent years have necessitated increasingly stringent outcome measurement. Although sometimes challenging to meet, these requirements have benefited the patient greatly by helping to hold PTs and PTAs to a higher standard of care.

The accurate reporting of the outcomes of your interventions with patients demonstrates the evidence that the patient is or is not improving. This information helps you decide whether to stay with the current interventions or try something else within the POC. It also helps the PT make decisions about continuing physical therapy or recommending withholding physical therapy altogether until further examination by the patient's physician.

When you measure or test a patient's impairment or function, provide an intervention, and then retest or measure, you are participating in outcomes research on an individual scale. On a much larger scale, we refer to this as evidence-based practice. This term refers to all the evidence we have that a specific intervention will or will not work for a select patient. This evidence includes

research articles such as those that report random controlled trials, or RCTs, in professional publications. Case studies found in professional journals also help clinicians determine which interventions are the best to use with a particular patient problem. Expert opinion, too, is considered a part of evidence-based practice. Finally, patient values and preferences related to various physical therapy interventions are used to determine appropriate interventions. For example, if both superficial heat and cold modalities can address a particular goal and both are included in the POC, the PTA may use patient preference of heat over ice to determine that moist heat packs may be the best choice in a given situation.

All of the above types of evidence are used at various points during each patient's episode of care by both PT and PTA. PTAs must be aware of current research and the effectiveness of various interventions on the different types of patients they work with; they must also use judgment and consider the other types of evidence when selecting interventions. Above all, they must choose interventions that are within the POC written by the PT.

You are probably learning within your technical program about the different resources available that provide access to research reports. The APTA has launched an initiative called "Hooked on Evidence" that provides opportunities for clinicians to review and post their findings on specific articles. The purposes are to compile a comprehensive review of the literature related to physical therapy and to assist clinicians with finding appropriate evidence for specific interventions used in physical therapy. There are also many search engines available to assist you in finding relevant research. Your school and public libraries can be valuable resources and should be used in addition to online resources.

What's the *Guide* All About?

You have already been introduced to the *Guide to Physical Therapist Practice*, another resource that helps PTs and PTAs decide how to approach patients. This document was written and revised by the APTA to "help physical therapists analyze their patient/client management and describe the scope of their practice." It describes four different "preferred practice patterns," which describe a variety of ways PTs manage patient problems. The language of the *Guide* is used throughout this text to promote improved communication and learning. Furthermore, each case presented in the text is listed according to the primary preferred practice pattern to assist you in connecting the cases to the practice patterns. Keep in mind that, often, the patient's diagnosis may fit more than one practice pattern. The *Guide* also provides a summary of tests and measures that are used in physical therapy to document progress as well as types of interventions. These are helpful to the PTA but can only be included in the interventions if they are a part of the POC written by the PT for the patient/client. Another purpose of the *Guide* is to help standardize terminology to improve communication between the physical therapy profession and third-party payers.

Clinical Problem Solving for the PTA

So, how do you put this all together to help learn to solve clinical problems as a PTA? Among other components, problem solving involves critical thinking. Many authors have described a variety of ways of understanding what critical thinking is and how to develop this crucial skill. Alfaro-LeFevre, in her book, *Critical Thinking and Clinical Judgment*, written for nursing students, summarizes various descriptions of traits that people have who are able to think critically.[3] Important traits for you, as the PTA, include the following:

- An understanding of your own limitations
- The ability to admit when you do not know something
- A willingness to ask questions and be open-minded to learning new things
- The ability and willingness to seek new knowledge through a variety of sources
- Creativity
- Flexibility
- The ability to engage in ongoing self-assessment and reflection on decisions made to learn from prior experiences

Alfaro-LeFevre also describes factors that usually enhance critical thinking. Factors that typically enhance critical thinking include the following:

- Moral development and fair-mindedness
- Being older with greater life experience (remember, this is typically true)
- Having some self-confidence and emotional intelligence
- Knowledge of problem-solving, decision-making, and research principles
- Effective communication and interpersonal skills
- Habitual evaluation
- Effective writing, reading, and learning skills
- Knowledge of related factors
- Awareness of resources

- Positive reinforcement
- Presence of motivating factors

However, those with the following characteristics will likely have a more difficult time thinking critically and making sound clinical decisions:

- Being prejudiced and biased
- Having an unhealthy lifestyle
- Undergoing a high level of anxiety, stress, or fatigue
- Having time limitations or environmental distractions

Students who wish to practice and improve their critical thinking skills and enhance their ability to make sound clinical decisions would do well to consider how these traits and characteristics can be developed in their own lives and in other areas outside of physical therapy.

The nursing profession has published the majority of clinical research in the field of critical thinking and decision making related to health care, much of which does apply to PTA students and the physical therapy profession. In addition to resources outside of the field of physical therapy, PT professionals also have studied critical thinking and clinical decision making, primarily in the setting of physical therapy education programs, not PTA programs. Again, the findings can be applied to all clinicians who want to improve in this critical area of professionalism. The APTA has developed resources to assist PTA students and graduates in improving their critical thinking and problem-solving skills. Figure 1-1 depicts a problem-solving algorithm developed by the Education Section of the APTA to help describe the process used by PTAs in patient/client interventions. Controlling assumptions are included to help understand and apply the information.

It is important to understand that the PTA is trained and able to make decisions at the level of intervention only. The PT performs all the other aspects of the patient and client management model. As you review this algorithm, notice the important instances in which the PTA will need to communicate with the supervising PT:

- To clarify, as needed, the interventions to be used in the POC
- When the patient's condition has changed from that when the POC was written
- If the patient or client is not safe or comfortable during the selected interventions and your modifications within the POC have not helped
- If there is no progress toward the goals and your modifications within the POC have not helped the patient to progress toward the goals
- When a goal or more than one goal has been met

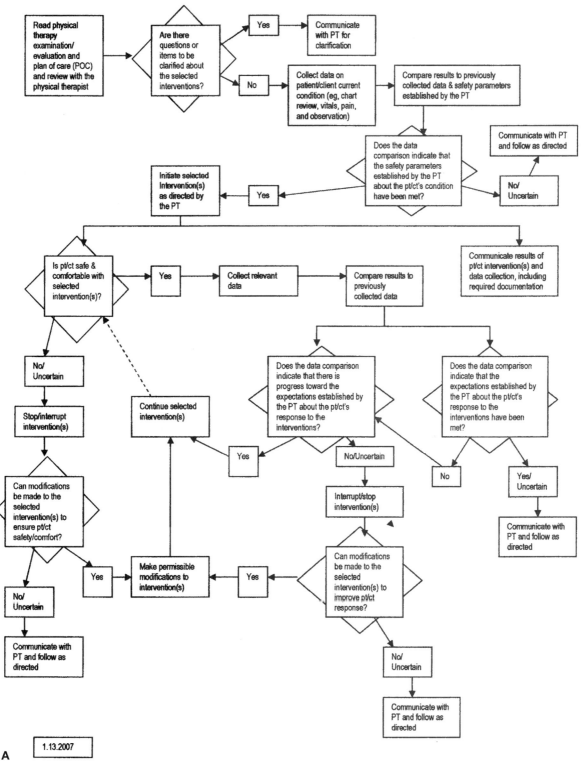

FIGURE 1-1 A problem solving algorithm. *Reprinted with permission from the American Physical Therapy Association. (cont'd)*

Problem Solving Algorithm Utilized by PTAs in Patient/Client Intervention

This algorithm, developed by APTA's Departments of Education, Accreditation, and Practice, is intended to reflect current policies and positions on the problem solving processes utilized by physical therapist assistants in the provision of selected interventions. The controlling assumptions are essential to understanding and applying this algorithm. (This document can be found in *A Normative Model of Physical Therapist Assistant Education: Version 2007.*)

Controlling Assumptions

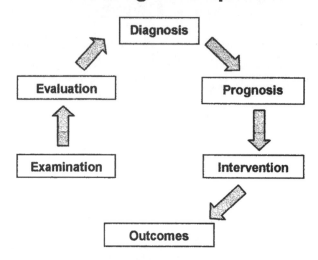

- The physical therapist integrates the five elements of patient/client management – examination, evaluation, diagnosis, prognosis, and intervention – in a manner designed to optimize outcomes. Responsibility for completion of the examination, evaluation, diagnosis, and prognosis is borne solely by the physical therapist. The physical therapist's plan of care may involve the physical therapist assistant to assist with selected interventions. This algorithm represents the decision making of the physical therapist assistant within the intervention element.

- The physical therapist will direct and supervise the physical therapist assistant consistent with APTA House of Delegates positions, including Direction and Supervision of the Physical Therapist Assistant (HOD P06-05-18-26); APTA core documents, including Standards of Ethical Conduct for the PTA; and federal and state legal practice standards; and institutional regulations.

- All selected interventions are directed and supervised by the physical therapist. Additionally, the physical therapist remains responsible for the physical therapy services provided when the physical therapist's plan of care involves the physical therapist assistant to assist with selected interventions.

- Selected intervention(s) includes the procedural intervention, associated data collection, and communication, including written documentation associated with the safe, effective, and efficient completion of the task.

- The algorithm may represent the thought processes involved in a patient/client interaction or episode of care. Entry into the algorithm will depend on the point at which the physical therapist assistant is directed by the physical therapist to provide selected interventions.

- Communication between the physical therapist and physical therapist assistant regarding patient/client care is ongoing. The algorithm does not intend to imply a limitation or restriction on
B   communication between the physical therapist and physical therapist assistant.

FIGURE 1-1 —cont'd

Anyone interested in developing critical thinking and clinical problem-solving skills would do well to first learn more about the topic, develop the ability to make careful observations and ask thoughtful questions, learn to use resources efficiently and regularly, and participate in self-assessment that includes reflection on the way one thinks. It is important to "think about thinking" and, thus, learn to think more critically. Above all, sticking with the process for the "long haul" is important to continue learning and growing; this is expected of everyone in the health-care professions by the patients and families that we serve. In fact, there is no greater reason to develop these skills than to be able to provide the highest-quality health care possible within each different setting or circumstance. Pursue excellence in all that you do. There is great satisfaction in knowing you are doing your best work and that your work with patients is changing lives forever.

References

1. American Physical Therapy Association: Policy and Procedures for the Outstanding Physical Therapist/Physical Therapist Assistant Team Award BOD Y06-08-02. Retrieved February 2010. Available at: http:www.apta.org.

2. American Physical Therapy Association: Guide to Physical Therapist Practice, Second Edition. Alexandria, VA: Author, 2001.

3. Alfaro-LeFevre R: Critical Thinking and Clinical Judgment: A Practical Approach. St. Louis: Saunders, 2004.

CHAPTER 2

Mr. Anderson: A Patient With Myocardial Infarction

 Preferred Practice Pattern: Cardiovascular/Pulmonary, Pattern D

CHAPTER OUTLINE

Introducing Mr. Anderson

Mr. Anderson is a patient who just suffered a myocardial infarction. According to the APTA's *Guide to Physical Therapist Practice* (the *Guide*), he could have a number of impairments, including the following:

- Abnormal heart rate or pulmonary response to increased oxygen demand
- Impaired aerobic capacity
- Flat or falling blood pressure in response to increased oxygen demand

He could have functional limitations such as decreased ability to perform ADLs because of symptoms.[1] Please refer to the *Guide* for a complete list of possible impairments and functional limitations. As you work through this case, think about which of these the patient is experiencing.

Vocabulary List

Diaphoresis	Gallops
Nitroglycerin	Hepatosplenomegaly
Auscultation	Ascites
Wheeze	ST elevation
Rales	Troponins
Rhonchi	Acute coronary syndrome
S1, S2, S3, S4	Acute ST segment elevation
Murmurs	Coronary angiography
Rubs	

PHYSICIAN'S HISTORY AND PHYSICAL

PATIENT NAME: Herbert F. Anderson
ADMIT DATE: March 7, 2010
BIRTH DATE: Jan. 14, 1959
SEX: Male
ROOM/BED: 418-02
MEDICAL RECORD #: 12345678
CHIEF COMPLAINT: Chest pain
ATTENDING: Dr. Janice Harvey, DO

HISTORY OF PRESENT ILLNESS: This 51-year-old male reports that about 4 hours earlier today he experienced sudden-onset chest pain, shortness of breath, and fatigue. He states he has been out of shape and decided to start an exercise program by running about 1 mile, during which he noted symptoms and returned home. He reports no loss of consciousness and that his wife called 9-1-1 when he experienced a crushing pain in his chest. He was worried he was having a heart attack and did take an aspirin. He complains of left shoulder and jaw aching. He denies any palpitations or lightheadedness leading up to this incident but did have **diaphoresis**, nausea, and a feeling he might vomit; otherwise, he had no other symptoms. He has not had any prior similar symptoms.

PAST MEDICAL HISTORY: The patient's medical history is significant for obesity, HTN, and appendectomy. He has not had any lipid studies and has not seen a doctor, he reports, in more than 10 years.

ALLERGIES: NKDA
No known Drug allergies

MEDICATIONS: The patient is not currently taking any medications.

FAMILY HISTORY: Both parents died in their early 60s of cardiac arrest, and the father also had DM II. A brother had an MI in his 50s.

SOCIAL HISTORY: The patient is married with two teenaged children living at home. He smokes 1 pack of cigarettes per day and drinks about 2 beers per day. He denies use of other drugs. He works as a car salesman.

REVIEW OF SYSTEMS: See HPI; otherwise, negative

PHYSICAL EXAMINATION: VITAL SIGNS: Temperature 36.6°C, pulse 71 BPM, respiratory rate 22 respirations per minute, blood pressure 99/72 mm Hg, O_2 saturation 98% on 2 LPM supplemental O_2 via nasal cannula. GENERAL: Alert and oriented, resting in exam room; chest pain has been relieved with **nitroglycerin.** SKIN: Warm and dry without rash or jaundice. Bruising at right shoulder and face. HEENT: Unremarkable NECK: Unremarkable LUNGS: Clear to **auscultation** bilaterally without **wheeze, rales,** or **rhonchi.** No dullness to percussion. Normal diaphragmatic excursion. CARDIAC: Normal S1, S2. No S3, no S4. No **murmurs, rubs,** or **gallops.** ABDOMEN: Nontender, nondistended with positive bowel sounds. No **hepatosplenomegaly** or **ascites.** EXTREMITIES: 2+ dorsalis pedis, posterior tibial, popliteal, femoral, and radial pulses bilaterally with good capillary refill. No evidence of lower extremity edema.

NEUROLOGICAL: No evidence of neurological dysfunction or pathology.

ELECTROCARDIOGRAM: An ECG demonstrates normal sinus rhythm with **ST elevation** of at least 5 mm in leads II, III, aVF, and V4 through V6.

LABORATORY DATA: Elevated **troponins;** lipid panel: total cholesterol 220, LDL 160, HDL 38, triglycerides 550; otherwise noncontributory

ASSESSMENT:
1. **Acute coronary syndrome**
2. Obesity

PLAN: The patient, with **acute ST segment elevation MI,** needs immediate cardiology consult and likely further testing in the way of **coronary angiography.** He is aware of the risks and benefits and wishes to proceed. Results of study will indicate further treatment. Currently, he will be treated with nitroglycerin and supplemental O_2. Begin nicotine cessation.

Medical Update

03/09/2010

Upon discharge from the acute setting on 3/9/10, the patient is s/p MI with 2 stent placements. New medications include: Plavix 75 mg daily, Crestor 20 mg daily, lisinopril 5 mg daily, hydrochlorothiazide 12.5 mg daily. The plan is to start an outpatient cardiac rehabilitation program and to follow up with a cardiologist in 1 week.

SEEING THE DIAGNOSIS IN ACTION 02-01

One of the first interventions to provide patients after experiencing an MI is instruction in breathing exercises. At times, the patient will need to know specific types of exercises, such as pursed-lip breathing, if he or she also has a disease such as COPD. The following images illustrate the progression of a typical treatment process of a patient with S/P MI and some of the precautions the PTA would want to be mindful of.

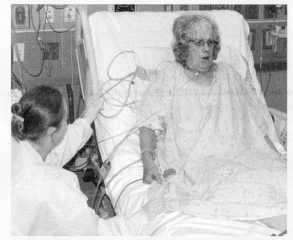

Figure 2-1 Often, the PTA will instruct in basic diaphragmatic breathing techniques and help the patient learn to breathe properly while performing ADLs and exercises.

continued

SEEING THE DIAGNOSIS IN ACTION 02-01 *continued*

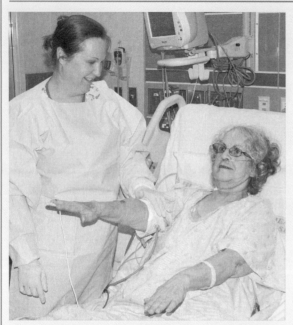

Figure 2-2 Although the patient with MI in the acute setting often progresses quickly to out-of-bed activities, many times the PTA will instruct the patient in bed exercises for the first session as well as in warm-up exercises in following sessions. This patient performs upper extremity exercises in bed very soon after MI to warm up her muscles before getting out of bed.

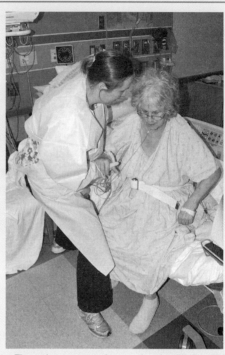

Figure 2-4 The patient prepares for transfer after MI. The PTA will need to monitor vital signs throughout the breathing and exercise session as well as during the functional activities to ensure that the patient is tolerating the activity well and that no adverse effects are observed. The patient may again experience some dizziness upon standing and should be permitted to adjust slowly to the new position before beginning ambulation.

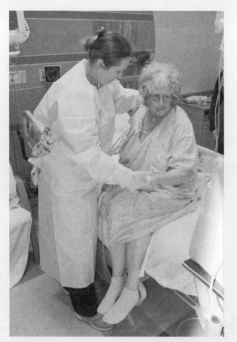

Figure 2-3 After warming up, the patient dangles her legs over the edge of the bed to prepare for transfer out of bed and ambulation. The patient may report symptoms of lightheadedness or dizziness, especially during the first attempt to sit up; the PTA will need to monitor the patient closely.

REVIEWING THE MEDICAL HISTORY

1. What do you already know about MI and other cardiac conditions?

_____

_____

_____

_____

_____

2. Review the vocabulary list and physician's notes. Look up the meanings of any terms you do not understand in a medical dictionary or other text.

_____

_____

_____

_____

_____

3. Review the diagnoses in the past medical history using a medical or pathology text, Internet resource, or other available resource.

_____

_____

_____

_____

_____

4. Which diagnoses in the past medical history would be significant and potentially affect the patient's response to the physical therapy interventions?

_____

_____

_____

_____

_____

5. List the purpose and potential side effects of each of the medications the patient is taking.

_____

_____

_____

_____

_____

6. Describe what each laboratory result measures and list considerations for physical therapy if the results for this patient were *not* in the normal range.

_____

_____

_____

_____

_____

BOX 2-1 | Physical Therapy Specialty: Cardiopulmonary

The American Physical Therapy Association, the national association for PTs and PTAs, promotes the field of physical therapy and provides many benefits to its members. Membership can also include up to 18 different sections, one of which is the Cardiovascular and Pulmonary Section. The APTA also provides specializations for PTs in different areas, one being cardiopulmonary. For more information, go to http://www.apta.org. The website for the Cardiovascular and Pulmonary Section is http://www.cardiopt.org. Treating patients with cardiovascular or pulmonary impairments is a specialty in and of itself. Although much of physical therapy addresses pain, ROM, and strength impairments in the outpatient setting or functional mobility impairments in the acute and subacute settings, patients with cardiopulmonary impairments typically need different types of interventions. Therapists and assistants need to monitor patients' vital signs and cardiopulmonary function while they gradually return to a normal level of activity and increase their endurance for those activities. Much of the intervention includes education. Often, patients follow up with a cardiac rehabilitation program after the initial acute phase of recovery.

Acute Care Physical Therapy Initial Evaluation

Patient History

NAME	Herbert Anderson
ROOM # & BED	B418-02
MEDICAL RECORD #	12345678
ATTENDING PHYSICIAN	Dr. Harvey
CHIEF COMPLAINT	Chest pain
AGE	51
DATE OF BIRTH	01/14/1959
SEX	Male
PRIMARY LANGUAGE	English
ISOLATION	No
HEIGHT (CM)	180
WEIGHT (KG)	99
MEDICATION ALLERGIES	NKDA
FOOD ALLERGIES	None
INITIATED BY	Donna Smith, PT
DATE	03/08/2010
TIME	12:37
TREATING DIAGNOSIS	Decreased mobility secondary to acute MI
ONSET DATE	03/07/2010
PERTINENT MEDICAL HISTORY	Per H & P, significant for obesity, HTN, and prior appendectomy; otherwise unremarkable

PRECAUTIONS	Monitor vital signs with activity; avoid Valsalva
WEIGHT-BEARING STATUS	WBAT
LIVING SITUATION	Home
PRIOR LEVEL OF FUNCTION	Independent with all mobility and care needs; works as a car salesman at local dealership.
ASSISTANCE AVAILABLE	Spouse helps with meals and household cleaning; she works full-time, and children are in school.
STAIRS TO ENTER HOME	6 + 8, plus 1 flight of stairs in home to upstairs bedrooms with 2 rails and another flight down to basement where he does not need to access
RAIL(S) ON STAIRS	One side
ASSISTIVE DEVICE USED PRIOR	None
EQUIPMENT PATIENT HAS	None
DRIVING PRIOR TO ADMIT	Yes
OCCUPATION/LIFE ROLE	Salesman

Systems Review

HEARING	Intact
VISION	Intact
SPEECH	Intact
PAIN SCALE	VPS
PAIN LEVEL	2
PAIN LOCATION	Chest
PAIN TYPE	Ache
PAIN INTERVENTION	Notified RN
RESTING HEART RATE (BPM)	70
RESTING RESPIRATORY RATE (respirations per minute)	21
RESTING BLOOD PRESSURE (mm Hg)	100/69

RESTING SpO_2	98% on 2 LPM supplemental O_2
ACTIVITY HEART RATE (BPM)	101 with ambulation 125 feet
ACTIVITY RESPIRATORY RATE (respirations per minute)	28
ACTIVITY BLOOD PRESSURE (mm Hg)	120/78
ACTIVITY SpO_2	98% on 2 LPM supplemental O_2
POSTACTIVITY HEART RATE (bPM)	85
POSTACTIVITY RESPIRATORY RATE (respirations per minute)	26

POSTACTIVITY BLOOD PRESSURE (mm Hg)	115/75	ORIENTATION	x4
POSTACTIVITY SpO₂	98% On 2 LPM supplemental O₂	SHORT-TERM MEMORY	Intact
LEVEL OF CONSCIOUSNESS	Alert		

Tests and Measures

ROM NECK/TRUNK	WNL	SUPINE TO SIT; SIT TO SUPINE	Min. A
ROM BUE	WNL	SIT TO STAND; STAND TO SIT	Min. A
ROM BLE	WNL except as noted; supine, bilateral SLR 60 degrees, hip extension to neutral and ankle dorsiflexion 0, plantarflexion 65 degrees	TRANSFERS	Min. A; stand pivot without device
		SITTING BALANCE	Good; at edge of bed
BUE STRENGTH	WFL during dressing and other ADLs but not tested with MMT because of Valsalva precaution	STANDING BALANCE	Fair
		TIMED GAIT	125 feet with occasional use of wall handrail in 5 minutes
BLE STRENGTH	WFL during dressing and other ADLs but not tested with MMT because of Valsalva precaution	STAIRS	Not tested
		SITTING TOLERANCE	60 minutes edge of bed
BED MOBILITY	Min. A		

Evaluation

DIAGNOSIS	Cardiovascular/pulmonary, pattern D
PROGNOSIS	Good potential to meet goals. Patient has a supportive family and has up until now been independent. He has the motivation to return home and to work when cleared medically. He expresses a desire now to improve his lifestyle and reduce his cardiac risk, stating he does not want to leave his children without a father as happened with him.

Plan of Care

PATIENT'S GOALS	He wants to return home and participate in a regular exercise program.	INTERVENTIONS	Balance training Gait training Home program Therapeutic exercise Therapeutic activities Family training
DISCHARGE GOALS	1. Bed mobility and transfers independent 2. Gait independent to 1000 feet in 5 minutes without assistive device 3. Stairs independent with rails per home situation 4. Performs home exercise program independently using written program	PATIENT EDUCATION TOPIC(S)	HR, RPE monitoring during activity Safety: call for help
		TAUGHT BY	PT
TIME TO ACHIEVE GOALS	By time of discharge	WHO WAS TAUGHT	Patient/spouse
PATIENT/FAMILY UNDERSTAND/AGREES WITH GOALS	Patient/spouse yes	METHOD OF INSTRUCTION	Verbal/demonstration
INTERVENTIONS	Bed mobility training Transfer training	EVALUATION OF LEARNING	Patient and wife demonstrated ability to monitor heart rate and RPE, using call light for help

---

Acute Care Nursing Note

03/08/2010   7:42 AM

The patient reports minimal discomfort overall, just a little "weak." The patient complains of dizziness and anxiety related to potential of another MI; BP is stable at 106/70 mm Hg, and no dysrhythmias are noted. He denies chest pain. He is continent of bowel and bladder and calls for help when needed. No loss of balance is noted. He is up walking with a PT before breakfast and plans to walk with his wife later in day. CNA will also ambulate him per activity orders for ambulation 4 times per day. He is eating about 75% of meals. He hopes to D/C home tomorrow but needs to try stairs first with the PT.

SEEING THE DIAGNOSIS IN ACTION 02-02

After the patient is discharged from the acute setting after an MI, he or she may be referred to the outpatient cardiac rehabilitation program, often held at the hospital. In the outpatient setting, patients will continue their rehabilitation using different equipment as they progress in strength and conditioning. PTs and PTAs may be involved in cardiac rehabilitation programs, but more often, these are operated by exercise physiologists and nurses with physician oversight.

After MI or other heart disease, it is very important for the patient to continue an exercise program designed to lower the risk for further complications and death. He or she will need to have regular physician checkups, monitor heart health, and follow any dietary or other lifestyle habits recommended by the physician. The PTA can play a role in the discharge planning of these patients by encouraging patient compliance and offering suggestions for making changes in old habits.

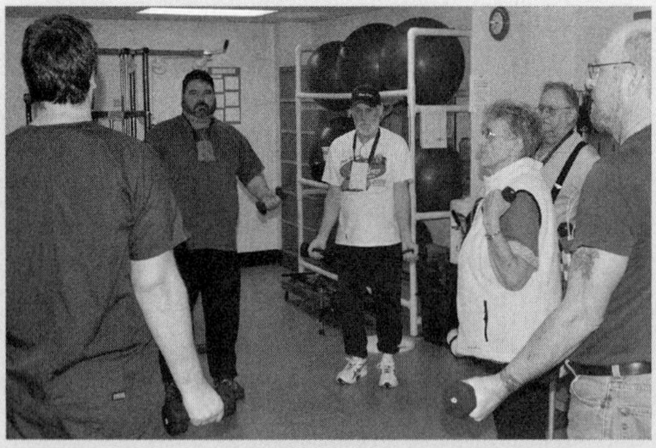

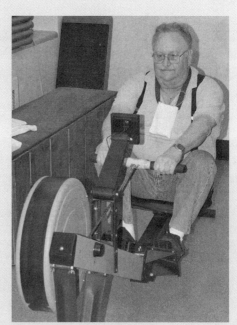

Figure 2-5 Here, patients participate in a group exercise class to warm up before other activities.

Figure 2-6 One patient performs exercise on a rowing machine. The purpose for most of these activities is to help the patient to exercise safely at a level that will strengthen the cardiovascular system. When the patient finishes the program, he or she should have the knowledge and skills to safely continue the cardiovascular rehabilitation program at home or in a gym setting independently.

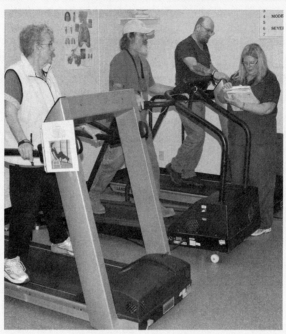

Figure 2-7 Other equipment often used in a cardiac rehabilitation program includes stationary bikes or ergometers and treadmills. Here, the RN monitors patients working out on treadmills, teaching them signs and symptoms to be aware of while exercising later on their own, after discharge from the program.

ACUTE CARE CRITICAL THINKING QUESTIONS

After reviewing the acute care physical therapy initial evaluation and other discipline notes, address the following:

1. What are the patient's impairments? Functional limitations? Is there a disability?

   Inability to work on leisure t
   _home at work + With _____

   _____

   _____

   _____

2. Find assessments of gait, strength, ROM, and balance if available from the initial evaluation and list.

   a. How could each potentially be used to assess function and demonstrate progress toward goals or show the patient's response to physical therapy interventions?

   _____ time t _____ Transfers

   _____ ROS

   care, ROM strength, balance,

b. What would be the most important items to document for this patient?

   _____ gait _____

   _____

   _____

3. After reviewing the plan of care, describe a possible next treatment session. List the activities/ exercises and your rationale for the order of treatment activities that you selected.

   _____

   _____

   _____

4. What subjective information will you gather during your session to help in your treatment of this patient and why?

   pain level c/o SOB tiredness

   _____

   _____

continued

ACUTE CARE CRITICAL THINKING QUESTIONS *continued*

5. What tests or measures will you use to assess the patient's progress and response to treatment?

HR & O2 Sat, tiled ambo.

_____

6. What subjective or objective information that you gather during the treatment might cause you to alter your treatment for this patient and why?

Events the low O2

_____

7. How would you document your treatment in the SOAP or Patient/Client Management format?

_____
_____
_____
_____

8. If the treatment goes as expected, what will you do for the next treatment?

Heel

_____

9. How would you expect this patient to progress over time?

_____

_____

10. If the patient does not progress as expected, what might be some reasons for a lack of progress?

_____
_____

11. What signs or symptoms, if observed or reported by the patient, would cause you to hold treatment and check with the nursing staff, primary PT, or MD?

_____
_____
_____

12. Are there any cultural, socioeconomic, or ethical issues presented in this case that might affect your interventions or communication with this patient? If so, how?

_____
_____
_____
_____

13. Re-review this case. Are there any coexisting medical diagnoses that might affect how this patient responds to physical therapy? If so, what are they, and how might they cause the patient to respond to physical therapy differently than you expected?

_____
_____
_____
_____
_____

14. After reviewing the other disciplines' notes regarding this patient, is there any other information that will help you to plan your treatment sessions?

_____
_____
_____
_____
_____

15. Compare your responses on this case with those of your classmates or instructors. What, if anything, would you change and why?

_____
_____
_____
_____

BOX 2-2 | Health-Care Team Member Role: Cardiac Rehabilitation

According to the American Heart Association, cardiac rehabilitation is a "medically supervised program to help patients recover quickly and improve their overall physical, mental and social functioning. The goal is to stabilize, slow or even reverse the progression of cardiovascular disease, thereby reducing the risk of heart disease, another cardiac event or death." Program elements include counseling to help the patient understand and manage the disease process, beginning an exercise program, nutrition counseling, help with modifications of risk factors, vocational counseling for return to work, information on physical limitations, emotional support, and medication counseling. Most programs include onsite exercise, although this is tailored to each person's needs. Exercise may be monitored with ECG or other monitoring devices or may be less structured with more infrequent monitoring, depending on the person's specific problems and needs. Nurses, along with exercise science professionals, often provide the services in a cardiac rehabilitation program. See the American Heart Association's website for more information at http://www.americanheart.org.

IMPLICATIONS OF PATHOLOGY FOR THE PTA[2]

1. Why would a patient with MI be instructed not to hold his breath or perform a Valsalva maneuver? What kinds of physical therapy interventions might cause a patient to do this?

2. What are signs of another MI that the PTA should watch for during intervention sessions?

3. What potential negative consequences should the PTA be alert for when working with a patient who has had an MI and is taking pain medications?

4. What are the potential negative consequences of aggressive physical handing, such as with scar massage or manual resistive exercise, in patients taking anticoagulant medications?

5. Why should a patient S/P MI avoid caffeine with exercise?

6. Why would it be important to provide for a gradual cool down of exercise for the patient who is S/P MI?

continued

IMPLICATIONS OF PATHOLOGY FOR THE PTA[2] *continued*

7. What are some specific contraindications to exercise in a patient who is S/P MI?

— *pain tightness in chest*

— *palpitations*

— *SOB*

— *dizzy*

— *leg claudication*

— *Δ in cognition / level of responsiveness*

— *pallor*

— *DVT*

8. What should the PTA be aware of when working with patients with the following cardiovascular conditions?
- Congestive heart failure
- S/P CABG
- Peripheral vascular disease
- Cardiac arrhythmias with and without pacemaker
- Cardiomyopathy
- Aneurysm
- Chronic venous insufficiency

BOX 2-3 | PTA Tip

PTAs should monitor vital signs before, during, and after working with patients who have had an MI. In general, the heart rate should not rise more than 25% above resting level. The BP should rise no more than 25 mm Hg above resting level. If the systolic BP does not rise as expected (normal is 7.5 mm Hg), then exercise intensity should be immediately reduced. Oxygen saturation should be maintained in the 90s with or without supplemental oxygen, as prescribed by the physician.[2]

References

1. American Physical Therapy Association: Guide to Physical Therapist Practice, Second Edition. Alexandria, VA: Author, 2001.

2. Goodman CC, Boissonnault FG, Fuller KS: Pathology: Implications for the Physical Therapist, Second Edition. Philadelphia: Saunders, 2003.

CHAPTER 3

Ms. Brown: A Patient With Chronic Obstructive Pulmonary Disease

Preferred Practice Pattern: Cardiovascular/Pulmonary, Pattern C

CHAPTER OUTLINE

Introducing Ms. Brown

Ms. Brown was just admitted to the hospital for COPD exacerbation. According to the APTA *Guide to Physical Therapist Practice* (the *Guide*), she could have any of the following impairments:

- **Dyspnea** at rest or with exertion
- Impaired airway clearance, cough, gas exchange
- Impaired ventilatory forces and flow
- Impaired ventilatory volumes

She could have functional limitations affecting her ability to perform self-care and work activities because of symptoms. Please refer to the *Guide* for a complete list of possible impairments and functional limitations.[1] As you work through this case, think about which of these the patient is experiencing.

Vocabulary List

Dyspnea	Tachycardic
Nebulizer	Hepatosplenomegaly
Heart catheterization	Guarding rebound
Tachypneic	Ascites
Wheezes	Hyperinflation
Rhonchi	Infiltrates
Murmur	Pneumothorax

PHYSICIAN'S HISTORY AND PHYSICAL

PATIENT NAME: Lila E. Brown
ADMIT DATE: October 4, 2010
BIRTH DATE: July 5, 1945
SEX: Female
ROOM/BED: 440-01
MEDICAL RECORD #: 12345678
CHIEF COMPLAINT: Increased shortness of breath
ATTENDING: Dr. Phillip Bloom, MD

HISTORY OF PRESENT ILLNESS: This 65-year-old Caucasian female with MS presented to the emergency department with increasing shortness of breath and cough for about 2 weeks prior. Symptoms have been worsening over the past week. She states she has been using 2 liters of supplemental oxygen at home for chronic COPD for the past year and leads a sedentary lifestyle. She does not have any lightheadedness or dizziness, nausea, or vomiting and has no other symptoms. In the emergency department, her O_2 saturation was 87%, which improved with **nebulizer** treatments.

PAST MEDICAL HISTORY: Medical history is significant for MS, anxiety disorder, depression, COPD, emphysema, recurrent bronchitis, and fibromyalgia syndrome with chronic back and neck pain, **heart**

catheterization 1 year ago with mild nonobstructive CAD, seasonal allergies.

PAST SURGICAL HISTORY: TAH

ALLERGIES: Latex, seasonal allergies

MEDICATIONS: Zoloft 100 mg PO daily
Spiriva 1 capsule daily
Advair Diskus 100/50 daily
albuterol nebulizer PRN for breakthrough
oxycodone with acetaminophen 5 mg/325 mg 1 to
2 tablets every 4 hours PRN
diazepam 5 mg PO twice daily
Allegra 180 mg PO daily
Nasacort one spray three times daily
vitamin D_3 4000 mg daily
oral prednisone 12 mg daily
Copaxone 20 mg daily subcutaneously
baclofen 10 mg three times daily

FAMILY HISTORY: The patient's mother died from breast cancer and had breathing problems, and her father had cardiovascular disease; the patient's sister died of breast cancer in her 50s.

SOCIAL HISTORY: Patient is divorced with three grown children who do not live in the area, and she does not speak to them often. She lives alone in a single-wide mobile home with a ramp and uses a wheelchair or walker for mobility. She receives Meals on Wheels but has no support network in the area. She uses public transportation. She does not have medical insurance and has applied for Medicaid. She smokes a pack of cigarettes a day and reports prior alcoholism but has not had a drink in more than 5 years.

REVIEW OF SYSTEMS: Patient reports occasional vaginal yeast infections; otherwise, she denies any symptoms other than those listed in HPI. She is able to ambulate independently with a walker.

PHYSICAL EXAMINATION: VITAL SIGNS: Temperature 36°C, pulse 104 BPM, respiratory rate 22 respirations per minute, blood pressure 125/82 mm Hg, O_2 saturation 86% on room air, 96% on 2 LPM supplemental O_2 via nasal cannula.

GENERAL: **Tachypneic** with conversation

SKIN: No rash, ulcerations, or nodules

HEENT: Unremarkable

NECK: Tenderness to palpation of cervical musculature

LUNGS: **Wheezes** and **rhonchi**; not using her accessory breathing musculature

CARDIAC: Regular rate and rhythm without **murmur** but **tachycardic** at rest

ABDOMEN: Soft, nontender, nondistended with bowel sounds in all four quadrants; no **hepatosplenomegaly, guarding rebound,** or **ascites**

EXTREMITIES: 2+ pitting edema BLE

NEUROLOGICAL: Hyperreflexic DTRs, hypertonic BLE with occasional muscle spasms

LABORATORY RESULTS: Sodium 142, potassium 3.9, BUN 11, creatinine 0.5, white blood cell count 6.8, hemoglobin 14.5, hematocrit 46, platelets 322,000

IMAGING RESULTS: Chest radiograph reveals **hyperinflation** without evidence of **infiltrates**; no **pneumothorax**

ASSESSMENT:
1. COPD exacerbation, end-stage
2. Relapsing-remitting MS
3. Depression and anxiety
4. Chronic nicotine addiction
5. Chronic pain

PLAN: The patient will be placed on a medical floor with telemetry monitoring and respiratory consult. She will start a nicotine cessation protocol and will be provided O_2 supplementation via nasal cannula to maintain O_2 saturation above 90%. She is classified as NO CODE at this time. Physical therapy, occupational therapy, and social work consultations will be provided for D/C planning.

Medical Update

10/08/2010

Upon discharge from the acute setting on 10/08/10, the patient is S/P COPD exacerbation with MS. IV Solu-Medrol 100 mg every 8 hours was started in hospital. The plan at discharge includes increasing oral prednisone to 40 mg and then tapering, the patient being able to ambulate short distances, and the cough being improved, with follow-up to an MD in 1 week. The patient declines short-term SNF or home health care. She is to be discharged to home.

SEEING THE DIAGNOSIS IN ACTION 3-1

Patients with COPD may often experience exacerbations of their disease process, which may lead to hospitalization. The physician will monitor especially the respiratory system and ensure that the patient is stable before discharging the patient. Often, patients have other underlying pathological processes that also must be considered. Depending on the medical history, age, and other factors of the patient, he or she may require short-term rehabilitation in an SNF before going home. When patients are able, they are discharged home and may or may not require outpatient physical therapy.

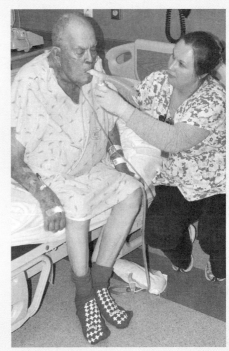

Figure 3-3 The patient with COPD now demonstrates breathing exercises. These may be the highest priority in terms of treatment interventions for many patients; they are often taught at the beginning of therapy and then incorporated into the remainder of the sessions.

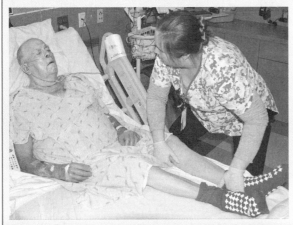

Figure 3-1 This patient with COPD prepares for a transfer to the edge of the bed. The PTA will need to monitor the patient's tolerance to initial activity and watch for signs of shortness of breath, blue coloring of the skin, and other signs that may require further monitoring of vital signs, including oxygen saturation.

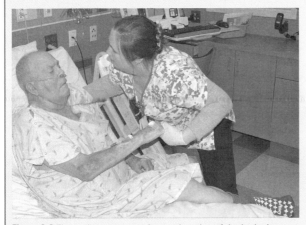

Figure 3-2 The patient now transfers to the edge of the bed where the PTA can take vital signs easily if needed based on prior observations of the patient.

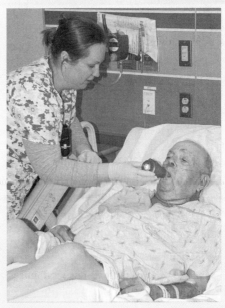

Figure 3-4 Patients are encouraged to use the various breathing exercises during the day and during other functional activities outside of therapy time.

REVIEWING THE MEDICAL HISTORY

1. What do you already know about COPD and other pulmonary conditions?

_____
_____
_____
_____

2. Review the vocabulary list and physician's notes. Look up the meanings of any terms you do not understand in a medical dictionary or other text.

_____
_____
_____
_____
_____

3. Review the diagnoses in the past medical history using a medical or pathology text, Internet resource, or other available resource.

_____
_____
_____
_____
_____

4. Which diagnoses in the past medical history would be significant and potentially affect the patient's response to the physical therapy interventions?

_____
_____
_____
_____
_____

5. List the purpose and potential side effects of each of the medications the patient is taking.

_____
_____
_____
_____
_____

6. Describe what each laboratory result measures and list considerations for physical therapy if the results for this patient were *not* in the normal range.

_____
_____
_____
_____
_____

(handwritten margin note: Purpose of the medication)

BOX 3-1 | Physical Therapy Specialty: Acute Care

Another section of the APTA is the Acute Care Section. This section focuses on physical therapy provided in the acute or hospital setting. Members can access information and take advantage of continuing education and other resources to learn more about the provision of physical therapy in hospitals. See http://www.acutept.org for further information. PTAs are utilized less in the acute setting, perhaps, than other settings for several reasons; one of the greatest may be the shortened length of hospital stays now compared with a number of years ago. Because PTs are responsible for the initial evaluations and for following patients whose medical status is changing frequently, PTAs are utilized less. For the appropriate patients, however, the PTA can provide a valuable service in this setting.

Acute Care Physical Therapy Initial Evaluation

Patient History

NAME	Lila Brown	PRECAUTIONS	Monitor vital signs with activity, maintain SpO_2 at 90%
ROOM # & BED	B440-01		
MEDICAL RECORD #	12345678	WEIGHT-BEARING STATUS	WBAT
ATTENDING PHYSICIAN	Dr. Bloom		
CHIEF COMPLAINT	Increased SOB	LIVING SITUATION	Mobile home
AGE	65	PRIOR LEVEL OF FUNCTION	Independent with all mobility and care needs using a FWW or manual W/C; has been on disability related to medical conditions
DATE OF BIRTH	07/05/1945		
SEX	Female		
PRIMARY LANGUAGE	English	ASSISTANCE AVAILABLE	Meals on Wheels, applying for Medicaid for medical insurance; very limited Social Security income, and no outside help readily available. States her daughter wants her to move close to her in another state but that she does not want to burden her daughter with her care needs.
ISOLATION	No		
HEIGHT (CM)	160		
WEIGHT (KG)	57.2		
MEDICATION ALLERGIES	Latex		
FOOD ALLERGIES	None		
INITIATED BY	Donna Smith, PT		
DATE	10/05/2010	STAIRS TO ENTER HOME	Ramp
TIME	10:42	RAIL(S) ON STAIRS	One side
ONSET DATE	10/04/2010	ASSISTIVE DEVICE USED PRIOR	FWW, W/C
PERTINENT MEDICAL HISTORY	Per H & P, significant for anxiety disorder, depression, COPD, emphysema, recurrent bronchitis, and fibromyalgia syndrome with chronic back and neck pain, mild non-obstructive CAD with heart catheterization 1 year ago, seasonal allergies	EQUIPMENT PATIENT HAS	FWW, W/C
		DRIVING PRIOR TO ADMIT	No
		OCCUPATION/LIFE ROLE	Disability

Systems Review

HEARING	Intact	RESTING SpO_2	98% on 3 LPM supplemental O_2
VISION	Intact	ACTIVITY HEART RATE (BPM)	118 with ambulation 40 feet
SPEECH	Intact		
PAIN SCALE	VPS	ACTIVITY RESPIRATORY RATE (respirations per minute)	32
PAIN LEVEL	9		
PAIN LOCATION	"All over"		
PAIN TYPE	Ache	ACTIVITY BLOOD PRESSURE (mm Hg)	138/83
PAIN INTERVENTION	Notified RN	ACTIVITY SpO_2	91% on 3 LPM supplemental O_2
RESTING HEART RATE (BPM)	98	POSTACTIVITY HEART RATE (BPM)	102
RESTING RESPIRATORY RATE (respirations per minute)	24	POSTACTIVITY RESPIRATORY RATE (respirations per minute)	26
RESTING BLOOD PRESSURE (mm Hg)	130/80	POSTACTIVITY BLOOD PRESSURE (mm Hg)	132/81

continued

Acute Care Physical Therapy Initial Evaluation *continued*

Systems Review

POSTACTIVITY SpO$_2$	96% on 3 LPM supplemental O$_2$	ORIENTATION	×4
LEVEL OF CONSCOUSNESS	Alert	SHORT-TERM MEMORY	Intact

Tests and Measures

ROM NECK/TRUNK	WNL	TRANSFERS	Min. A; stand pivot with FWW
ROM BUE	WNL	SITTING BALANCE	Good; at edge of bed
ROM BLE	WNL except as noted; supine, bilateral SLR 55 degrees, hip extension to neutral, ankle plantarflexion 5 to 60 degrees	STANDING BALANCE	Fair
		TIMED GAIT	CGA; 40 feet with FWW and SOB in 3 minutes including 1 standing rest break of 30 seconds
BUE STRENGTH	4/5		
BLE STRENGTH	4/5	WHEELCHAIR MOBILITY	Independent on level surfaces × 100 feet; Mod. A for up ramp, Min. A for down ramp
BED MOBILITY	Min. A		
SUPINE TO SIT; SIT TO SUPINE	Min. A	STAIRS	Not tested
SIT TO STAND; STAND TO SIT	Min. A	SITTING TOLERANCE	45 minutes edge of bed

Evaluation

DIAGNOSIS	Cardiovascular/pulmonary, pattern C	PROGNOSIS	will do any good. She wants to return home alone and feels she is doing "alright," although she could use some help with housekeeping. Outpatient physical therapy was recommended to her at discharge, but the patient states she is not interested. If unable to meet goals, she would need short-term SNF placement at discharge.
PROGNOSIS	Good potential to meet goals. Patient has been independent, but according to MSW notes, it is unclear whether she has been able to provide herself adequate nutrition and hygiene. She states she will not stay on smoking cessation once she returns home; she states her medical condition is already bad and doesn't think quitting now		

Plan of Care

PATIENT'S GOALS	Home	TIME TO ACHIEVE GOALS	By time of discharge
DISCHARGE GOALS	1. Bed mobility and transfers independently 2. Gait: independent with FWW, 100 feet in 3 minutes without rest break 3. Wheelchair mobility: independent up and down ramp as well as 200 feet on level, outdoor surface to access bus for transportation 4. Home exercise program: independent with written program	PATIENT/FAMILY UNDERSTAND/AGREES WITH GOALS	Patient yes
		INTERVENTIONS	Bed mobility training Transfer training Balance training Gait training Home program Therapeutic exercise Therapeutic activities

FREQUENCY	BID		WHO WAS TAUGHT	Patient
PATIENT EDUCATION TOPIC(S)	HR, RPE monitoring during activity, pursed-lip breathing; using call light for safety		METHOD OF INSTRUCTION	Verbal/demonstration
			EVALUATION OF LEARNING	Needs reinforcement
TAUGHT BY	PT			

BOX 3-2 | Health-Care Team Member Role: Nurse

Nursing staff are critical team members in a patient's recovery, especially in a hospital or other inpatient setting. Nurses may be LPNs (licensed practical nurses) with a 1-year degree or RNs (registered nurses) with either a 2- or 4-year degree. In educational and sometimes clinical settings, you will encounter master's degree–trained nurses. Nurses have many roles, including dispensing medications, performing invasive procedures such as starting IV lines and delivering medications through injections, and managing a wide variety of tubes and lines for the purpose of gathering data about the patient or providing needed treatments such as oxygen or tube feeding. They communicate with the MD (or other prescribing health professional) when medical changes warrant and follow new orders to provide high-quality care to patients. CNAs (certified nursing assistants) provide critical functions as well, such as assist with feeding, bathing, toileting, dressing, and other ADLs. All nursing staff must document their treatments for and assessments of patients, and their notes are helpful to the PTA in determining current patient status. Usually, the PTA will read the nursing notes and then check in with the CNA or nurse to obtain recent information, especially when the patient is more acutely ill. For more information about the nursing profession and its role in health care, see http://www.nursingworld.org.

Acute Care Nursing Note

10/04/2010   9:22 PM

The patient is not using a call light to walk to the bathroom. Some loss of balance is noted. The patient is encouraged to use the light; the bed alarm and chair alarm are now in use. Physical therapy, occupational therapy, and social work consults are pending. The patient wants D/C to home but states she is not sure the "doctor will let her." She expresses anger related to her situation and makes demanding requests frequently. She has generalized pain at 8/10 and requests pain medications every 4 hours, noting some relief. The patient is using a nebulizer for respiratory distress with good results. She is continent of bowel and bladder. A dietitian assessment is pending. The patient's airway clearance is adequate.

Acute Care Social Work Note

10/05/2010   3:14 PM

The patient has acute exacerbation of COPD. PMH includes MS, anxiety disorder, depression, COPD, emphysema, recurrent bronchitis, and fibromyalgia syndrome with chronic back and neck pain, mild nonobstructive CAD, TAH, heart catheterization, and seasonal allergies. The patient reports past alcoholism and current nicotine addiction. She states that she needs help with housekeeping but is unable to afford to pay for help and is unwilling to live closer to any of her children. Her daughter is "too busy" to help much, and she is estranged from her 2 sons. Her ex-husband lives locally, but they have not spoken in years. An adult protective services report was filed during a prior admission here because of unclean living conditions and a neighbor's concern that she wasn't taking her medications properly and having frequent falls in the home. Will follow up with D/C planning after PT and OT recommendations.

Acute Care Occupational Therapy Summary

10/05/2010   4:45 PM

The patient needs minimal assistance for toileting hygiene and bathing BLE, back, and perineal region and has limited standing endurance and balance for meal preparation. She is able to safely dress herself while seated and is able to retrieve her clothing from the closet but needs minimal assistance for balance while ambulatory. She is independent with grooming, oral hygiene, and feeding and is continent of bowel and bladder. BID occupational therapy services are recommended to work toward independence in all ADLs before D/C. She may need a short-term SNF stay but states she is unwilling to "go to one of those places. I would rather die."

SEEING THE DIAGNOSIS IN ACTION 3-2

Patients with COPD may need outpatient physical therapy as a follow-up to their hospital admission for COPD exacerbation. Alternatively, many patients with COPD will receive outpatient physical therapy for another problem, perhaps musculoskeletal, and the PTA will need to monitor the patient's respiratory system while performing interventions specifically for the other problem.

Patients are encouraged to continue a home exercise program to maintain and improve their function after discharge from the inpatient or outpatient setting. They may need encouragement from the PT/PTA team to help them focus on any lifestyle changes the physician recommends, such as smoking cessation, dietary changes, and medication compliance.

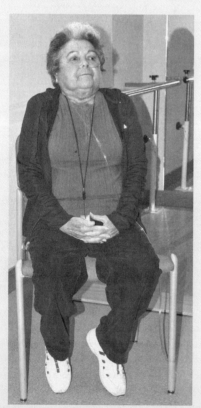

Figure 3-5 This patient with COPD performs breathing exercises in the outpatient setting. No matter what are the physical therapy diagnosis and problems, all patients with COPD can benefit from further training in breathing exercises to promote overall improved function of the respiratory system.

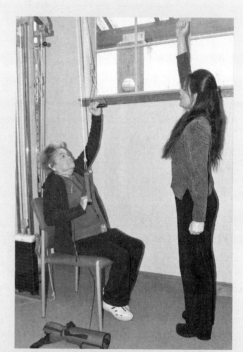

Figure 3-6 Often, patients with COPD need upper body strengthening to maximize their respiratory function. Here, a patient performs upper extremity exercises using pulleys.

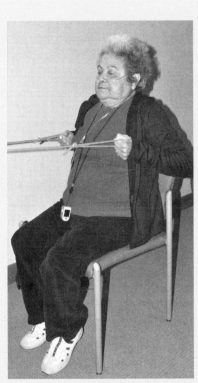

Figure 3-7 This patient with COPD performs rowing exercises to strengthen the upper back.

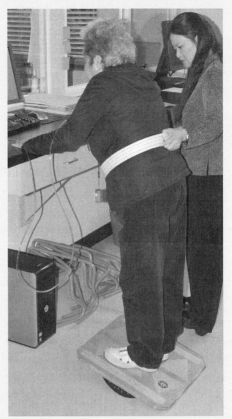

Figure 3-8 Patients with COPD are often older and may also benefit from balance training to reduce fall risk. This patient demonstrates this type of activity.

ACUTE CARE CRITICAL THINKING QUESTIONS

After reviewing the acute care physical therapy initial evaluation and other discipline notes, address the following:

1. What are the patient's impairments? Functional limitations? Is there a disability?

_____

_____

2. Find assessments of gait, strength, ROM, and balance if available from the initial evaluation and list.

   a. How could each potentially be used to assess function and demonstrate progress toward goals or show the patient's response to physical therapy interventions?

_____

_____

_____

b. What would be the most important items to document for this patient?

_____

_____

_____

3. After reviewing the POC, describe a possible next treatment session.

   a. List the activities and exercises and your rationale for the order of treatment activities that you selected.

_____

_____

_____

_____

continued

ACUTE CARE CRITICAL THINKING QUESTIONS *continued*

4. What subjective information will you gather during your session to help in your treatment of this patient and why?

_____

_____

_____

5. What tests or measures will you use to assess the patient's progress and response to treatment?

_____

_____

_____

6. What subjective or objective information that you gather during the treatment might cause you to alter your treatment for this patient and why?

_____

_____

_____

7. How would you document your treatment in the SOAP or Patient/Client Management format?

_____

_____

_____

_____

8. If the treatment goes as expected, what will you do for the next treatment?

_____

_____

_____

9. How would you expect this patient to progress over time?

_____

_____

_____

10. If the patient does not progress as expected, what might be some reasons for a lack of progress?

_____

_____

_____

11. What signs or symptoms, if observed or reported by the patient, would cause you to hold treatment and check with the nursing staff, primary PT, or MD?

_____

_____

_____

_____

12. Are there any cultural, socioeconomic, or ethical issues presented in this case that might affect your interventions or communication with this patient? If so, how?

_____

_____

_____

13. Re-review this case. Are there any coexisting medical diagnoses that might affect how this patient responds to physical therapy? If so, what are they, and how might they cause the patient to respond to physical therapy differently than you expected?

_____

_____

_____

14. After reviewing the other disciplines' notes regarding this patient, is there any other information that will help you to plan your treatment sessions?

_____

_____

_____

15. Compare your responses on this case with those of your classmates or instructors. What, if anything, would you change and why?

_____

_____

_____

IMPLICATIONS OF PATHOLOGY FOR THE PTA[2]

1. Describe how instruction on pacing and energy conservation is incorporated in the intervention sessions for patients with COPD.

_____

_____

_____

_____

_____

_____

2. Explain when breathing and coughing techniques could be incorporated into the intervention sessions.

_____

_____

_____

_____

_____

_____

3. How is upper extremity strength and conditioning (or weakness) related to functional capacity in the patient with COPD?

_____

_____

_____

_____

_____

4. Even though exercise does not appear to improve lung function, why is it important and how does it benefit the patient with COPD? How would you explain this to the patient who often does not feel like exercising and may not see the importance?

_____

_____

_____

_____

_____

5. What should the PTA be aware of when working with patients with the following respiratory conditions?
   - Pneumonia
   - Asthma
   - Tuberculosis
   - Sleep apnea
   - Cystic fibrosis
   - Pulmonary edema
   - Acute respiratory distress syndrome
   - Pulmonary embolism
   - Pulmonary hypertension

_____

_____

_____

_____

_____

References

1. American Physical Therapy Association: Guide to Physical Therapist Practice, Second Edition. Alexandria, VA: Author, 2001.

2. Goodman CC, Boissonnault FG, Fuller KS: Pathology: Implications for the Physical Therapist, Second Edition. Philadelphia: Saunders, 2003.

Mr. Davis: A Patient With Rotator Cuff Repair

 Preferred Practice Pattern: Musculoskeletal, Pattern I

CHAPTER OUTLINE

Introducing Mr. Davis
Vocabulary List
Physician's History and Physical
Reviewing the Medical History
Acute Care Physical Therapy Initial
    Evaluation

Acute Care Nursing Note
Acute Care Critical Thinking Questions
Medical Update
Outpatient Physical Therapy Evaluation
Outpatient Critical Thinking Questions

Continuum of Care Critical Thinking
    Questions
Implications of Pathology for the PTA

Introducing Mr. Davis

Mr. Davis is a 38-year-old man who injured his shoulder on the job and underwent rotator cuff repair. According to the APTA's *Guide to Physical Therapist Practice* (the *Guide*), he could have the following impairments:

- Decreased ROM, strength, and endurance
- Impaired joint mobility
- Pain and swelling

Functional limitations may include limited independence in ADLs. Please refer to the *Guide* for a complete list of possible impairments and functional limitations.[1] As you work through this case, think about which of these the patient is experiencing.

Vocabulary List
- Auscultation
- Wheeze
- Rales
- Rhonchi
- Hepatosplenomegaly

PHYSICIAN'S HISTORY AND PHYSICAL

PATIENT NAME: Richard M. Davis
ADMIT DATE: July 14, 2010
BIRTH DATE: Feb. 10, 1972
SEX: Male
ROOM/BED: 310-02
MEDICAL RECORD #: 12345678

CHIEF COMPLAINT: Right shoulder pain after a fall
ATTENDING: Dr. Patricia Jefferson, DO

HISTORY OF PRESENT ILLNESS: This is a 38-year-old male who was working as a roofer and fell 10 feet from a ladder, landing on the right shoulder. He attempted to break the fall with an outstretched right arm. He heard a loud popping sound and experienced immediate pain in his right shoulder. He reports pain at 10/10 with any movement and less at rest, as well as mild nausea associated with the pain. MRI reveals full-thickness rotator cuff tear, and he now has decided to have it surgically repaired. He has been informed of the risks, including blood clots, infection, cardiac arrest, stroke, and death. He is admitted for rotator cuff repair.

PAST MEDICAL HISTORY: The patient's medical history is significant for hypothyroidism, high cholesterol, and depression.

PAST SURGICAL HISTORY: Appendectomy

ALLERGIES: Seasonal allergies to grass and weeds

MEDICATIONS: Zocor 20 mg daily
Zoloft 10 mg daily
Synthroid 75 mcg daily

FAMILY HISTORY: HTN and DM II on mother's side of family

SOCIAL HISTORY: The patient is married with three school-aged children and is the primary wage earner. His wife works part-time as a paralegal. He denies smoking and drinks occasionally.

BOX 4-1 | Health-Care Team Member Role: Physician

The physician is responsible for overseeing the care of the patient in the acute setting and monitors the patient after discharge. The physician writes orders for medications and other treatments needed, such as physical therapy and occupational therapy, for tests needed, such as laboratory work and imaging, and assesses the patient at regular intervals to ensure that the patient is making reasonable progress. The physician decides when the patient is ready for discharge from the hospital, using information from all medical team members to make an appropriate discharge decision. In many cases, the patient is admitted to the hospital by a family doctor who has hospital privileges. In some hospitals, the primary care provider may delegate the care of the patient to a hospitalist, who is a physician hired by the hospital, often one who specializes in internal medicine. In many orthopedic or other surgical cases, the surgeon will oversee the patient both in the hospital and afterward with outpatient follow-up appointments. See the website of the American Medical Association for more information on the role of the physician in health care: http://www.ama-assn.org. Other health-care practitioners who may provide these services include physicians assistants, osteopathic doctors, and in outpatient settings, chiropractors.

REVIEW OF SYSTEMS: See HPI.

PHYSICAL EXAMINATION:

VITAL SIGNS: Temperature 36.8°C, pulse 68 BPM, respiratory rate 15 respirations per minute, blood pressure 119/69 mm Hg, O_2 saturation 98% on room air.

GENERAL: Uncomfortable with right shoulder pain, Dilaudid given in the emergency department with good effect but still reports pain at 8/10 with any movement.

SKIN: Warm and dry. Abrasion on right elbow and knee.

HEENT: Unremarkable

NECK: Tenderness to palpation at base of the skull; cervical AROM 50% of normal.

CARDIAC: Regular rate and rhythm

LUNGS: Clear to **auscultation** bilaterally without **wheeze, rales,** or **rhonchi.**

ABDOMEN: Bowel sounds present, nontender, nondistended. No **hepatosplenomegaly.**

EXTREMITIES: Tenderness to palpation of right anterior and posterior shoulder.

NEUROLOGICAL: Alert and oriented. Moving his right shoulder slowly due to pain. Cranial nerves intact.

LABORATORY DATA: Noncontributory

IMAGING STUDIES: MRI of right shoulder shows complete rotator cuff tear. Radiographs are negative for fracture, with no evidence of acromioclavicular joint separation.

ASSESSMENT: Right rotator cuff full-thickness tear

PLAN: The plan is to admit the patient to the surgical floor for rotator cuff repair and to continue his medications. A physical therapy consult is recommended for exercise and discharge planning, and his sling should stay on at all times other than therapy.

SEEING THE DIAGNOSIS IN ACTION 4-1

After rotator cuff surgery, patients receive initial instruction on ROM exercises and other functional mobility in the acute setting. They are often discharged home within about 2 days, depending on their age and overall physical condition. Typically, they will follow up with outpatient physical therapy according to the protocol used by the surgeon.

Patients will need to continue a home exercise program in order to continue strengthening after discharge from the outpatient setting. They may need additional follow-up visits several weeks or months afterward to ensure they are progressing toward their goals, which will typically include a return to work.

continued

SEEING THE DIAGNOSIS IN ACTION 4-1 *continued*

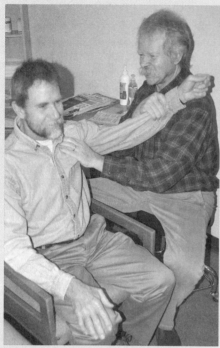

Figure 4-1 The PT provides soft tissue mobilization and AAROM exercise to a patient after rotator cuff repair. These interventions are useful in the beginning of recovery to help the patient regain motion needed to perform work and leisure activities.

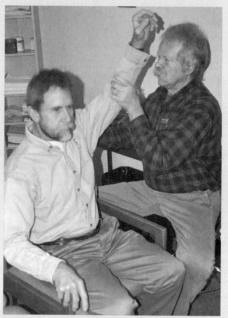

Figure 4-3 Here, the PT reassesses shoulder flexion ROM in the patient after rotator cuff repair to demonstrate the effectiveness of the prior treatment interventions.

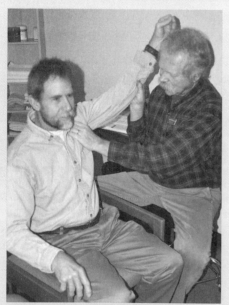

Figure 4-2 Manual therapy techniques such as soft tissue and joint mobilization may also be incorporated with passive or active motions to help the patient regain full motion.

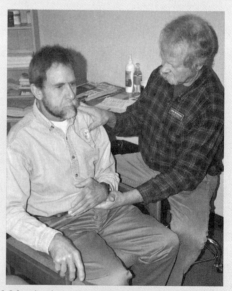

Figure 4-4 Another important motion the patient will need to perform functional activities is rotation. Often, external rotation is limited by the surgeon for a period of time after surgery in order to promote proper healing. The PTA will need to be aware of any restrictions in this and other motions when providing therapeutic exercise.

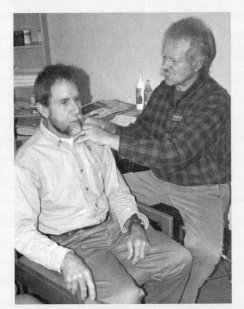

Figure 4-5 Often, acromioclavicular joint motion is impaired in patients after rotator cuff repair. The PT assesses this motion as part of an overall picture of the patient's problems.

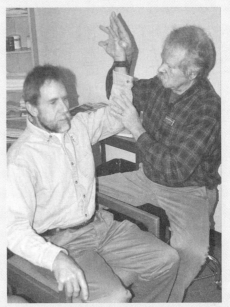

Figure 4-6 After gaining some, but perhaps not all, of the ROM, and while continuing to address flexibility, the patient begins strengthening within the surgeon's protocol. Here, the patient performs exercises while the PT gives manual resistance. Often, PNF exercises are used as well to help improve function and mobility. Strengthening with other types of resistance, such as weights, pulleys, and resistance bands, are all ways that the patient may further strengthen the shoulder after surgical repair.

REVIEWING THE MEDICAL HISTORY

1. What do you already know about rotator cuff injuries, surgical repair, and other shoulder injuries?

_____

_____

_____

_____

_____

2. Review the vocabulary list and physician's notes. Look up the meanings of any terms you do not understand in a medical dictionary or other text.

_____

_____

_____

_____

_____

3. Review the diagnoses in the past medical history using a medical or pathology text, Internet resource, or other available resource.

_____

_____

_____

_____

_____

4. Which diagnoses in the past medical history would be significant and potentially affect the physical therapy intervention?

_____

_____

_____

_____

_____

continued

REVIEWING THE MEDICAL HISTORY *continued*

5. List the purpose and potential side effects of each of the medications the patient is taking.

_____

_____

_____

_____

_____

6. Describe what each laboratory result measures and list considerations for physical therapy if the results for this patient were *not* in the normal range.

_____

_____

_____

_____

_____

Acute Care Physical Therapy Initial Evaluation

Patient History

NAME	Rick Davis		PERTINENT MEDICAL HISTORY	Per H & P, significant for hypothyroidism, high cholesterol, depression, and appendectomy
ROOM # & BED	B310-02			
MEDICAL RECORD #	12345678		SURGERY	Right RCR
ATTENDING PHYSICIAN	Dr. Jefferson		SURGERY DATE	07/14/2010
CHIEF COMPLAINT	Right rotator cuff tear		PRECAUTIONS	Right sling on at all times when up; out for exercises per protocol
AGE	38			
DATE OF BIRTH	02/10/1972		WEIGHT-BEARING STATUS	NWB RUE
SEX	Male			
PRIMARY LANGUAGE	English		LIVING SITUATION	Home
ISOLATION	No		PRIOR LEVEL OF FUNCTION	Independent
HEIGHT (CM)	178			
WEIGHT (KG)	75.5		ASSISTANCE AVAILABLE	Spouse; works part-time during school hours
MEDICATION ALLERGIES	NKDA			
FOOD ALLERGIES	None		STAIRS TO ENTER HOME	5 plus 1 flight of stairs in home to upstairs bedrooms and 1 rail
INITIATED BY	Donna Smith, PT			
DATE	07/14/2010		RAIL(S) ON STAIRS	Both sides
TIME	5:52		ASSISTIVE DEVICE USED PRIOR	None
TREATING DIAGNOSIS	Decreased mobility secondary to right rotator cuff tear from fall off 10-foot ladder at work		EQUIPMENT PATIENT HAS	None
			DRIVING PRIOR TO ADMIT	Yes
ONSET DATE	07/13/2010			
			OCCUPATION/LIFE ROLE	Roofer

Systems Review

HEARING	Intact		PAIN LEVEL	8
VISION	Intact		PAIN LOCATION	RUE
SPEECH	Intact		PAIN TYPE	Surgical
PAIN SCALE	VPS		PAIN INTERVENTION	Notified RN

RESTING HEART RATE (BPM)	65		RESTING SpO$_2$	100% on room air
			LEVEL OF CONSCIOUSNESS	Alert but drowsy from medications
RESTING RESPIRATORY RATE (respirations per minute)	20		ORIENTATION	x 4
			SHORT-TERM MEMORY	Intact
RESTING BLOOD PRESSURE (mm Hg)	117/68			

Tests and Measures

ROM NECK/TRUNK	Impaired; active cervical ROM: right rotation 60 degrees, left rotation 45 degrees, both with pain at end range		BED MOBILITY	Min. A
			SUPINE TO SIT/SIT TO SUPINE	Mod. A
ROM RUE	WNL except as noted; PROM shoulder flexion to 48 degrees, abduction to 30 degrees, both with pain		SIT TO STAND/STAND TO SIT	CGA with some lightheadedness upon standing; stable BP
			TRANSFERS	CGA stand pivot holding onto IV pole with LUE
ROM LUE	WNL			
ROM BLE	WNL		SITTING BALANCE	Good; at edge of bed
RUE STRENGTH	4/5 for elbow, wrist, hand; shoulder not tested		STANDING BALANCE	Fair with IV pole
			GAIT	CGA; 20 feet with IV pole
LUE STRENGTH	5/5		STAIRS	Not tested
BLE STRENGTH	5/5		SITTING TOLERANCE	60 minutes in chair
SENSATION	Intact			

Evaluation

DIAGNOSIS	Musculoskeletal, pattern I		PROGNOSIS	Good; patient is S/P right rotator cuff repair with residual pain, limited motion, and an inability to perform functional mobility tasks. He is slightly lightheaded upon standing but able to safely support himself using IV pole.

Plan of Care

PATIENT'S GOALS	To resume premorbid activities at home and return to work as soon as possible		INTERVENTIONS.(con't)	Gait training Stair training Home program Therapeutic exercise Therapeutic activities Family training PRN
DISCHARGE GOALS	1. Bed mobility and transfers: independent 2. Gait: independent without assistive device >500 feet 3. Stairs: independent, 1 flight with 1 rail per home situation 4. Home exercise program: independent with written program			
			FREQUENCY	BID
			PATIENT EDUCATION TOPIC(S)	Sling use, donning and doffing
TIME TO ACHIEVE GOALS	By time of discharge		TAUGHT BY	PT
PATIENT/FAMILY UNDERSTAND/AGREES WITH GOALS	Patient/spouse yes		WHO WAS TAUGHT	Patient/spouse
			METHOD OF INSTRUCTION	Verbal/demonstration
INTERVENTIONS	Bed mobility training Transfer training Balance training		EVALUATION OF LEARNING	Needs reinforcement

Acute Care Nursing Note

07/14/2010   3:30 PM

The patient arrived from the PACU at 1500; he reports nausea without emesis and pain of 7/10. Zofran was ordered for nausea and has been given with good effect. Educated regarding using the call light and taking Percocet for pain. It is recommended that he don a sling for RUE and that he go up to the bathroom with SBA for safety. He is able to sip ginger ale. His wife is at the bedside. The patient reports no increase in depressive symptoms but is glad his shoulder surgery is done. The suture line has been approximated, and the dressing is clean, dry, and intact.

ACUTE CARE CRITICAL THINKING QUESTIONS

After reviewing the acute care physical therapy initial evaluation and other discipline notes, address the following:

1. What are the patient's impairments? Functional limitations? Is there a disability?

_____

_____

2. Find assessments of gait, strength, ROM, and balance if available from the initial evaluation and list.

   a. How could each potentially be used to assess function and demonstrate progress toward goals or show the patient's response to physical therapy interventions?

   _____

   _____

   _____

   b. What would be the most important items to document for this patient?

   _____

   _____

   _____

3. After reviewing the POC, describe a possible next treatment session.

   a. List the activities/exercises and your rationale for the order of treatment activities that you selected.

   _____

   _____

   _____

4. What subjective information will you gather during your session to help in your treatment of this patient and why?

   _____

   _____

5. What tests or measures will you use to assess the patient's progress and response to treatment?

   _____

   _____

6. What subjective or objective information that you gather during the treatment might cause you to alter your treatment for this patient and why?

   _____

   _____

   _____

7. How would you document your treatment in the SOAP or Patient/Client Management format?

   _____

   _____

   _____

8. If the treatment goes as expected, what will you do for the next treatment?

   _____

   _____

   _____

9. How would you expect this patient to progress over time?

   _____

   _____

   _____

10. If the patient does not progress as expected, what might be some reasons for a lack of progress?

   _____

   _____

11. What signs or symptoms, if observed or re-ported by the patient, would cause you to hold treatment and check with the nursing staff, pri-mary PT, or MD?

_____

_____

12. Are there any cultural, socioeconomic, or ethi-cal issues presented in this case that might af-fect your interventions or communication with this patient? If so, how?

_____

_____

13. Re-review this case. Are there any coexisting medical diagnoses that might affect how this patient responds to physical therapy? If so, what are they, and how might they cause the patient to respond to physical therapy differ-ently than you expected?

_____

_____

_____

14. After reviewing the other disciplines' notes regarding this patient, is there any other information that will help you to plan your treatment sessions?

_____

_____

_____

_____

_____

15. Compare your responses on this case with those of your classmates or instructors. What, if anything, would you change and why?

_____

_____

_____

_____

_____

_____

Medical Update

_07/16/2010_

Upon discharge from the acute setting on 07/16/2010, the patient is S/P right rotator cuff repair. He has no new laboratory results or imaging studies and one new medication: Percocet 5 mg/325 mg 1 to 2 tablets by mouth every 4 hours as needed for pain. His other medications are unchanged. The plan is for him to follow up with an MD in 1 week and start outpatient physical therapy after that.

BOX 4-2 | Physical Therapy Specialty: Orthopedics

Orthopedics, another specialty area in physical therapy, specializes in the treatment of orthopedic conditions (generally, conditions of the bones, joints, muscles, and other soft tissue), both surgical and nonsurgical. The Orthopaedic section of the APTA supports members who wish to learn more about and treat orthopedic in-juries. See http://www.orthopt.org. Within the area of orthopedics, the specialty of work hardening is some-times used when patients need extensive therapy and conditioning in order to return to work. Work hardening is highly specific to the particular job tasks and gradu-ally increases the workload until the patient is able to perform close to the expectations of the work site. Some companies now provide physical therapy care on site for larger companies to reduce time off work for keeping physical therapy appointments. Therapists who work in this type of setting also provide extensive education to employees that is intended to help reduce on-the-job injuries and reduce company expense due to injuries.

Outpatient Physical Therapy Evaluation

NAME	Rick Davis
DATE	August 18, 2010
DIAGNOSIS	Right rotator cuff repair
SUBJECTIVE INFORMATION	Patient is about 4½ weeks S/P right rotator cuff repair. Has been doing pendulum exercises at home as well as active assistive flexion and abduction using a dowel. He does these once per day and uses ice PRN for pain. Pain is generally at about 4/10 but increases after exercises or other light use. He is not using his sling and has increased pain after being up and having the arm dangle up to an hour at a time. He hopes to return to work soon and questions when that might be possible. He also wants to know when he can return to some light yard work such as weeding and using a lawn mower. At this time, he cannot use his right arm for any lifting or reaching overhead or out to the side to do things such as washing his hair. He cannot lift his 4-year-old daughter or jog yet, both of which he did before surgery. He is walking about a mile per day for exercise and wants to get back to jogging and the gym for weight training. He started driving independently a week ago.
OBJECTIVE INFORMATION	
Posture	Right shoulder elevated compared with left, mildly kyphotic thoracic spine
Strength	Right shoulder flexion, abduction 3–/5; internal rotation and extension 2–/5; external rotation not tested. Elbow and hand 5/5. LUE 5/5.
AROM	In supine position, right shoulder flexion 32 degrees, abduction 25 degrees, external rotation not tested because of limitations per protocol, internal rotation 50 degrees. In sitting, extension 30 degrees.
PROM	In supine position, right shoulder flexion 90 degrees, abduction 85 degrees, external rotation not tested, internal rotation 70 degrees. In sitting position, extension 50 degrees.
Palpation/scar	Tender to palpation of right rotator cuff insertions and scar area; scar healed with some immobility present from adhesions; increased muscular tension and pain palpated in right upper and middle trapezius, scalenes, cervical and thoracic paraspinals, and upper cervical musculature greater than left side
ASSESSMENT	Patient is about 4½ weeks S/P rotator cuff tear and surgical repair with resulting impairments of pain, decreased strength, and ROM. Functional limitations include reaching overhead, out to the side and behind and lifting anything greater than 5 pounds. These limitations affect his ability to drive, help with housework and yard work, perform basic car maintenance, and lift his youngest child, age 4. He is unable to return to work as a roofer at this time. He will benefit from physical therapy interventions to address these impairments and limitations and facilitate his ability to return to work as a roofer. Since he is young and in relatively good health as well as motivated to return to his prior work environment, he has good potential to reach his goals.
STG (in 2 weeks)	1. Increase PROM right shoulder flexion and abduction to 100 degrees to allow reaching overhead and to the side; increase extension to 60 degrees to reach backward. 2. Decrease pain level to 5/10 during and after physical therapy sessions to allow greater functional mobility in reaching and to perform exercises. 3. Patient will be independent with home exercise program per RCR protocol.
LTG	Independent with home exercise program for strengthening and ROM to allow patient to return to full household and part-time or modified yard work and work activities.
PLAN	3 times per week for 8 weeks for physical modalities to decrease pain and increase ROM, soft tissue mobilization, ROM and strengthening exercise program per protocol, and functional movement training to simulate return to household and work activities.

BOX 4-3 | Surgical Protocols

Often, surgeons develop protocols to be used with their patients after surgery, and hospitals may use standard protocols that all physicians who perform surgeries there agree to. Protocols allow for consistency in rehabilitation and communication between surgeon and the physical therapy staff. Typically, after rotator cuff surgery, protocols include limiting shoulder external rotation for a period of time, usually 3 to 4 weeks after surgery. It will include timing for progression from PROM to AAROM to AROM and then resistance training. Finally, it will give parameters for sling or brace use after surgery. Even though a surgeon has developed a set protocol to follow, the PTA must be observant of changes in the patient's status that might require a slowing down of the progression through the phases of the protocol. Any questions that arise should be directed to the PT, who can communicate concerns to the surgeon and determine how to proceed with the individual patient.

OUTPATIENT CRITICAL THINKING QUESTIONS

After reviewing the outpatient physical therapy evaluation, address the following:

1. What are the patient's impairments? Functional limitations? Is there a disability?

_____

_____

_____

_____

_____

2. Find assessments of gait, strength, ROM, and balance if available from the initial evaluation and list.

   a. How could each potentially be used to assess function and demonstrate progress toward goals or show the patient's response to physical therapy interventions?

   _____

   _____

   b. What would be the most important items to document for this patient?

   _____

   _____

   _____

3. After reviewing the POC, describe a possible next treatment session.

   a. List the activities/exercises and your rationale for the order of treatment activities that you selected.

   _____

   _____

   _____

4. What subjective information will you gather during your session to help in your treatment of this patient and why?

_____

5. What tests or measures will you use to assess the patient's progress and response to treatment?

_____

_____

_____

_____

6. What subjective or objective information that you gather during the treatment might cause you to alter your treatment for this patient and why?

_____

_____

7. How would you document your treatment in the SOAP or Patient/Client Management format?

_____

_____

_____

_____

8. If the treatment goes as expected, what will you do for the next treatment?

_____

_____

_____

continued

OUTPATIENT CRITICAL THINKING QUESTIONS *continued*

9. How would you expect this patient to progress over time?

_____

_____

_____

_____

10. If the patient does not progress as expected, what might be some reasons for a lack of progress?

_____

_____

_____

_____

11. What signs or symptoms, if observed or reported by the patient, would cause you to hold treatment and check with the nursing staff, primary PT, or MD?

_____

_____

_____

_____

12. Are there any cultural, socioeconomic, or ethical issues presented in this case that might affect your interventions or communication with this patient? If so, how?

_____

_____

_____

_____

13. Re-review this case. Are there any coexisting medical diagnoses that might affect how this patient responds to physical therapy? If so, what are they, and how might they cause the patient to respond to physical therapy differently than you expected?

_____

_____

_____

_____

_____

14. After reviewing the other disciplines' notes regarding this patient, is there any other information that will help you to plan your treatment sessions?

_____

_____

_____

_____

_____

15. Compare your responses on this case with those of your classmates or instructors. What, if anything, would you change and why?

_____

_____

_____

_____

CONTINUUM OF CARE CRITICAL THINKING QUESTIONS

After reviewing the continuum of care for this patient, consider the following:

1. How did the patient's problems change over the month after his initial injury and surgery?

_____

_____

_____

_____

_____

2. How did this affect the interventions that were chosen?

_____

_____

_____

_____

_____

CONTINUUM OF CARE CRITICAL THINKING QUESTIONS *continued*

3. How were the same interventions modified over time to progress the patient according to his changing needs?

_____

_____

_____

_____

_____

4. What are some potential community resources that this patient might like to participate in and how would these help him to more quickly reach his ultimate goal of returning to work as soon as possible?

_____

_____

_____

_____

IMPLICATIONS OF PATHOLOGY FOR THE PTA[2]

1. What is the normal timing for healing of soft tissue injury and how will this knowledge affect your approach to this patient in the acute setting as well as later in the outpatient setting?

_____

_____

_____

_____

2. What are the effects of the various physical therapy modalities on soft tissue healing?

_____

_____

_____

_____

_____

3. What are the effects of the various types of exercise on soft tissue healing?

_____

_____

_____

_____

_____

4. What should the PTA be aware of when working with patients with the following soft tissue injuries or surgical repairs?

   a. Lateral or medial epicondylitis

   b. Carpal tunnel syndrome with or without surgical repair

   c. Arthroscopic knee surgery

   d. Anterior cruciate ligament injury and surgical repair

   e. Plantar fasciitis

   f. Bunionectomy

_____

_____

_____

_____

_____

_____

_____

_____

_____

_____

_____

_____

References

1. American Physical Therapy Association: Guide to Physical Therapist Practice, Second Edition. Alexandria, VA: Author, 2001.

2. Goodman CC, Boissonnault FG, Fuller KS: Pathology: Implications for the Physical Therapist, Second Edition. Philadelphia: Saunders, 2003.

CHAPTER 5

Mr. Garcia: A Patient With Laminectomy

 Preferred Practice Pattern: Musculoskeletal, Pattern I

CHAPTER OUTLINE

Introducing Mr. Garcia

Mr. Garcia is a 45-year-old man who had experienced severe lower back pain for several years before his lumbar laminectomy. According to the APTA's *Guide to Physical Therapist Practice* (the *Guide*), he could have the following impairments:

- Decreased ROM, strength, and endurance
- Impaired joint mobility
- Pain and swelling

Functional limitations may be related to his ability to perform ADLs. Please refer to the *Guide*[1] for a complete list of possible impairments and functional limitations. As you work through this case, think about which of these the patient is experiencing.

Vocabulary List

- Arthroscopy
- Murmurs
- Auscultation
- Wheeze
- Rales
- Rhonchi
- Hepatosplenomegaly

PHYSICIAN'S HISTORY AND PHYSICAL

PATIENT NAME: Carlos H. Garcia
ADMIT DATE: October 21, 2010
BIRTH DATE: July 9, 1965
SEX: Male

ROOM/BED: 320-01
MEDICAL RECORD #: 12345678
CHIEF COMPLAINT: Low back pain with right lower extremity radiating pain, weakness, and numbness
ATTENDING: Dr. Patricia Jefferson, DO

HISTORY OF PRESENT ILLNESS: This is a 45-year-old male who has had several recurrences of low back pain over the past 3 years and has now had an exacerbation of pain since lifting and moving a heavy desk on the job. He has unremitting back pain that shoots down his right lower extremity, now with numbness and tingling to the ankle. He elects to receive lumbar laminectomy with lateral resections and has been informed of the risks, including blood clots, infection, cardiac arrest, stroke, and death. He is admitted for the procedure.

PAST MEDICAL HISTORY: His medical history is significant for HTN, DM II under fair control with Hg A_{1C} at 6.8, and epilepsy.

PAST SURGICAL HISTORY: **Arthroscopy** of left knee 3 years ago for medial meniscus tear; right ankle fracture with ORIF 2 years ago. *Not significant now*

ALLERGIES: Sulfa, penicillin

MEDICATIONS: propranolol 40 mg twice daily - *HTN*
glipizide 10 mg twice daily - *Diabetes*
phenobarbital 150 mg daily — *epilepsy*
Flexeril 5 mg three times daily PRN for spasms

Percocet 5 mg/325 mg 1 to 2 tablets every 4 hours PRN for pain

FAMILY HISTORY: HTN and DM II on father's side of family; strokes and cardiovascular disease on mother's side of family.

SOCIAL HISTORY: Patient is married with three preteen to teenaged children. He works as a janitor at the local elementary school evenings and nights; he speaks Spanish and very little English. His wife works as a caregiver at night. His mother-in-law lives with the family. He smokes 1 pack of cigarettes per day and drinks about 1 beer per day.

REVIEW OF SYSTEMS: See HPI.

PHYSICAL EXAMINATION: VITAL SIGNS: Temperature 37°C, pulse 72 BPM, respiratory rate 18 respirations per minute, blood pressure 132/84 mm Hg, O_2 saturation 99% on room air.
GENERAL: Experiencing low back pain radiating into RLE; unable to sit or walk comfortably.
SKIN: Warm and dry.
HEENT: Unremarkable.
NECK: Unremarkable.

CARDIAC: Regular rate and rhythm, no **murmurs.**
LUNGS: Clear to **auscultation** bilaterally without **wheeze, rales,** or **rhonchi.**
ABDOMEN: Bowel sounds present, nontender, nondistended. No **hepatosplenomegaly.**
EXTREMITIES: Tenderness to palpation of lumbar musculature. Straight-leg raise positive at 30 degrees on the right.
NEUROLOGICAL: Alert and oriented. Cranial nerves intact. Light-touch sensation impaired RLE in L4 dermatome. Sluggish right patellar tendon reflex.

LABORATORY DATA: CMP normal except for fasting blood glucose of 183. Hg A_{1C} 6.8, creatinine 1.4.

IMAGING STUDIES: MRI of lumbar spine shows lateral disc herniation at L4. No lateral recess narrowing and minimal arthritic changes.

ASSESSMENT: L4 lateral disc herniation.

PLAN: The plan is to admit the patient to the surgical floor for laminectomy. Continue medications, except D/C glipizide, and start metformin 500 mg twice daily. Monitor glucose levels. A physical therapy consult is planned for exercise and discharge planning.

SEEING THE DIAGNOSIS IN ACTION 5-1

After laminectomy, patients typically need to stay in the hospital for 1 to 2 days to recuperate from surgery and stabilize medically. The PTA will work with the PT to instruct the patient in appropriate techniques, such as log roll for bed mobility to protect the back as it heals from surgery.

After discharge home, the patient will likely receive follow-up outpatient physical therapy that includes a variety of interventions designed to promote return of mobility, strength, and balance. Often, the ultimate goal is for the patient to return to work. The PTA will also likely instruct the patient in proper body mechanics and back care to help the patient prevent further back injury. A long-term exercise program will be encouraged after discharge to promote full recovery and prevention of further injury.

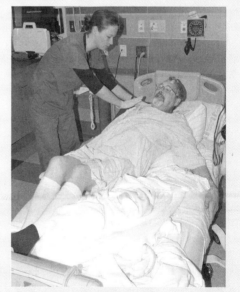

Figure 5-1 Often, a first activity is sitting at the edge of the bed, dangling the legs and allowing the blood pressure to stabilize before getting up to walk. Here, a patient prepares to sit at the edge of the bed after laminectomy.

continued

SEEING THE DIAGNOSIS IN ACTION 5-1 *continued*

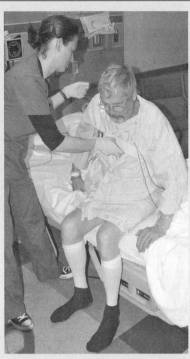

Figure 5-2 While the patient is sitting on the edge of the bed, the PTA can monitor for any signs that the patient is not tolerating the activity. Blood pressure and other vital signs are important to monitor, especially if the patient complains of lightheadedness or dizziness upon sitting up. Often, the patient only needs a few minutes to stabilize, but sometimes the patient must lie down again in order to stabilize the blood pressure and prevent syncope.

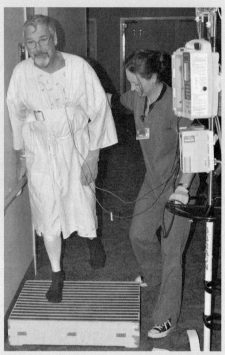

Figure 5-4 Before the patient is discharged, especially if the patient will have to negotiate stairs at home, the PT/PTA team should address stair training and ensure that the patient can manage safely at home.

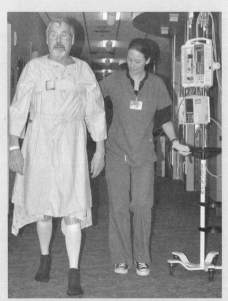

Figure 5-3 Once the patient is stabilized, the PTA can provide appropriate gait training according to the PT plan of care. Severe gait deviations are not typical, but the patient may need an assistive device for a short time after surgery.

REVIEWING THE MEDICAL HISTORY

1. What do you already know about laminectomy and other back injuries and surgeries?

_____

_____

_____

_____

_____

2. Review the vocabulary list and physician's notes. Look up the meanings of any terms you do not understand in a medical dictionary or other text.

_____

_____

_____

_____

_____

3. Review the diagnoses in the past medical history using a medical or pathology text, Internet resource, or other available resource.

_____

_____

_____

_____

_____

4. Which diagnoses in the past medical history would be significant and potentially affect the physical therapy intervention?

_____

_____

_____

_____

_____

5. List the purpose and potential side effects of each of the medications the patient is taking.

_____

_____

_____

_____

_____

6. Describe what each laboratory result measures and list considerations for physical therapy if the results for this patient were *not* in the normal range.

_____

_____

_____

_____

_____

BOX 5-1 | Health-Care Team Member Role: Cultural Awareness

It is important for all health-care professionals and para-professionals to be aware of cultural, religious, socioeconomic, and lifestyle similarities and differences when working with patients. Whatever your own background, you should first observe your own biases and prejudices toward other groups and try to become aware of how you may interact differently with persons within those groups. One of the most important principles to keep in mind is to treat all persons with respect. One way to begin with someone of a different background than yourself is to establish a rapport. To begin developing a rapport with that person, ask one or two questions about the culture. Listen to the person and make eye contact, showing that you are truly interested. As you work with people, try to think about where they are coming from so that you can be more effective with your interventions. I remember a time early in my career when giving a home program to a homeless person. The program was modified somewhat after the patient expressed his concern for privacy. Situations that often arise when working with people of different cultures have to do with privacy, body awareness, pain, family participation in the process, the role of the injured or sick person, and language barriers, as well as many others. To summarize, keeping an open mind to others with the mindset that you are learning from each individual is a great way to build rapport with patients and to provide them with the best of care. Many resources are available to help with learning cultural awareness and diversity.

Acute Care Physical Therapy Initial Evaluation

Patient History

NAME	Carlos Garcia	PERTINENT MEDICAL HISTORY	Per H & P, significant for HTN, DM II, epilepsy, prior left knee arthroscopy, right ankle fracture, and ORIF
ROOM # & BED	B320-01		
MEDICAL RECORD #	12345678	SURGERY	Lumbar laminectomy L3-5
ATTENDING PHYSICIAN	Dr. Jefferson	SURGERY DATE	10/21/2010
CHIEF COMPLAINT	Lumbar pain and laminectomy	PRECAUTIONS	Spinal precautions; log roll
AGE	45	WEIGHT-BEARING STATUS	WBAT
DATE OF BIRTH	07/09/1965		
SEX	Male	LIVING SITUATION	Home
PRIMARY LANGUAGE	Spanish	PRIOR LEVEL OF FUNCTION	Independent
ISOLATION	No		
HEIGHT (CM)	185	ASSISTANCE AVAILABLE	Spouse, works nights; children ages 12, 14, and 17 at home
WEIGHT (KG)	86		
MEDICATION ALLERGIES	Sulfa, penicillin	STAIRS TO ENTER HOME	17 steps plus 12 steps inside to bedrooms
FOOD ALLERGIES	None	RAIL(S) ON STAIRS	One side (right side) ascending outside and 2 rails inside
INITIATED BY	Donna Smith, PT		
DATE	10/21/2010	ASSISTIVE DEVICE USED PRIOR	None
TIME	3:52		
TREATING DIAGNOSIS	Decreased mobility secondary to lumbar laminectomy with fusion due to low back pain	EQUIPMENT PATIENT HAS	None
		DRIVING PRIOR TO ADMIT	Yes
ONSET DATE	10/02/2010	OCCUPATION/LIFE ROLE	Janitor

Systems Review

HEARING	Intact	RESTING RESPIRATORY RATE (respirations per minute)	21
VISION	Intact		
SPEECH	Intact		
PAIN SCALE	VPS	RESTING BLOOD PRESSURE (mm Hg)	140/86
PAIN LEVEL	6		
PAIN LOCATION	Low back	RESTING SpO$_2$	100% on room air
PAIN TYPE	Surgical	LEVEL OF CONSCIOUSNESS	Alert
PAIN INTERVENTION	Notified RN; cold pack end of session		
		ORIENTATION	x 4
RESTING HEART RATE (BPM)	70	SHORT-TERM MEMORY	Intact

Tests and Measures

ROM NECK/TRUNK	Cervical ROM WNL; lumbar ROM impaired all directions with about 50% of normal	BUE STRENGTH	5/5
		BLE STRENGTH	LLE 5/5; right quadriceps, hamstrings, ankle dorsiflexion all 3–/5 with atrophy apparent; others not tested
ROM BUE	WNL		
ROM BLE	WNL except as noted: right SLR 45 degrees, left SLR 55 degrees; bilateral ankle plantarflexion 5 to 65 degrees	SENSATION	Light touch impaired in L3, L4, L5 dermatomes on the right

BED MOBILITY	Mod. A for rolling and scooting up in bed	SITTING BALANCE	Fair at edge of bed because of slight dizziness
SUPINE TO SIT/SIT TO SUPINE	Mod. A with bed flat; using log roll	STANDING BALANCE	Fair with FWW
SIT TO STAND/STAND TO SIT	Min. A with some lightheadedness upon standing; stable BP	GAIT	CGA; 15 feet with FWW
		STAIRS	Not tested
TRANSFERS	Min. A stand pivot with FWW	SITTING TOLERANCE	10 minutes edge of bed

(handwritten annotations: dehydration, loss of blood, medication, blood sugar, ↓H&H)

Evaluation

DIAGNOSIS	Musculoskeletal, pattern I		present during evaluation. He appears motivated to return to his home and work but will need further outpatient physical therapy to address long-term rehabilitation goals and education.
PROGNOSIS	Good; patient is S/P lumbar laminectomy with residual pain, limited motion, and inability to perform functional mobility tasks. He is supported by wife who is		

Plan of Care

PATIENT'S GOALS	To return home and return to work as soon as possible		Gait training
			Stair training
DISCHARGE GOALS	1. Bed mobility and transfers: independent		Home program
	2. Gait: independent greater than 500 feet with assistive device to be determined if needed		Therapeutic exercise
			Therapeutic activities
			Family training PRN
	3. Stairs: independent 17 steps with 1 rail per home situation	FREQUENCY	BID
	4. Home exercise program: independent with written program	PATIENT EDUCATION TOPIC(S)	Log roll
TIME TO ACHIEVE GOALS	By time of discharge	TAUGHT BY	PT
PATIENT/FAMILY UNDERSTAND/AGREES WITH GOALS	Patient/spouse yes	WHO WAS TAUGHT	Patient/spouse
		METHOD OF INSTRUCTION	Verbal/demonstration
INTERVENTIONS	Bed mobility training Transfer training Balance training	EVALUATION OF LEARNING	Needs reinforcement

---

Acute Care Nursing Note

10/21/2010   12:30 PM

The patient arrived from PACU at 1100 and reports nausea with pain of 7/10. Educated regarding using the call light. Percocet is planned for pain management and Zofran for nausea, with regular insulin on a sliding scale. The patient is continent of bladder but has not had a BM yet. He started a stool softener per MD order, with instruction to avoid Valsalva maneuver with BM. The patient's sensation and circulation are intact BLE. A small amount of oozing of serosanguineous fluid is occurring at the top 0.5 cm of the incision. The lungs are clear with cough and deep breath. The PT is to evaluate the patient. The patient is unsteady on his feet, with lightheadedness when he gets up to go to the bathroom. He is able to take ice chips and should be offered crackers and soda when ready. His wife is at his bedside.

ACUTE CARE CRITICAL THINKING QUESTIONS

After reviewing the acute care physical therapy initial evaluation and other discipline notes, address the following:

1. What are the patient's impairments? Functional limitations? Is there a disability?

_____

_____

2. Find assessments of gait, strength, ROM, and balance if available from the initial evaluation and list.

   a. How could each potentially be used to assess function and demonstrate progress toward goals or show the patient's response to physical therapy interventions?

   _____

   _____

   _____

   b. What would be the most important items to document for this patient?

   _____

   _____

   _____

3. After reviewing the POC, describe a possible next treatment session.

   a. List the activities/exercises and your rationale for the order of treatment activities that you selected.

   _____

   _____

   _____

4. What subjective information will you gather during your session to help in your treatment of this patient and why?

   _____

   _____

5. What tests or measures will you use to assess the patient's progress and response to treatment?

   _____

   _____

6. What subjective or objective information that you gather during the treatment might cause you to alter your treatment for this patient and why?

   _____

   _____

7. How would you document your treatment in the SOAP or Patient/Client Management format?

   _____

   _____

   _____

   _____

8. If the treatment goes as expected, what will you do for the next treatment?

   _____

   _____

9. How would you expect this patient to progress over time?

   _____

   _____

10. If the patient does not progress as expected, what might be some reasons for a lack of progress?

    _____

    _____

11. What signs or symptoms, if observed or reported by the patient, would cause you to hold treatment and check with the nursing staff, primary PT, or MD?

    _____

    _____

12. Are there any cultural, socioeconomic, or ethical issues presented in this case that might affect your interventions or communication with this patient? If so, how?

    _____

    _____

13. Re-review this case. Are there any coexisting medical diagnoses that might affect how this patient responds to physical therapy? If so, what are they, and how might they cause the patient to respond to physical therapy differently than you expected?

_____

_____

14. After reviewing the other disciplines' notes regarding this patient, is there any other information that will help you to plan your treatment sessions?

_____

_____

15. Compare your responses on this case with those of your classmates or instructors. What, if anything, would you change and why?

_____

_____

_____

_____

_____

_____

_____

_____

_____

_____

_____

Medical Update

10/22/2010

Upon discharge from the acute setting on 10/22/2010, the patient is S/P lumbar laminectomy. Discontinue glipizide and start metformin 500 mg twice daily. The plan is to follow up in 1 week with the surgeon and for the patient to receive outpatient physical therapy per the surgeon's recommendation.

BOX 5-2 | Physical Therapy Specialty: Back Classes and Education

Most people experience some form of back pain at some point in their lives. Besides a great deal of physical pain and inability to participate in normal activities, patients are often unable to work, creating significant financial loss. Furthermore, after a back injury (and this is true of most injuries), patients are at risk for developing compensatory movement strategies and dysfunction that can contribute to further injury in the same region or elsewhere. Effective physical therapy interventions and best practices for any condition include patient education to prevent further injury and dysfunction. For patients with a back injury, specialized programs have been developed to help educate patients and reduce the risk for further injury. Back classes are often held in group settings in either a hospital or outpatient setting. Some clinics offer this education in the form of video or printed materials that can be reviewed in the clinic or at home. This more formalized education augments the one-on-one instruction in the physical therapy sessions. PTs and PTAs encourage patients to ask questions and will give further information or refer patients to information sources as needed. Back care classes and education typically cover a variety of topics, including common back injuries and surgical procedures; common lifestyle and other risk factors for back problems; basic information to care for the back, including body mechanics and overall health strategies; and finally, basic exercises that will be useful for most patients with back injuries. Specific instruction that is tailored to the individual patient, especially in the area of exercise, is crucial so that the patient's particular problems are addressed.

Two well-known companies that provide patient education materials regarding not only back problems but also other problems are Krames and Visual Health Information. Through their websites, http://www.krames.com and http://www.vhikits.com, one can purchase written or software materials that can be used for patient education. The U.S. National Library of Medicine's National Institute of Health Medline Plus web page at http://www.nlm.nih.gov/medlineplus/backpain.html offers free information about back pain, including its causes and treatments. Many additional resources are available for patient education materials.

Outpatient Physical Therapy Evaluation

NAME	Carlos Garcia
DATE	November 16, 2010
DIAGNOSIS	Lumbar laminectomy L3-5
SUBJECTIVE INFORMATION	Patient reports laminectomy for severe back pain nearly 1 month ago. He does not speak English and has his son here today to translate, but his son will be unable to attend any further sessions because of his school and work schedule. He states, through translation, that his pain is at about 6/10, even with his pain medications, and that it does not allow him to stand or sit longer than 30 minutes. He has trouble bending or lifting anything and cannot drive his car yet because of discomfort when getting in and out of the car and sitting for very long. He drives a Toyota Corolla. He works as a janitor and hopes to return to work soon. He is afraid of losing his job because he supports family in Mexico as well as his family here. He has lived in the United States for 3 years.
OBJECTIVE INFORMATION	
POSTURE	Forward head and lumbar spine flat; slouching in chair with forward shoulders
GAIT	Slight foot drop RLE; uses cane on right side; without cane, he demonstrates Trendelenburg on right side
STRENGTH	Right quadriceps, hamstrings 3/5; dorsiflexors 3–/5; hip abductors 3–/5, extensors 2–/5; LLE 5/5
AROM	RLE limited because of decreased strength per above
PROM	Right SLR 48 degrees; left SLR 55 degrees Bilateral ankle dorsiflexion with knees straight: 5 degrees from neutral; bilateral ankle dorsiflexion with knees bent to neutral
PALPATION/SCAR	Tender to palpation in paraspinals from T8 to S1; gluteals, piriformis, iliotibial band, and hip flexors all right greater than left; spasms in right piriformis
SENSATION	Impaired but still intact RLE L3-5 dermatomes
DIABETIC FOOT EVALUATION	Callus formation bilateral heels and metatarsal heads; no history of ulcer; dry skin; hammertoes; protective sensation; bilateral heels absent

ASSESSMENT	Patient is S/P lumbar laminectomy with fusion and has considerable pain and movement dysfunction related to weakness in RLE. He is unable to perform his normal, daily duties at home, including helping with house or yard work, driving a car, and making a bed. He will benefit from skilled physical therapy services to address the following problems: • Back pain • Decreased ROM and strength • Risk for diabetic foot ulcers • Impaired functional mobility • Inability to return to work
STG (in 2 weeks)	1. Decrease back pain levels to 3/10 to allow him to get in and out of car and sit or stand up to 1 hour. 2. Increase passive bilateral SLR to 70 degrees; ankle dorsiflexion with knees straight to neutral and knees bent to 5 degrees, both to allow normalized gait pattern 3. Increase RLE strength to 3+/5 to allow normalized movement pattern 4. Patient will be able to perform home exercise program of lumbar stabilization and BLE flexibility and strength as well as walking program independently. 5. Patient will demonstrate ability to care for his feet using written diabetic foot protocol.
LTG	Patient will use proper body mechanics for all simulated job duties and yard and house work activities. He will be able to manage his pain levels at home with heat/ice and exercise program. He will be able to walk indoors and outdoors on a variety of surfaces, small hills, and a flight of steps without assistive device and decrease in gait deviations of Trendelenburg and foot drop as a result of increased strength and ROM RLE.
PLAN	Three times per week for 6 weeks for ice and heat modalities to reduce pain and increase ROM, diabetic foot care education, body mechanics training using back care education materials, soft tissue mobilization, ROM and strengthening exercise program, and functional movement training to simulate return to household and work activities.

OUTPATIENT CRITICAL THINKING QUESTIONS

After reviewing the outpatient physical therapy evaluation, address the following:

1. What are the patient's impairments? Functional limitations? Is there a disability?

_____

_____

_____

2. Find assessments of gait, strength, ROM, and balance if available from the initial evaluation and list.

   a. How could each potentially be used to assess function and demonstrate progress toward goals or show the patient's response to physical therapy interventions?

   _____

   _____

   _____

   b. What would be the most important items to document for this patient?

   _____

   _____

3. After reviewing the POC, describe a possible next treatment session.

   a. List the activities/exercises and your rationale for the order of treatment activities that you selected.

   _____

   _____

   _____

4. What subjective information will you gather during your session to help in your treatment of this patient and why?

_____

_____

_____

5. What tests or measures will you use to assess the patient's progress and response to treatment?

_____

_____

_____

6. What subjective or objective information that you gather during the treatment might cause you to alter your treatment for this patient and why?

_____

_____

_____

7. How would you document your treatment in the SOAP or Patient/Client Management format?

_____

_____

_____

8. If the treatment goes as expected, what will you do for the next treatment?

_____

_____

_____

9. How would you expect this patient to progress over time?

_____

_____

10. If the patient does not progress as expected, what might be some reasons for a lack of progress?

_____

_____

_____

11. What signs or symptoms, if observed or reported by the patient, would cause you to hold treatment and check with the nursing staff, primary PT, or MD?

_____

_____

_____

12. Are there any cultural, socioeconomic, or ethical issues presented in this case that might affect your interventions or communication with this patient? If so, how?

_____

_____

_____

continued

OUTPATIENT CRITICAL THINKING QUESTIONS *continued*

13. Re-review this case. Are there any coexisting medical diagnoses that might affect how this patient responds to physical therapy? If so, what are they, and how might they cause the patient to respond differently than you expected?

_____

_____

_____

_____

14. After reviewing the other disciplines' notes regarding this patient, is there any other information that will help you to plan your treatment sessions?

_____

_____

_____

_____

15. Compare your responses on this case with those of your classmates or instructors. What, if anything, would you change and why?

_____

_____

_____

_____

_____

_____

_____

_____

_____

_____

_____

CONTINUUM OF CARE CRITICAL THINKING QUESTIONS

After reviewing the continuum of care for this patient, consider the following:

1. How did the patient's problems change over the month after his initial injury and surgery?

_____

_____

_____

_____

_____

2. How did this affect the interventions that were chosen?

_____

_____

_____

_____

_____

3. How were the same interventions modified over time to progress the patient according to his changing needs?

_____

_____

_____

_____

4. What are some potential community resources that this patient might like to participate in and how would these help him to more quickly reach his ultimate goal of returning to work as soon as possible?

_____

_____

_____

IMPLICATIONS OF PATHOLOGY FOR THE PTA[2]

1. What is the normal timing for healing of soft tissue injury and how will this knowledge affect your approach to this patient in the acute setting as well as later in the outpatient setting?

_____

_____

_____

_____

_____

_____

_____

_____

2. What are the effects of the various physical therapy modalities on soft tissue healing?

_____

_____

_____

_____

_____

_____

_____

_____

_____

3. What are the effects of the various types of exercise on soft tissue healing?

_____

_____

_____

_____

_____

_____

_____

_____

4. What should the PTA be aware of when working with patients with the following soft tissue injuries or surgical repairs?

   a. Degenerative disc disease

   b. Spondylolisthesis

   c. Disc protrusion without surgery

   d. Cervical fusion

   e. Vertebral fracture with and without vertebroplasty

_____

_____

_____

_____

_____

_____

_____

_____

_____

_____

_____

_____

_____

_____

_____

_____

_____

_____

References

1. American Physical Therapy Association: Guide to Physical Therapist Practice, Second Edition. Alexandria, VA: Author, 2001.

2. Goodman CC, Boissonnault FG, Fuller KS: Pathology: Implications for the Physical Therapist, Second Edition. Philadelphia: Saunders, 2003.

Ms. Harper: A Patient With Bilateral Total Knee Replacement

 Preferred Practice Pattern: Musculoskeletal, Pattern H

CHAPTER OUTLINE

Introducing Ms. Harper

Ms. Harper is a 57-year-old woman who has had osteoarthritis in both knees for a number of years and just underwent bilateral total knee replacement (TKR). According to the APTA's *Guide to Physical Therapist Practice* (the *Guide*), she could have the following impairments:

- Decreased ROM
- Muscle weakness
- Muscle guarding
- Pain

Functional limitations may include an inability to access transportation and pain with functional movements and activities. Please refer to the *Guide*[1] for a complete list of possible impairments and functional limitations. As you work through this case, think about which of these the patient is experiencing.

Vocabulary List
- Analgesics
- Narcotics
- NSAIDs
- Auscultation
- Wheeze
- Rales
- Rhonchi
- Hepatosplenomegaly
- Effusion
- Physiatry
- Genu valgus

PHYSICIAN'S HISTORY AND PHYSICAL

PATIENT NAME: Brenda A. Harper
ADMIT DATE: March 22, 2010
BIRTH DATE: April 10, 1952
SEX: Female
ROOM/BED: 314-02
MEDICAL RECORD #: 12345678
CHIEF COMPLAINT: Bilateral knee pain
ATTENDING: Dr. Wayne Smith, MD

HISTORY OF PRESENT ILLNESS: This 57-year-old female is being admitted for bilateral TKR because of a long history of bilateral knee pain due to osteoarthritis. She describes pain with walking, sitting too long, going up and down stairs, and golfing. She has recurrent swelling of the right knee joint. She has tried **analgesics** and **narcotics** as well as **NSAIDs** with only temporary relief. Physical therapy regimen was also unsuccessful in relieving her pain. A steroid injection about 3 months ago to the right knee provided good relief for about 5 weeks. She now opts for surgical intervention. She has been informed of the benefits as well as the potential risks, including blood clot, cardiac arrest, stroke, and death, and chooses to proceed.

PAST MEDICAL HISTORY: The patient's medical history includes the following: bladder cystocele with stress urinary incontinence; anxiety; chronic osteoarthritis of knees, hips, and spine; borderline diabetes; and obesity.

PAST SURGICAL HISTORY: TAH, appendectomy

ALLERGIES: Penicillin *[handwritten: Total abdominal Hysrectomy]*

MEDICATIONS: venlafaxine 50 mg three times daily *[handwritten: Nerve pain, antidepressant]* naproxen 250 mg twice daily *[handwritten: NSaid]*

FAMILY HISTORY: Mother with cardiac history; father with diabetes and stroke.

SOCIAL HISTORY: Patient is divorced with two grown children and two grandchildren, who all live outside the area. She denies smoking and drinking.

REVIEW OF SYSTEMS: See HPI; otherwise negative

PHYSICAL EXAMINATION: VITAL SIGNS: Temperature 37°C, pulse 70 BPM, respiratory rate 20 respirations per minute, blood pressure 120/78 mm Hg, O_2 saturation 100% on room air.
GENERAL: Comfortable
SKIN: Warm and dry without rash or jaundice
HEENT: Unremarkable
SPINE: Tenderness along paraspinals bilaterally from neck to sacrum
CARDIAC: Regular rate and rhythm

LUNGS: Clear to **auscultation** bilaterally without **wheeze, rales,** or **rhonchi**
ABDOMEN: Bowel sounds present, nontender, nondistended. No **hepatosplenomegaly.** *[handwritten: swelling]*
EXTREMITIES: Both knees with **effusion;** no specific tenderness; stable joint without laxity; decreased flexion on the right knee.
NEUROLOGICAL: Alert and oriented. Cranial nerves intact.

LABORATORY DATA: Fasting blood glucose 126

IMAGING STUDIES: Bilateral knee radiography demonstrates severe osteoarthritis, mostly of medial compartments.

ASSESSMENT:
1. Severe bilateral knee osteoarthritis
2. Borderline diabetes

PLAN: The patient will be admitted to the surgical floor for bilateral TKR. The patient will be monitored for sugars and evaluated using the sliding scale of regular insulin for diabetes. **Physiatry,** physical therapy, occupational therapy, and social work consults will be provided, along with discharge planning.

SEEING THE DIAGNOSIS IN ACTION 6-1

Patients who elect to have TKR often need replacement of both knees. If they opt for bilateral surgeries, they often will need more extensive rehabilitation in a rehabilitation facility or skilled nursing facility. They may also need this more intensive rehabilitation if they are in poor physical condition or have coexisting health conditions or other complications while in the hospital.

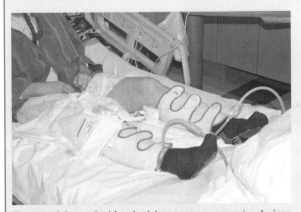

Figure 6-1 It is standard for physicians to use compression devices in the hospital to help improve circulation, prevent increased edema, and prevent DVT. The PTA will remove these devices during the intervention session and replace them when finished.

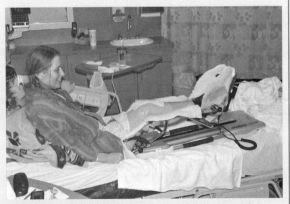

Figure 6-2 Another intervention often used in the acute setting is the continuous passive motion machine to increase knee ROM after surgery. The early use of this device often helps decrease the patient's pain and discomfort with further stretching performed by the PT or PTA.

continued

SEEING THE DIAGNOSIS IN ACTION 6-1 *continued*

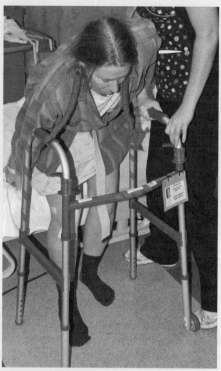

Figure 6-3 Early mobility is important after a TKR, just as after any other surgical procedure. Here, the patient performs sit to stand using a FWW.

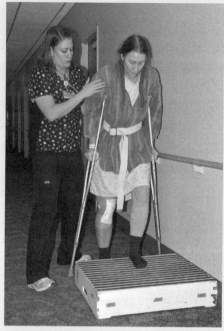

Figure 6-4 Once the patient is ambulating well and before discharge home, especially if there are steps to enter the patient's home, instruction in step training is necessary. Here, the patient performs step training with crutches, but other devices may also be used.

REVIEWING THE MEDICAL HISTORY

1. What do you already know about knee replacements and other knee injuries and surgeries?

_____

_____

_____

_____

_____

2. Review the vocabulary list and physician's notes. Look up the meanings of any terms you do not understand in a medical dictionary or other text.

_____

_____

_____

_____

_____

3. Review the diagnoses in the past medical history using a medical or pathology text, Internet resource, or available other resource.

_____

_____

_____

_____

_____

4. Which diagnoses in the past medical history would be significant and potentially affect the physical therapy intervention?

_____

_____

_____

_____

_____

5. List the purpose and potential side effects of each of the medications the patient is taking.

_____

_____

_____

_____

_____

_____

6. Describe what each laboratory result measures and list considerations for physical therapy if the results for this patient were *not* in the normal range.

_____

_____

_____

_____

_____

Acute Care Physical Therapy Initial Evaluation
Patient History

NAME	Brenda Harper	SURGERY	Bilateral TKR
ROOM # & BED	B314-02	SURGERY DATE	03/22/2010
MEDICAL RECORD #	12345678	PRECAUTIONS	Respiratory MRSA
ATTENDING PHYSICIAN	Dr. Smith	WEIGHT-BEARING STATUS	WBAT
CHIEF COMPLAINT	Bilateral knee pain		
AGE	57	LIVING SITUATION	Home in her apartment
DATE OF BIRTH	04/10/1952	PRIOR LEVEL OF FUNCTION	Independent with ambulation without assistive device but has a cane
SEX	Female		
PRIMARY LANGUAGE	English	ASSISTANCE AVAILABLE	Boyfriend can bring some meals but works full-time
ISOLATION	Yes; MRSA		
HEIGHT (CM)	168	STAIRS TO ENTER HOME	8 + 6, plus 6 steps up to living area and bedrooms
WEIGHT (KG)	98		
MEDICATION ALLERGIES	Penicillin	RAIL(S) ON STAIRS	One side, outside and inside
FOOD ALLERGIES	None	ASSISTIVE DEVICE USED PRIOR	None
INITIATED BY	Donna Smith, PT		
DATE	03/22/2010	EQUIPMENT PATIENT HAS	Cane
TIME	15:25		
TREATING DIAGNOSIS	Decreased mobility S/P bilateral TKR	DRIVING PRIOR TO ADMIT	YES
ONSET DATE	03/22/2010		
PERTINENT MEDICAL HISTORY	Per H & P, significant for the following: bladder prolapse; stress urinary incontinence; anxiety; chronic osteoarthritis of knees, hips, and spine; borderline DM II, TAH, appendectomy, and obesity.	OCCUPATION/LIFE ROLE	Bookkeeper; enjoys gardening, cooking, entertaining, and travel

continued

Acute Care Physical Therapy Initial Evaluation *continued*

Systems Review

HEARING	HOH		RESTING RESPIRATORY RATE (respirations per minute)	22
VISION	Intact			
SPEECH	Normal		RESTING BLOOD PRESSURE (mm Hg)	120/82
PAIN SCALE	VPS			
PAIN LEVEL	8		RESTING SpO$_2$	99% on room air
PAIN LOCATION	Bilateral knees		LEVEL OF CONSCIOUSNESS	Alert
PAIN TYPE	Surgical			
PAIN INTERVENTION	Notified RN and was medicated before mobility assessments		ORIENTATION	x 4
			SHORT-TERM MEMORY	Intact
RESTING HEART RATE (BPM)	78			

Tests and Measures

ROM NECK/TRUNK	WFL		SUPINE TO SIT/SIT TO SUPINE	Max. A with head flat; Min. A with head of bed elevated
ROM BUE	WNL			
ROM RLE	PROM knee flexion 15 to 65 degrees		SIT TO STAND/STAND TO SIT	Mod. A
ROM LLE	PROM knee flexion 16 to 69 degrees			
BUE STRENGTH	WNL		TRANSFERS	Mod. A stand pivot with FWW
RLE STRENGTH	Hip flexion, knee extension 3–/5; ankle 4/5		SITTING BALANCE	Fair; edge of bed using BUE to support self
			STANDING BALANCE	Fair with FWW
LLE STRENGTH	Hip flexion, knee extension 3–/5; ankle 4/5		GAIT	4 feet with FWW, Mod. A and extreme anxiety because of pain
SENSATION	Intact light-touch BLE			
BED MOBILITY	Mod. A to roll; Min. A to scoot up in bed but needs overhead trapeze		STAIRS	Unable
			SITTING TOLERANCE	5 minutes edge of bed

Evaluation

DIAGNOSIS	Musculoskeletal, pattern H		years and worries it may be worse after getting the catheter out because she cannot move quickly enough to get to the bathroom. Recommend inpatient rehabilitation stay before D/C home, and outpatient follow-up with a women's health specialist who can also address urinary incontinence problems.
PROGNOSIS	Good. Patient is S/P bilateral TKR. She has been fairly active with gardening but is generally deconditioned and is having a difficult time managing the postsurgical pain. Pain limits participation; she needs premedication before treatments. She reports stress urinary incontinence for		

Plan of Care

PATIENT'S GOALS	To return home, but she agrees to additional rehabilitation before going home; she wants to be able to return to gardening, driving, housekeeping, and working part-time.		Home program Therapeutic exercise Therapeutic activities
		FREQUENCY	BID
DISCHARGE GOALS	Bed mobility and transfers: Min. A Gait: Min. A 30 feet with FWW Home exercise program: Min. A	PATIENT EDUCATION TOPIC(S)	Activity; use of ankle pumps to increase circulation to legs. Call for help with transfers for safety.
TIME TO ACHIEVE GOALS	By time of discharge	TAUGHT BY	PT
PATIENT/FAMILY UNDERSTAND/AGREES WITH GOALS	Patient yes	WHO WAS TAUGHT	Patient
		METHOD OF INSTRUCTION	Verbal/demonstration
INTERVENTIONS	Bed mobility training Transfer training Balance training Gait training	EVALUATION OF LEARNING	Needs reinforcement

---

Acute Care Nursing Note

03/22/2010   3:15 PM

The patient is on respiratory MRSA precautions and reports pain of 5/10. The patient has received instruction regarding pain pump. Her dressings are clean, dry, and intact. The Foley catheter is draining amber urine. She has not had a BM but has mild nausea. She is able to sip 7-Up and eat a cracker but is still nauseous. Her boyfriend is visiting. The patient plans to D/C to inpatient rehabilitation unit if a bed is available. The plan is to start diabetic education tomorrow. She is on a diabetic diet. FBG is taken twice daily, and her current blood glucose level is 164. The patient's anxiety level is increased, according to the patient and boyfriend, because of uncertainty about going home. A dietitian consult is pending for diet and weight loss.

Acute Care Social Work Note

3/23/2010   11:35 AM

Patient is S/P bilateral TKR. Patient would prefer inpatient rehabilitation unit if a bed is available; otherwise, she would prefer SNF close to home. Admissions coordinator for the rehabilitation unit states that a bed should be available for possible D/C on 03/25/2010. The patient is on Medicaid. No other social work needs have been identified at this time, but will follow-up as needed.

Acute Care Occupational Therapy Summary

3/23/2010   2:27 PM

Patient is S/P bilateral TKR with decreased mobility, pain, and difficulty with all ADLs. She needs Mod. A to dress lower body, Min. A for upper body, Max. A for toilet transfer, and Mod. A for toileting, including pulling pants down/up and hygiene for BM. She still has a Foley catheter. She needs setup for grooming and oral care from W/C level. Shower has not been assessed yet. Goals for the patient include increasing to Min. A for dressing lower body, Mod. A for toilet transfer, and Min. A for toileting as well as independent dressing of upper body, grooming, and oral care all before D/C. D/C to inpatient rehabilitation unit recommended.

SEEING THE DIAGNOSIS IN ACTION 6-2

When stabilized medically and discharged from the acute and subacute settings, the patient will likely need outpatient physical therapy to ensure progress toward goals of returning to work and leisure activities. Typically, patients still do not have full ROM or strength in the affected extremity and need progressive ROM and strengthening activities as well as balance and a safe return to a general exercise program if applicable.

As with most patients, those who have had TKR will need to continue with a home exercise program after they are discharged from all therapies. The program will likely include progressive strengthening, flexibility, and balance exercise as well as a return to prior activities and a general exercise program.

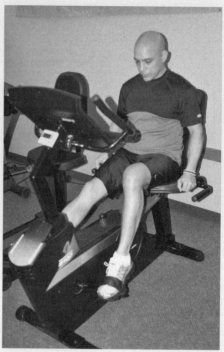

Figure 6-6 Patients may also use a recumbent bike to increase ROM. Here, the patient works to increase ROM on the left knee after TKR.

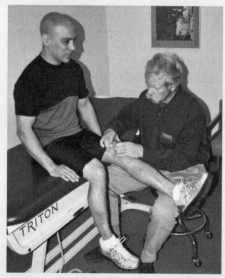

Figure 6-5 Once the incision is healed, the physical therapy POC may include patellar mobilization to help increase ROM and decrease pain.

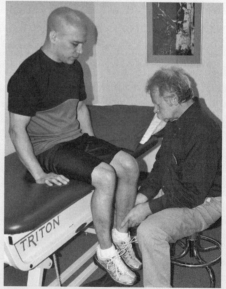

Figure 6-7 After providing interventions, the PT remeasures knee flexion ROM in order to document progress.

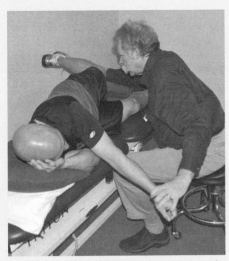

Figure 6-8 Here, the PT uses proprioceptive neuromuscular facilitation techniques to promote full recovery of strength and coordinated movement after left TKR.

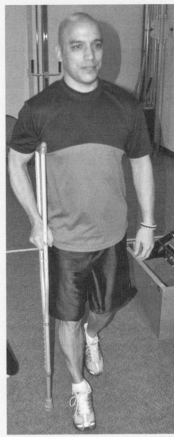

Figure 6-9 Gait training is still important in these later phases of rehabilitation in order to correct or prevent further dysfunction caused by gait deviations. Here, the patient progresses to using a single crutch and may or may not use a cane before being able to walk independently without a device.

ACUTE CARE CRITICAL THINKING QUESTIONS

After reviewing the acute care physical therapy initial evaluation and other discipline notes, address the following:

1. What are the patient's impairments? Functional limitations? Is there a disability?

_____

_____

_____

_____

_____

2. Find assessments of gait, strength, ROM, and balance if available from the initial evaluation and list.

   a. How could each potentially be used to assess function and demonstrate progress toward goals or show the patient's response to physical therapy interventions?

_____

_____

_____

continued

ACUTE CARE CRITICAL THINKING QUESTIONS *continued*

b. What would be the most important items to document for this patient?

_____

_____

_____

3. After reviewing the POC, describe a possible next treatment session.

a. List the activities/exercises and your rationale for the order of treatment activities that you selected.

_____

_____

_____

4. What subjective information will you gather during your session to help in your treatment of this patient and why?

_____

_____

5. What tests or measures will you use to assess the patient's progress and response to treatment?

_____

_____

6. What subjective or objective information that you gather during the treatment might cause you to alter your treatment for this patient and why?

_____

_____

7. How would you document your treatment in the SOAP or Patient/Client Management format?

_____

_____

_____

_____

8. If the treatment goes as expected, what will you do for the next treatment?

_____

_____

9. How would you expect this patient to progress over time?

_____

_____

_____

10. If the patient does not progress as expected, what might be some reasons for a lack of progress?

_____

_____

11. What signs or symptoms, if observed or reported by the patient, would cause you to hold treatment and check with the nursing staff, primary PT, or MD?

_____

_____

12. Are there any cultural, socioeconomic, or ethical issues presented in this case that might affect your interventions or communication with this patient? If so, how?

_____

_____

13. Re-review this case. Are there any coexisting medical diagnoses that might affect how this patient responds to physical therapy? If so, what are they, and how might they cause the patient to respond to physical therapy differently than you expected?

_____

_____

14. After reviewing the other disciplines' notes regarding this patient, is there any other information that will help you to plan your treatment sessions?

_____

_____

15. Compare your responses on this case with those of your classmates or instructors. What, if anything, would you change and why?

_____

_____

Medical Update

03/25/2010

Upon discharge from the acute setting on 03/25/2010, the patient is S/P bilateral TKR. Her blood sugars have been less than 200. PT/INR is 1.2. The plan includes inpatient rehabilitation with monitoring of blood sugars, removal of the Foley catheter when ready, and starting Coumadin 5 mg daily.

BOX 6-1 | Health-Care Team Member Role: Patient

PTAs must always remember that the patient is the most important member of the health-care team. If we, as professionals, will listen to what patients have to say, we will usually be able to learn how best to help them. PTAs can practice active listening skills to determine the patient's understanding of the POC as well as their perception of progress being made or not made. Doing so will help uncover questions patients may have but don't know how to articulate. If PTs and PTAs will encourage patients to participate more in their therapy plan, from goal setting to discharge planning, and if patients are active in this way, they will usually have a better outcome. If patients are not participating as well or as actively as we think they should be, we can take a step back to try to understand where the patient is coming from. Perhaps there are outside issues, such as finances, emotional disturbance, interpersonal conflicts or even grieving over their losses (even if they are temporary), that are affecting their ability to focus on physical therapy. The PT and PTA team can listen and offer reassurances, make appropriate referrals to other resources if needed, and generally encourage patients to come along and participate as best they can. Increased patient participation, in the end, enables patients to progress more easily through the stages of healing, helping to prevent them from getting "stuck" in the rehabilitation process.

Inpatient Rehabilitation Physical Therapy Initial Evaluation
Patient History

NAME	Brenda Harper		new diagnosis of DM II; TAH; appendectomy; and obesity.
ROOM # & BED	B364-02		
MEDICAL RECORD #	12345678	SURGERY	Bilateral TKR
ATTENDING PHYSICIAN	Dr. Gordon	SURGERY DATE	03/22/2010
CHIEF COMPLAINT	Bilateral knee pain	PRECAUTIONS	Respiratory MRSA
AGE	57	WEIGHT-BEARING STATUS	WBAT
DATE OF BIRTH	04/10/1952		
SEX	Female	LIVING SITUATION	Apartment
PRIMARY LANGUAGE	English	PRIOR LEVEL OF FUNCTION	Independent with ambulation without assistive device but has a cane. No fall risk.
ISOLATION	Yes; respiratory MRSA		
HEIGHT (CM)	168		
WEIGHT (KG)	96	ASSISTANCE AVAILABLE	Boyfriend is minimally available; he works full-time.
MEDICATION ALLERGIES	Penicillin	STAIRS TO ENTER HOME	8 + 6, plus 6 steps up to living area and bedrooms
FOOD ALLERGIES	No food allergies		
INITIATED BY	Roger Lee, PT	RAIL(S) ON STAIRS	One side, outside and inside
DATE	03/25/2010	ASSISTIVE DEVICE USED PRIOR	None
TIME	11:21		
TREATING DIAGNOSIS	Decreased mobility S/P bilateral TKR	EQUIPMENT PATIENT HAS	Cane
ONSET DATE	03/22/2010	DRIVING PRIOR TO ADMIT	Yes
PERTINENT MEDICAL HISTORY	Per H & P, significant for the following: bladder cystocele; stress urinary incontinence; anxiety; chronic osteoarthritis of knees, hips, and spine;	OCCUPATION/LIFE ROLE	Bookkeeper; enjoys gardening, cooking, entertaining, travel

continued

Inpatient Rehabilitation Physical Therapy
Initial Evaluation *continued*

Systems Review

HEARING	HOH	RESTING HR (BPM)	75
VISION	Intact	RESTING RESPIRATORY RATE (respirations per minute)	22
SPEECH	Normal		
PAIN SCALE	VPS	RESTING BP (mm Hg)	122/78
PAIN LEVEL	6	RESTING SpO$_2$	100% on room air
PAIN LOCATION	Bilateral knees	LEVEL OF CONSCIOUSNESS	Alert
PAIN TYPE	Surgical/ache		
PAIN INTERVENTION	Notified RN and was medicated before mobility assessments	ORIENTATION	x 4
		SHORT-TERM MEMORY	Intact

Tests and Measures

ROM NECK/TRUNK	WFL	SIT TO STAND/STAND TO SIT	Contact guard assist
ROM BUE	WNL		
ROM RLE	PROM knee flexion 10 to 75 degrees Ankle dorsiflexion 5 degrees from neutral	TRANSFERS	Min. A stand pivot with FWW
		SITTING BALANCE	Fair at edge of bed using BUE to support self
ROM LLE	PROM knee flexion 12 to 82 degrees Ankle dorsiflexion 8 degrees from neutral	STANDING BALANCE	Fair with FWW; BERG score 39/56
BUE STRENGTH	WNL	GAIT	20 feet with FWW, Min. A and lateral trunk lean, decreased step lengths bilaterally and minimal knee flexion with bilateral circumduction to compensate
BLE STRENGTH	Hip flexion 3–/5 limited by obesity; knee extension 3–/5; hamstring takes minimal resistance in sitting; ankle plantarflexion, dorsiflexion, eversion, inversion 4/5		
		STAIRS	4 steps with 2 rails, Min. A
SENSATION	Intact light-touch BLE; intact temperature and pain sensation BLE	SITTING TOLERANCE (MIN)	20 minutes edge of bed; 2 hours in chair
BED MOBILITY	Min. A to roll; Mod. I to scoot up in bed with overhead trapeze; Mod. A without trapeze	DIABETIC FOOT EVALUATION	Protective sensation intact; hammer toes; dry skin
SUPINE TO SIT/SIT TO SUPINE	Min. A with head flat		

Evaluation

DIAGNOSIS	Musculoskeletal, pattern H
PROGNOSIS	Good. Patient is S/P bilateral TKR and needs skilled physical therapy services to enable her to return to her prior level of function both in the home and at work. She demonstrates motivation to participate in inpatient rehabilitation program and has emotional support from boyfriend and other friends who visit regularly. Pain control has improved since acute admit but still limits participation; she needs premedication before treatments. Her boyfriend can bring food over but works full-time and cannot be there during the day after D/C. Can stay at night to help if needed at D/C. Progress with ROM has been slow thus far because of pain control, but steady, gradual progress is expected until ready for D/C home and can begin rehabilitation in outpatient setting. The patient will need FWW at D/C.

Plan of Care			
PATIENT'S GOALS	Return to home and work ASAP. Wants to walk better and be independent with dressing, bathing, cooking, and driving. Enjoys gardening, driving, housekeeping.	INTERVENTIONS	Bed mobility training Transfer training Balance training Gait training Home program Therapeutic exercise Therapeutic activities Electrical stimulation Physical modalities Family training PRN Diabetic foot care training
DISCHARGE GOALS	1. Bed mobility, transfers, car transfers: Mod. I 2. Gait: Mod. I x 300 feet indoors; 100 feet outdoors on sidewalk and grass surfaces with FWW or cane 3. Home exercise program: Mod. I		
TIME TO ACHIEVE GOALS	By time of discharge		
PATIENT/FAMILY UNDERSTAND/AGREES WITH GOALS	Patient yes		

Inpatient Rehabilitation Nursing Note

3/25/2010   12:55 PM

The resident was admitted today S/P bilateral TKR. She has a new diagnosis of DM II and has a history of stress urinary incontinence. She was transferred from W/C onto bed with one-person assist. She is able to make her needs known. Foley is draining light amber urine. She is continent of bowel. Her vital signs are as follows: temperature 37.1°C, resting pulse 72 BPM, respiratory rate 20 respirations per minute, BP 120/72 mm Hg, SpO$_2$ 99% on room air at rest. She complains of bilateral knee pain at 8/10 and was given one Percocet with good relief 1 hour later. Blood sugars are at 239, and the patient has been given insulin. She is on an ADA diet.

Inpatient Rehabilitation Social Work Summary

3/29/2010   10:18 AM

The patient was admitted 03/25/2010 S/P bilateral TKR. A team conference took place today, 03/29/2010, with the patient, boyfriend, MD, PT, OT, RN, and MSW present. The MD reports following laboratory results and blood work to make sure blood sugars are within normal limits. She is also recommending a urology consult for incontinence problems. Staples are to be removed in 2 weeks. Therapists report patient needing minimal assist for most mobility tasks. She is participating well but is limited by pain and anxiety. The PT is using ice and electrical stimulation for enhanced pain control before or after therapy. The patient expresses concern about urinary incontinence, hoping to keep the Foley in as long as possible. Nursing staff are to address this issue with a bladder program once the Foley is out; the PT and OT will begin pelvic floor strengthening. Nursing staff are working toward improved pain control with medication schedule to follow therapy schedule and also following blood sugars and beginning diabetic teaching; a nutrition consult is planned. The current plan is to D/C home with outpatient physical therapy follow-up and assistive device and other equipment to be determined. D/C is tentatively planned for 2 weeks from today, depending on progress. Family training is set for one day, 04/05/2010, with her boyfriend.

Inpatient Rehabilitation Occupational Therapy Summary

03/30/2010   9:15 AM

The patient is S/P bilateral TKR with new diagnosis of DM II. She uses a reacher to retrieve things out of reach and toileting aid for hygiene after BM. Her Foley was just removed, and she has a history of urinary stress incontinence; I will work with nursing staff on a bladder program. Goals for discharge home include the following: Mod. I status with all dressing, toileting, grooming, oral hygiene needs, cooking, light meal preparation, and showering.

INPATIENT REHABILITATION CRITICAL THINKING QUESTIONS

After reviewing the inpatient rehabilitation physical therapy initial evaluation and other discipline notes, address the following:

1. What are the patient's impairments? Functional limitations? Is there a disability?

_____

_____

_____

2. Find assessments of gait, strength, ROM, and balance if available from the initial evaluation and list.

   a. How could each potentially be used to assess function and demonstrate progress toward goals or show the patient's response to physical therapy interventions?

_____

_____

_____

   b. What would be the most important items to document for this patient?

_____

_____

_____

3. After reviewing the POC, describe a possible next treatment session.

   a. List the activities/exercises and your rationale for the order of treatment activities that you selected.

_____

_____

_____

4. What subjective information will you gather during your session to help in your treatment of this patient and why?

_____

_____

5. What tests or measures will you use to assess the patient's progress and response to treatment?

_____

_____

6. What subjective or objective information that you gather during the treatment might cause you to alter your treatment for this patient and why?

_____

_____

7. How would you document your treatment in the SOAP or Patient/Client Management format?

_____

_____

8. If the treatment goes as expected, what will you do for the next treatment?

_____

_____

9. How would you expect this patient to progress over time?

_____

_____

10. If the patient does not progress as expected, what might be some reasons for a lack of progress?

_____

_____

_____

11. What signs or symptoms, if observed or reported by the patient, would cause you to hold treatment and check with the nursing staff, primary PT, or MD?

_____

_____

_____

12. Are there any cultural, socioeconomic, or ethical issues presented in this case that might affect your interventions or communication with this patient? If so, how?

_____

_____

_____

13. Re-review this case. Are there any co-existing medical diagnoses that might affect how this patient responds to physical therapy? If so, what are they, and how might they cause the patient to respond to physical therapy differently than you expected?

_____

_____

14. After reviewing the other disciplines' notes regarding this patient, is there any other information that will help you to plan your treatment sessions?

_____

_____

_____

15. Compare your responses on this case with those of your classmates or instructors. What, if anything, would you change and why?

_____

_____

Outpatient Physical Therapy Evaluation

NAME	Brenda Harper
DATE	April 9, 2010
DIAGNOSIS	Bilateral TKR
SUBJECTIVE INFORMATION	Patient is S/P bilateral TKR and was discharged from inpatient rehabilitation unit 1 day ago. She has pain in bilateral knees at 4/5 at rest and at 8/10 with exercises when pushed by therapist. She has difficulty going up/down her stairs at home and standing long enough to prepare a light meal, about 10 minutes. She would like to be able to go grocery shopping, drive her car, and start doing some gardening again. She and her boyfriend are planning an RV trip out of state in 2 months; she needs to do the driving. In addition to her knees, she reports urinary incontinence with stress whenever lifting or otherwise exerting herself. It can happen at least 4 times in the average day. The urologist tried her on a medication, but it did not help, and she did not return, but she is interested in learning exercises that may help.

OBJECTIVE INFORMATION	
POSTURE	Slightly kyphotic with forward head; right pelvis elevated compared with left, with apparent leg-length discrepancy; measured 1.5-cm leg-length difference with LLE shorter; bilateral **genu valgus** and pronated feet
GAIT	Slow, short but equal length steps that do not pass the opposite foot; lacks full knee and hip extension during stance phase bilaterally; uses FWW; trunk leans ipsilaterally with each step; on treadmill able to walk at 1 mile per hour
BALANCE	BERG balance scale 44/56
STRENGTH	Bilateral hip flexors, quads 3/5; hamstrings 3–/5; hip abduction 2–/5; hip extension 2–/5; ankle dorsiflexors/plantarflexors/eversion and inversion 4/5

continued

Outpatient Physical Therapy Evaluation *continued*

PROM	Right knee flexion 5 to 103 degrees with pain Left knee flexion 0 to 105 degrees with pain Bilateral ankle dorsiflexion to neutral with knees straight; 5 degrees from neutral with knees bent
PALPATION	Tenderness to palpation bilateral patellar tendons; myofascial restrictions of quadriceps and hamstrings both distally greater than proximally
SENSATION	Intact light-touch, temperature, and pain sensation BLE; impaired proprioception in bilateral great toes and ankles but intact knees and hips
KNEE CIRCUMFERENCES	Right: mid patella: 51.25 cm Left: mid patella: 49.5 cm
ASSESSMENT	Patient has impaired strength, PROM, balance, and pain as well as residual edema from bilateral TKR about 3 weeks ago. These impairments affect her ability to ambulate, especially outdoors and on stairs. Gait deviations are likely due to weakness, especially in hip extension and abduction, decreased knee ROM, and quadriceps and hamstring strength and pain. She still cannot drive comfortably, stand longer than 10 minutes to prepare a meal, or work in her garden because of her limitations. She will benefit from skilled therapy to address the following goals:
STG (2 weeks)	1. Decrease resting pain level to 2/10 and activity pain level to 3/10 in order to participate fully in a home exercise program. 2. Increase BERG balance scale total score to 50/56 to increase safety with ambulation and progress to a cane then no assistive device.

	3. Increase PROM bilateral knee flexion to 0 to 120 degrees to allow her to drive comfortably for at least 30 minutes at a time. 4. Increase PROM bilateral ankle dorsiflexion with knees straight to 5 degrees to enable her to walk with decreased gait deviations. 5. Increase bilateral quadriceps and hamstring strength to 4/5 to achieve improved gait with decreased deviations.
LTG	1. Ambulate at 3 mile per hour on treadmill for at least 20 minutes with decreased gait deviations of lateral trunk lean and short step length. 2. Independent with written home exercise program for ROM, strength, balance, and cardiovascular endurance as well as pelvic floor exercise program to allow her to return to light gardening and other prior activities with decreased frequency of urinary incontinence to once per day. 3. Able to manage pain bilateral knees with home ice/heat and exercises.
PLAN	The plan includes orthotic assessment and fabrication for feet to improve biomechanical alignment and decrease risk for further pain and dysfunction BLE and to address leg-length discrepancy. Also planned are ice and heating modalities to increase ROM and decrease pain; soft tissue and joint mobilization; stretching, strengthening, balance, and cardiovascular exercise; body mechanics training for household tasks such as cooking, cleaning, and gardening; and electrical stimulation two or three times per week for 6 weeks, along with a pelvic floor retraining program.

OUTPATIENT CRITICAL THINKING QUESTIONS

After reviewing the outpatient physical therapy evaluation, address the following:

1. What are the patient's impairments? Functional limitations? Is there a disability?

_____

_____

_____

_____

2. Find assessments of gait, strength, ROM and balance if available from the initial evaluation and list.

   a. How could each potentially be used to assess function and demonstrate progress toward goals or show the patient's response to physical therapy interventions?

_____

_____

_____

_____

   b. What would be the most important items to document for this patient?

_____

_____

_____

_____

3. After reviewing the POC, describe a possible next treatment session.

   a. List the activities/exercises and your rationale for the order of treatment activities that you selected.

_____

_____

_____

4. What subjective information will you gather during your session to help in your treatment of this patient and why?

_____

_____

_____

5. What tests or measures will you use to assess the patient's progress and response to treatment?

_____

_____

_____

6. What subjective or objective information that you gather during the treatment might cause you to alter your treatment for this patient and why?

_____

_____

_____

7. How would you document your treatment in the SOAP or Patient/Client Management format?

_____

_____

_____

_____

8. If the treatment goes as expected, what will you do for the next treatment?

_____

_____

9. How would you expect this patient to progress over time?

_____

_____

_____

10. If the patient does not progress as expected, what might be some reasons for a lack of progress?

_____

_____

11. What signs or symptoms, if observed or reported by the patient, would cause you to hold treatment and check with the nursing staff, primary PT, or MD?

_____

_____

continued

OUTPATIENT CRITICAL THINKING QUESTIONS *continued*

12. Are there any cultural, socioeconomic, or ethical issues presented in this case that might affect your interventions or communication with this patient? If so, how?

_____

_____

_____

13. Re-review this case. Are there any co-existing medical diagnoses that might affect how this patient responds to physical therapy? If so, what are they, and how might they cause the patient to respond to physical therapy differently than you expected?

_____

_____

_____

14. After reviewing the other disciplines' notes regarding this patient, is there any other information that will help you to plan your treatment sessions?

_____

_____

_____

_____

15. Compare your responses on this case with those of your classmates or instructors. What, if anything, would you change and why?

_____

_____

_____

_____

CONTINUUM OF CARE CRITICAL THINKING QUESTIONS

After reviewing the continuum of care for this patient, consider the following:

1. How did the patient's problems change over the months after her surgery?

_____

_____

_____

_____

_____

_____

_____

2. How did this affect the interventions that were chosen?

_____

_____

_____

_____

_____

_____

3. How were the same interventions modified over time to progress the patient according to her changing needs?

_____

_____

_____

_____

_____

_____

4. What are some potential community resources that this patient might like to participate in and how would these help her to maintain and improve her physical fitness?

_____

_____

_____

_____

IMPLICATIONS OF PATHOLOGY FOR THE PTA[2]

1. What might be the cause of the following signs/symptoms in a patient with osteoarthritis or S/P joint replacement and what should the PTA do if he/she encounters these with a patient:
   - Indigestion, nausea, vomiting, thoracic pain or melena (black, tarry stools)?
   - Unexplained back or shoulder pain or excessive bruising?
   - LE pain that may or may not include swelling and redness?
   - Chest pain or trouble breathing?
   - Excessive or new warmth to touch and/or edema in the area of surgery?

   _____

   _____

   _____

   _____

   _____

   _____

   _____

   _____

   _____

   _____

2. What should the PTA be aware of when working with patients with the following?
   - Anterior cruciate ligament injury/surgical repair
   - S/P knee arthroscopy
   - Meniscus tear
   - Patellar tendonitis
   - Chondromalacia patella

   _____

   _____

   _____

   _____

   _____

   _____

   _____

   _____

   _____

   _____

   _____

   _____

References

1. American Physical Therapy Association: Guide to Physical Therapist Practice, Second Edition. Alexandria, VA: Author, 2001.

2. Goodman CC, Boissonnault FG, Fuller KS: Pathology: Implications for the Physical Therapist, Second Edition. Philadelphia: Saunders, 2003.

Mr. Jenkins: A Patient With Total Hip Replacement

Preferred Practice Pattern: Musculoskeletal, Pattern H

CHAPTER OUTLINE

Introducing Mr. Jenkins

Mr. Jenkins is a 74-year-old man who has had osteoarthritis in the right hip for more than 5 years and just underwent right THR. According to the APTA's *Guide to Physical Therapist Practice* (the *Guide*), he could have the following impairments:

- Limited ROM
- Muscle weakness
- Muscle guarding
- Pain

Functional limitations may include the following:

- Inability to access transportation
- Pain with functional movements and activities

Please refer to the *Guide*[1] for a complete list of possible impairments and functional limitations. As you work through this case, think about which of these the patient is experiencing.

Vocabulary List

Analgesics	Arthroscopy
Narcotics	Jaundice
NSAIDs	Scoliosis
Murmur	Physiatry
Wheezes	Foley
Rhonchi	Trendelenburg
Hepatosplenomegaly	Antalgic
Osteophytes	

PHYSICIAN'S HISTORY AND PHYSICAL

PATIENT NAME: Harold P. Jenkins
ADMIT DATE: May 14, 2010
BIRTH DATE: March 12, 1936
SEX: Male
ROOM/BED: 304-02
MEDICAL RECORD #: 12345678
CHIEF COMPLAINT: Right hip pain
ATTENDING: Dr. Wayne Smith, MD

HISTORY OF PRESENT ILLNESS: This 74-year-old male is being admitted for right THR because of a long history of right hip pain due to osteoarthritis. He describes pain with walking, driving, going up and down stairs, and doing work on his boat and car. He has tried **analgesics,** including **narcotics** and **NSAIDs,** with minimal pain relief. He now opts for surgical intervention. He has been informed of the benefits and potential risks, including blood clot, cardiac arrest, stroke, and death, and chooses to proceed.

PAST MEDICAL HISTORY: His medical history includes prostate cancer, treated with chemotherapy and radiation therapy 5 years ago, and recent PSA of less than 0.1; atrial fibrillation on Coumadin; COPD; smoking; and early dementia.

PAST SURGICAL HISTORY: Back surgery twice; left knee **arthroscopy**, then TKR 7 years ago

ALLERGIES: Dairy

MEDICATIONS: Coumadin 2.5 mg daily
digoxin 0.125 mg daily
Spiriva HandiHaler 1 capsule daily
Aricept 5 mg daily
Tylenol 325 mg 1 to 2 tablets every 4 hours PRN for pain

FAMILY HISTORY: Father with heart problems; mother died at age 50 with uterine cancer

SOCIAL HISTORY: Widowed with two grown sons who live out of state

REVIEW OF SYSTEMS: See HPI; otherwise negative

PHYSICAL EXAMINATION:

VITAL SIGNS: Temperature 36.9°C, pulse 68 BPM, respiratory rate 21 respirations per minute, blood pressure 116/68 mm Hg, O_2 saturation 96% on 3 liters.

GENERAL: Comfortable other than right hip pain

SKIN: Warm and dry without rash or **jaundice**

HEENT: Unremarkable

SPINE: Scar from prior surgeries in lumbar spine; mild **scoliosis**

CARDIAC: Irregularly irregular rhythm without **murmur**

LUNGS: Expiratory **wheezes** and **rhonchi**

ABDOMEN: Bowel sounds present, nontender, nondistended. No **hepatosplenomegaly.**

EXTREMITIES: Normal appearing with decreased ROM in external rotation of right hip; nontender over trochanter.

NEUROLOGICAL: Alert and oriented. Cranial nerves intact.

LABORATORY DATA: Coumadin stopped 4 days ago, INR 1.2 today.

IMAGING STUDIES: Right hip radiograph demonstrates severe osteoarthritis with marked loss of joint cartilage and **osteophytes.**

ASSESSMENT: Severe right hip osteoarthritis

PLAN: The plan is to admit the patient to the surgical floor for right posterior approach THR. **Physiatry**, physical therapy, occupational therapy, and social work consults are planned, along with discharge planning. Coumadin will be reinstituted on second postoperative day.

SEEING THE DIAGNOSIS IN ACTION 7-1

Patients may elect for a THR due to osteoarthritis, or they may need one after a hip fracture, often due to a fall. Especially in the latter case, the physical therapy POC will probably include education in fall prevention strategies as well as the exercises and functional mobility training needed to return to the prior level of function. The PTA must remember to follow and teach the patient to follow the appropriate hip precautions that help prevent a dislocation.

When the patient begins outpatient physical therapy, it is usually appropriate to progress the patient, and a variety of equipment can be used to help the patient gain progress. The PTA must still help the patient adhere to the hip precautions; this can be difficult on certain types of equipment, especially if the patient must not flex the hip past 90 degrees.

continued

SEEING THE DIAGNOSIS IN ACTION 7-1 *continued*

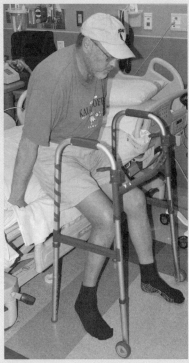

Figure 7-1 As is true after other surgical procedures, early mobility will help to decrease further complications such as DVT and pain with stiffness. Here, a patient with right THR performs sit to stand using a FWW.

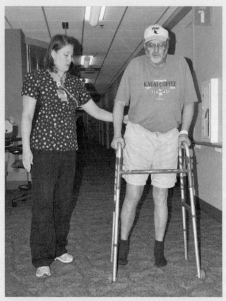

Figure 7-2 Gait training often begins in the hospital with a FWW to give the patient added stability and security. Later, the patient will progress to using a cane and then to no device at all if that was the prior level of function.

REVIEWING THE MEDICAL HISTORY

1. What do you already know about THR and other hip injuries and surgeries?

_____

_____

_____

_____

_____

2. Review the vocabulary list and physician's notes. Look up the meanings of any terms you don't understand in a medical dictionary or other text.

_____

_____

_____

_____

_____

_____

3. Review the diagnoses in the past medical history using a medical or pathology text, Internet resource, or other available resource.

_____

_____

_____

_____

_____

4. Which diagnoses in the past medical history would be significant and potentially affect the patient's respsonse to the physical therapy interventions?

_____

_____

_____

_____

_____

5. List the purpose and potential side effects of each of the medications the patient is taking.

_____

_____

_____

_____

_____

_____

6. Describe what each laboratory result measures and list considerations for physical therapy if the results for this patient were *not* in the normal range.

_____

_____

_____

_____

_____

BOX 7-1 | Physical Therapy Specialty: Geriatrics

The Geriatrics Section of the APTA is concerned with the provision of physical therapy services to the older individual, typically considered over the age of 65 years. The geriatric population is growing in number, and their needs are unique. When working with geriatric patients, it is important to show respect even in sometimes difficult circumstances. Understanding the normal effects of aging and the difference between those and the effects of disease processes helps the PTA to provide respectful care. End-of-life issues may also become a factor for this population and affect how physical therapy is delivered. For more information, see the website for the Geriatrics Section, http://www.geriatricspt.org. The American Geriatrics Society is also a good resource for health-care providers working with this population; see http://www.americangeriatrics.org.

Acute Care Physical Therapy Initial Evaluation
Patient History

NAME	Harold Jenkins	TREATING DIAGNOSIS	Decreased mobility S/P right THR
ROOM # & BED	B304-02	ONSET DATE	05/14/2010
MEDICAL RECORD #	12345678	PERTINENT MEDICAL HISTORY	Per H & P: prostate cancer treated with radiation/chemotherapy; left TKR; atrial fibrillation on Coumadin; COPD; smoker; beginning dementia
ATTENDING PHYSICIAN	Dr. Smith		
CHIEF COMPLAINT	Right hip pain		
AGE	74	SURGERY	Right THR
DATE OF BIRTH	03/12/1936	SURGERY DATE	05/14/2010
SEX	Male	PRECAUTIONS	Posterior total hip precautions
PRIMARY LANGUAGE	English	WEIGHT-BEARING STATUS	WBAT
ISOLATION	No		
HEIGHT (CM)	183	LIVING SITUATION	Assisted living facility
WEIGHT (KG)	84	PRIOR LEVEL OF FUNCTION	Independent with ambulation with cane inside and outdoors on sidewalks and level grass; two noninjury falls in past 6 months. Independent with bathing and all ADLs.
MEDICATION ALLERGIES	NKDA		
FOOD ALLERGIES	Dairy		
INITIATED BY	Donna Smith, PT		
DATE	05/14/2010	ASSISTANCE AVAILABLE	Staff for meals, cleaning, laundry
TIME	17:05	STAIRS TO ENTER HOME	Elevator; lives on second floor

continued

Acute Care Physical Therapy Initial Evaluation *continued*

Patient History

RAIL(S) ON STAIRS	Not applicable	DRIVING PRIOR TO ADMIT	No
ASSISTIVE DEVICE USED PRIOR	Cane	OCCUPATION/LIFE ROLE	Retired boat builder
EQUIPMENT PATIENT HAS	Cane		

Systems Review

HEARING	Intact with hearing aids	ACTIVITY RESPIRATORY RATE (respirations per minute)	20
VISION	Wears glasses		
SPEECH	Normal		
PAIN SCALE	VPS	ACTIVITY BLOOD PRESSURE (mm Hg)	126/80
PAIN LEVEL	6		
PAIN LOCATION	RLE	ACTIVITY SpO$_2$	97% on 3 LPM
PAIN TYPE	Surgical	POSTACTIVITY HEART RATE (BPM)	72
PAIN INTERVENTION	Notified RN and was medicated before mobility assessments	POSTACTIVITY RESPIRATORY RATE (respirations per minute)	19
RESTING HEART RATE (BPM)	70		
RESTING RESPIRATORY RATE (respirations per minute)	17	POSTACTIVITY BLOOD PRESSURE (mm Hg)	125/80
		POSTACTIVITY SpO$_2$	98% on 3 LPM
RESTING BLOOD PRESSURE (mm Hg)	120/78	LEVEL OF CONSCIOUSNESS	Lethargic
RESTING SpO$_2$	98% on 3 LPM; 86% on 2 LPM	ORIENTATION	x 2
ACTIVITY HEART RATE (BPM)	75	SHORT-TERM MEMORY	Impaired

Tests and Measures

ROM NECK/TRUNK	WFL	BED MOBILITY	Max. A to roll; total assist to scoot up in bed, but with trapeze Mod. A
ROM BUE	WNL		
ROM RLE	PROM knee flexion 5 to 120 degrees AROM hip flexion to 90 degrees (limited by precautions) and extension to neutral	SUPINE TO SIT/SIT TO SUPINE	Max. A with head of bed elevated
		SIT TO STAND/STAND TO SIT	Mod. A
ROM LLE	PROM knee flexion 5 to 125 degrees AROM hip flexion to 110 degrees, extension to neutral	TRANSFERS	Mod. A stand pivot with FWW
		SITTING BALANCE	Fair; edge of bed
BUE STRENGTH	WNL	STANDING BALANCE	Fair with FWW
RLE STRENGTH	Hip flexion not tested, knee extension 3/5; ankle 4/5	GAIT	2 side steps to the left at bedside with FWW, Mod. A
LLE STRENGTH	Hip flexion, knee extension 3/5; ankle 4/5	STAIRS	Unable
SENSATION	Intact light-touch, kinesthesia, and temperature sensation BLE	SITTING TOLERANCE	2 minutes edge of bed

Evaluation

DIAGNOSIS	Musculoskeletal, pattern H		cognitive impairments and pain at this time. He will benefit from skilled physical therapy services to address his impairments and functional limitations so that he will be able to return to his prior living situation. Two sons are out of state and have not contacted the patient yet according to the RN. He is a good candidate for and will need inpatient rehabilitation stay before D/C back to the assisted living facility.
PROGNOSIS	Good. Patient is S/P right THR with beginning dementia and prior left knee surgery. He is still lethargic from anesthesia with some short-term memory loss and not totally oriented but is able to participate and follow one- or two-step directions. It is unclear whether his cognitive impairments now are due to the dementia or anesthesia. He has difficulty maintaining hip precautions because of		

Plan of Care

PATIENT'S GOALS	He is unable to discuss goals but agrees he wants to feel better and walk better; he is willing to participate in therapy.		Home program Therapeutic exercise Therapeutic activities Caregiver training as needed
DISCHARGE GOALS	1. Bed mobility and transfers: Min. A 2. Gait: Mod. A, 30 feet with FWW 3. Home exercise program: Min. A	FREQUENCY	BID
TIME TO ACHIEVE GOALS	By time of discharge	PATIENT EDUCATION TOPIC(S)	Activity and posterior hip precautions; call for help with transfers for safety
PATIENT/FAMILY UNDERSTAND/AGREES WITH GOALS	Patient yes	TAUGHT BY	PT
		WHO WAS TAUGHT	Patient
INTERVENTIONS	Bed mobility training Transfer training Balance training Gait training	METHOD OF INSTRUCTION	Verbal/demonstration
		EVALUATION OF LEARNING	Needs reinforcement

Acute Care Nursing Note

05/14/2010   4:45 PM

The patient has been trying to get out of bed; an alarm has been placed for safety. **Foley** *catheter is draining amber urine. The patient's O_2 saturation is 97% on 2 LPM; he is coughing up clear sputum. IV Dilaudid is given for pain. MD reports that the patient was more lucid before surgery and expects cognition to improve. Sensation and circulation are intact RLE. The suture line is approximated, and dressing is clean, dry, and intact.*

Acute Care Social Work Note

05/16/2010   3:45 PM

Patient is S/P right THR with postsurgical complication of disorientation and hallucinations. Nursing notes reflect this has cleared. Physical therapy and occupational therapy notes state that the patient is a good candidate for inpatient rehabilitation and good potential to return to assisted living facility. Two sons from out of state have been contacted and state they cannot help their father at all, that he is not including them in his will and that they do not wish to come and visit. Rehabilitation unit admissions coordinator states there will be a bed available for expected D/C on 05/17/2010. The patient is on Medicare with Blue Cross Blue Shield supplemental.

Acute Care Occupational Therapy Summary

5/16/2010   3:10 PM

The patient has improved cognition and is oriented 4 times today; he is able to remember 4/5 items for a short-term memory test. He follows hip precautions about 50% of the time, needing many cues to remember during dressing, toileting, and bathing activities. Inpatient rehabilitation is recommended so that the patient can maximize his function before returning to the assisted living facility.

SEEING THE DIAGNOSIS IN ACTION 7-2

The home exercise program for this patient will include a variety of exercises that the patient has been working on in the clinic and may include the use of resistance band or tubing, exercise equipment the patient has available, and/or cuff weights. If appropriate, the patient should also continue with a walking program or other form of general exercise to maintain health.

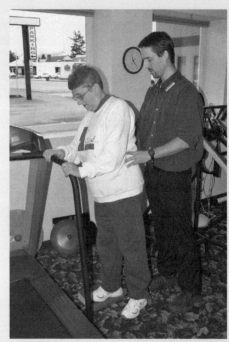

Figure 7-4 Balance exercises are important to help the patient regain full and safe mobility, especially if there is a history of falls.

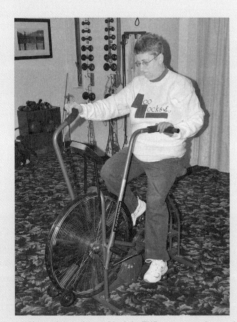

Figure 7-3 Here, the patient with right THR uses a stationary bike for strengthening and endurance training. These are also used as a warmup to other exercises.

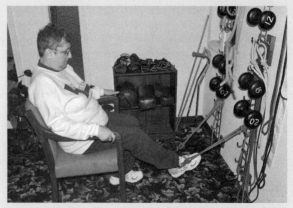

Figure 7-5 A variety of strengthening exercises are appropriate for the patient after THR. Here, the patient uses tubing for resistance.

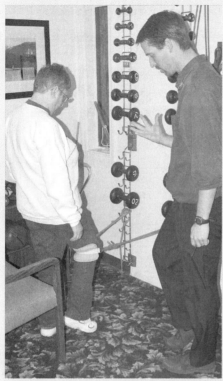

Figure 7-6 Here is another exercise using tubing for resistance and strengthening.

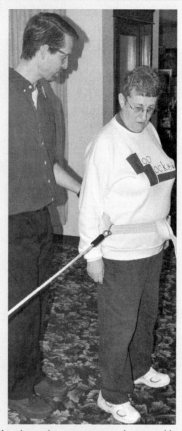

Figure 7-8 Here is another way to use resistance tubing to promote lateral stability and strengthening after THR.

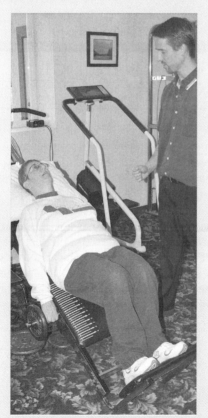

Figure 7-7 Here is a good example of a closed-chain lower body strengthening exercise that is functional for a patient after THR.

ACUTE CARE CRITICAL THINKING QUESTIONS

After reviewing the acute care physical therapy initial evaluation and other discipline notes, address the following:

1. What are the patient's impairments? Functional limitations? Is there a disability?

_____

_____

_____

2. Find assessments of gait, strength, ROM, and balance if available from the initial evaluation and list.

   a. How could each potentially be used to assess function and demonstrate progress toward goals or show the patient's response to physical therapy interventions?

   _____

   _____

   _____

   b. What would be the most important items to document for this patient?

   _____

   _____

   _____

3. After reviewing the POC, describe a possible next treatment session.

   a. List the activities/exercises and your rationale for the order of treatment activities that you selected.

   _____

   _____

   _____

4. What subjective information will you gather during your session to help in your treatment of this patient and why?

   _____

   _____

5. What tests or measures will you use to assess the patient's progress and response to treatment?

   _____

   _____

6. What subjective or objective information that you gather during the treatment might cause you to alter your treatment for this patient and why?

   _____

   _____

7. How would you document your treatment in the SOAP or Patient/Client Management format?

   _____

   _____

   _____

   _____

8. If the treatment goes as expected, what will you do for the next treatment?

   _____

   _____

9. How would you expect this patient to progress over time?

   _____

   _____

10. If the patient does not progress as expected, what might be some reasons for a lack of progress?

   _____

   _____

11. What signs or symptoms, if observed or reported by the patient, would cause you to hold treatment and check with the nursing staff, primary PT, or MD?

   _____

   _____

12. Are there any cultural, socioeconomic, or ethical issues presented in this case that might affect your interventions or communication with this patient? If so, how?

   _____

   _____

13. Re-review this case. Are there any coexisting medical diagnoses that might affect how this patient responds to physical therapy? If so, what are they, and how might they cause the patient to respond to physical therapy differently than you expected?

_____

_____

14. After reviewing the other disciplines' notes regarding this patient, is there any other information that will help you to plan your treatment sessions?

_____

_____

15. Compare your responses on this case with those of your classmates or instructors. What, if anything, would you change and why?

_____

_____

_____

_____

_____

_____

_____

_____

_____

_____

_____

Medical Update

05/17/2010

Upon discharge from the acute setting May 17, 2010, the patient is S/P right THR using posterior approach and will take Vicodin 5/500 mg every 4 to 6 hours PRN for pain. The patient still needs 2 LPM O_2 to maintain SpO_2 higher than 91%. The plan includes inpatient rehabilitation for physical and occupational therapy and nursing to follow INR, continuing O_2 as needed.

Inpatient Rehabilitation Physical Therapy Initial Evaluation
Patient History

NAME	Harold Jenkins	TIME	12:10
ROOM # & BED	B304-02	TREATING DIAGNOSIS	Decreased mobility S/P right THR
MEDICAL RECORD #	12345678	ONSET DATE	05/14/2010
ATTENDING PHYSICIAN	Dr. Gordon	PERTINIENT MEDICAL HISTORY	Per H & P: prostate cancer treated with radiation/chemotherapy; left TKR; atrial fibrillation on Coumadin; COPD; smoker; beginning dementia.
CHIEF COMPLAINT	Right hip pain		
AGE	74		
DATE OF BIRTH	03/12/1936		
SEX	Male	SURGERY	Right THR
PRIMARY LANGUAGE	English	SURGERY DATE	05/14/2010
ISOLATION	No	PRECAUTIONS	Posterior total hip precautions
HEIGHT (CM)	183	WEIGHT-BEARING STATUS	WBAT
WEIGHT (KG)	84		
MEDICATION ALLERGIES	NKDA	LIVING SITUATION	Assisted living facility
FOOD ALLERGIES	Dairy	PRIOR LEVEL OF FUNCTION	Independent with ambulation with cane inside and outdoors on sidewalks and level grass; two falls in past 6 months. Independent with bathing and all ADLs; quit driving a year ago.
INITIATED BY	Roger Lee, PT		
DATE	05/17/2010		

continued

Inpatient Rehabilitation Physical Therapy Initial Evaluation *continued*

Patient History

ASSISTANCE AVAILABLE	Staff for meals, cleaning, laundry	EQUIPMENT PATIENT HAS	Cane
STAIRS TO ENTER HOME	Elevator; lives on second floor 250 feet from apartment to dining room	DRIVING PRIOR TO ADMIT	No
RAIL(S) ON STAIRS	Not applicable		
ASSISTIVE DEVICE USED PRIOR	Cane	OCCUPATION/LIFE ROLE	Retired boat builder

Systems Review

HEARING	Intact with hearing aids	ACTIVITY BLOOD PRESSURE (mm Hg)	126/78
VISION	Wears glasses		
SPEECH	Normal	ACTIVITY SpO$_2$	98% on 2 LPM
PAIN SCALE	VPS	POSTACTIVITY HEART RATE (BPM)	74
PAIN LEVEL	3		
PAIN LOCATION	RLE	POSTACTIVITY RESPIRATORY RATE (respirations per minute)	19
PAIN TYPE	Ache		
PAIN INTERVENTION	Notified RN		
RESTING HR (BPM)	72	POSTACTIVITY BLOOD PRESSURE (mm Hg)	120/78
RESTING RESPIRATORY RATE (respirations per minute)	18		
		POSTACTIVITY SpO$_2$	98% on 2 LPM
		LEVEL OF CONSCIOUSNESS	Alert
RESTING BP (mm Hg)	118/76		
RESTING SpO$_2$	98% on 2 LPM	ORIENTATION	x 4
ACTIVITY HEART RATE (BPM)	82	SHORT-TERM MEMORY	Mildly impaired
ACTIVITY RESPIRATORY RATE (respirations per minute)	22		

Tests and Measures

ROM NECK/TRUNK	WFL	LLE STRENGTH	Hip flexion 3+/5, hip abduction 2–/5, hip extension 2–/5, knee extension 3+/5; ankle 4/5
ROM BUE	WNL		
ROM RLE	PROM knee flexion 5 to 115 degrees AROM hip flexion to 90 degrees (limited by precautions) and extension to neutral	SENSATION	Intact light-touch, temperature, and proprioception sensation BLE
ROM LLE	PROM knee flexion 5 to 120 degrees AROM hip flexion to 110 degrees, extension to neutral	BED MOBILITY	Mod. A to roll and cues to maintain hip precautions; Mod. A to scoot up in bed, but with trapeze Mod.
BUE STRENGTH	WNL	SUPINE TO SIT/SIT TO SUPINE	Mod. A with head of bed flat and cues to maintain hip precautions
RLE STRENGTH	Hip flexion not tested, hip abduction 2–/5, hip extension 2–/5, knee extension 3+/5; ankle 4/5	SIT TO STAND/STAND TO SIT	Min. A and cues to maintain hip precautions

TRANSFERS	Min. A stand pivot with FWW and cues to maintain hip precautions	GAIT	12 feet with FWW, Mod. A and cues to avoid pivoting on RLE during turn
SITTING BALANCE	Good; edge of bed	STAIRS	Unable
STANDING BALANCE	BERG balance score: 32/56	SITTING TOLERANCE	20 minutes edge of bed; 2 hours in W/C

Evaluation

DIAGNOSIS	Musculoskeletal, pattern H		mobility tasks are limited, and he moves impulsively. However, there is some carryover of learning and the need to work toward independent, safe mobility so that he can return to assisted living facility.
PROGNOSIS	Good. Patient is S/P right THR with strength, ROM, balance impairments, and pain that all affect his functional mobility. His safety awareness and judgment during		

Plan of Care

PATIENT'S GOALS	Wants to return to assisted living facility	INTERVENTIONS	Bed mobility training
DISCHARGE GOALS	1. Bed mobility, transfers: Mod. I 2. Gait: Mod. I x 300 feet with FWW 3. Home exercise program: Mod. I		Transfer training Balance training Gait training Home program Therapeutic exercise
TIME TO ACHIEVE GOALS	By time of discharge		Therapeutic activities
PATIENT/FAMILY UNDERSTAND/AGREES WITH GOALS	Patient yes		Caregiver training PRN
		FREQUENCY	BID

BOX 7-2 | Health-Care Team Member Role: Recreational Therapist

Recreational therapists work with patients and clients in a variety of settings. They incorporate the patient's interests in activities into therapy to assist the patient's return to full and independent leisure and recreational activities as much as possible. They often try to plan activities that will complement what PTs, OTs, and SLPs are doing with the patients. Activities may range from more sedentary ones, such as watching movies, playing computer games, or listening to favorite music, to more active ones, such as gardening or participating in off-campus trips to the bank or shopping excursions. Often, these are coordinated with the OT, PT, or SLP in order to address functional goals within those disciplines. For more information, see the following website: http://www.atra-online.com.

Inpatient Rehabilitation Nursing Note

05/18/2010   *11:13 AM*

The patient continues to attempt getting out of bed or chair, setting off alarms. He has had no visitors yet and states he has no friends who will come to see him. He shows signs of depression, including no interest in eating, sadness, and difficulty sleeping. He states he wants to smoke and has been agitated, although he is using the nicotine patch. When offered a chance to watch a movie in the recreation room, he declined. He has been referred to Recreation Therapist for trial of activities, and MD has been consulted regarding the patient's mood.

Inpatient Rehabilitation Social Work Summary

05/21/2010   9:30 AM

A Team Conference was held today with the patient and his oldest son, Bill, by phone. Bill states he cannot come to assist his dad and does not wish to have any further contact with the hospital. The patient had an outburst during the meeting regarding his stay here and his need to meet certain requirements before D/C. He states he feels he is nearly ready to go home independently now. He appears to be in denial regarding deficits. The MD reports she will prescribe a new medication for depression, Zoloft, and the patient is agreeable. Nursing staff report that he is still setting off alarms, but not as often. He also has had some incontinence of bladder since the Foley was removed. The PT reports he is making progress, and the goals are still to be independent at D/C. The PT and OT report that he still needs Min. A to Mod. A for all activities. The rehabilitation psychologist introduced himself to the patient and will make a visit later today. D/C is planned for assisted living facility on about June 1, 2010.

Inpatient Rehabilitation Occupational Therapy Summary

05/19/2010

The patient needs cues to follow hip precautions about 25% of time because of forgetfulness. He needs Mod. A for bathing in shower with a shower bench and Min. A for dressing. He is using a reacher to assist with lower body dressing. He is confused at times and demonstrates poor sequencing during dressing tasks.

INPATIENT REHABILITATION CRITICAL THINKING QUESTIONS

After reviewing the inpatient rehabilitation physical therapy initial evaluation and other discipline notes, address the following:

1. What are the patient's impairments? Functional limitations? Is there a disability?

_____

_____

2. Find assessments of gait, strength, ROM, and balance if available from the initial evaluation and list.

   a. How could each potentially be used to assess function and demonstrate progress toward goals or show the patient's response to physical therapy interventions?

_____

_____

_____

   b. What would be the most important items to document for this patient?

_____

_____

3. After reviewing the POC, describe a possible next treatment session.

   a. List the activities/exercises and your rationale for the order of treatment activities that you selected.

_____

_____

_____

4. What subjective information will you gather during your session to help in your treatment of this patient and why?

_____

_____

5. What tests or measures will you use to assess the patient's progress and response to treatment?

_____

_____

_____

6. What subjective or objective information that you gather during the treatment might cause you to alter your treatment for this patient and why?

_____

_____

_____

7. How would you document your treatment in the SOAP or Patient/Client Management format?

_____

_____

_____

_____

8. If the treatment goes as expected, what will you do for the next treatment?

_____

_____

9. How would you expect this patient to progress over time?

_____

_____

_____

10. If the patient does not progress as expected, what might be some reasons for a lack of progress?

_____

_____

11. What signs or symptoms, if observed or reported by the patient, would cause you to hold treatment and check with the nursing staff, primary PT, or MD?

_____

_____

_____

12. Are there any cultural, socioeconomic, or ethical issues presented in this case that might affect your interventions or communication with this patient? If so, how?

_____

_____

_____

_____

13. Re-review this case. Are there any coexisting medical diagnoses that might affect how this patient responds to physical therapy? If so, what are they, and how might they cause the patient to respond to physical therapy differently than you expected?

_____

_____

_____

_____

14. After reviewing the other disciplines' notes regarding this patient, is there any other information that will help you to plan your treatment sessions?

_____

_____

_____

_____

15. Compare your responses on this case with those of your classmates or instructors. What, if anything, would you change and why?

_____

_____

_____

_____

Outpatient Physical Therapy Evaluation

NAME	Harold Jenkins
DATE	June 3, 2010
DIAGNOSIS	S/P Right THR
SUBJECTIVE INFORMATION	The patient reports pain in the right hip at 4/10 during the day. Pain increases at night when he is trying to get comfortable to sleep and with some of his exercises

and walking, as well as sitting for more than 1 hour. He is unable to walk comfortably outdoors on uneven ground and hopes to be able to return to walking a loop around his assisted living facility that includes a trail through woods for about 2 miles.

continued

Outpatient Physical Therapy Evaluation *continued*

OBJECTIVE INFORMATION	
Posture	Hips flexed about 10 degrees, rounded shoulders
Gait	**Trendelenburg** on right, **antalgic** pattern with right stance phase shorter, using cane for support on right side, and ambulates with supports on treadmill at 2 miles per hour for 5 minutes.
Balance	BERG balance score 41/56
Strength	BLE: Hip flexors 3+/5, extensors 2+/5, abductors 2+/5; quadriceps 4−/5; hamstrings 4−/5
AROM	WFL
Palpation	Pain with spasms in right piriformis, quadratus lumborum, and tensor fascia lata
Sensation	Intact light-touch, temperature, kinesthesia, and proprioception BLE
ASSESSMENT	Patient is S/P right THR and continues to have weakness, decreased balance, and pain, with muscle spasms affecting his

ability to return to full activities, including walking a fairly level 2-mile trail. He uses this activity to help him maintain strength and function as he ages. He will benefit from skilled therapy services to address the following goals:

STG (2 WEEKS)	1. Pain will be decreased to 2/10 or less during all activities. 2. BERG balance score 50/56 in order to decrease fall risk. 3. Increase bilateral hip extensor and abduction strength to 3+/5; hip flexors, quadriceps and hamstrings to 4/5.
LTG	Able to walk 2-mile trail without assistive device in 45 minutes with minimal fall risk. Independent with a written home exercise program.
PLAN	Three times per week for 4 weeks for soft tissue mobilization, heat/cold modalities, and electrical stimulation to decrease pain and increase ROM, therapeutic exercise, body mechanics training, and home exercise program.

OUTPATIENT CRITICAL THINKING QUESTIONS

After reviewing the outpatient physical therapy evaluation, address the following:

1. What are the patient's impairments? Functional limitations? Is there a disability?

_____

_____

2. Find assessments of gait, strength, ROM, and balance if available from the initial evaluation and list.

   a. How could each potentially be used to assess function and demonstrate progress toward goals or show the patient's response to physical therapy interventions?

_____

_____

_____

_____

b. What would be the most important items to document for this patient?

_____

_____

_____

3. After reviewing the POC, describe a possible next treatment session.

   a. List the activities/exercises and your rationale for the order of treatment activities that you selected.

_____

_____

_____

4. What subjective information will you gather during your session to help in your treatment of this patient and why?

_____

_____

5. What tests or measures will you use to assess the patient's progress and response to treatment?

_____

_____

6. What subjective or objective information that you gather during the treatment might cause you to alter your treatment for this patient and why?

_____

_____

7. How would you document your treatment in the SOAP or Patient/Client Management format?

_____

_____

_____

_____

8. If the treatment goes as expected, what will you do for the next treatment?

_____

_____

9. How would you expect this patient to progress over time?

_____

_____

10. If the patient does not progress as expected, what might be some reasons for a lack of progress?

_____

_____

11. What signs or symptoms, if observed or reported by the patient, would cause you to hold treatment and check with the nursing staff, primary PT, or MD?

_____

_____

12. Are there any cultural, socioeconomic, or ethical issues presented in this case that might affect your interventions or communication with this patient? If so, how?

_____

_____

13. Re-review this case. Are there any coexisting medical diagnoses that might affect how this patient responds to physical therapy? If so, what are they, and how might they cause the patient to respond to physical therapy differently than you expected?

_____

_____

14. After reviewing the other disciplines' notes regarding this patient, is there any other information that will help you to plan your treatment sessions?

_____

_____

_____

15. Compare your responses on this case with those of your classmates or instructors. What, if anything, would you change and why?

_____

_____

_____

CONTINUUM OF CARE CRITICAL THINKING QUESTIONS

After reviewing the continuum of care for this patient, consider the following:

1. How did the patient's problems change over the weeks after his surgery?

_____

_____

_____

_____

2. How did this affect the goals and the interventions that the PT included in the POC?

_____

_____

_____

_____

_____

continued

CONTINUUM OF CARE CRITICAL THINKING QUESTIONS *continued*

3. How were the same interventions modified over time to progress the patient according to his changing needs?

_____

_____

_____

_____

_____

4. What are some potential community resources that this patient might like to participate in and how would these help him to maintain and improve his physical fitness?

_____

_____

_____

_____

_____

IMPLICATIONS OF PATHOLOGY FOR THE PTA[2]

1. What might be the cause of the following signs/symptoms in a patient with osteoarthritis or S/P joint replacement and what should the PTA do if he/she encounters these with a patient?

   a. Indigestion, nausea, vomiting, thoracic pain, or melena (black, tarry stools)

   b. Unexplained back or shoulder pain or excessive bruising

   c. LE pain that may or may not include swelling and redness

   d. Chest pain or trouble breathing

   e. Excessive or new warmth to touch and/or edema in the area of surgery

_____

_____

_____

_____

_____

2. What should the PTA be aware of when working with patients with the following?
   • Trochanteric bursitis
   • Hip fracture
   • Hip dislocation
   • Piriformis syndrome

_____

_____

_____

_____

_____

_____

_____

_____

_____

_____

References

1. American Physical Therapy Association: Guide to Physical Therapist Practice, Second Edition. Alexandria, VA: Author, 2001.

2. Goodman CC, Boissonnault FG, Fuller KS: Pathology: Implications for the Physical Therapist, Second Edition. Philadelphia: Saunders, 2003.

CHAPTER 8

Mrs. Martin: A Patient With Diabetes Type II and Transtibial Amputation

 Preferred Practice Patterns: Musculoskeletal, Pattern J, and Integumentary, Pattern C

CHAPTER OUTLINE

Introducing Mrs. Martin

Mrs. Martin is a 66-year-old woman who has had diabetes for more than 10 years. She had an open wound that would not heal on her great toe, which turned **gangrenous** and required a left forefoot amputation; now, she has had a transtibial amputation of the left leg. According to the APTA's *Guide to Physical Therapist Practice* (the *Guide*), this patient could have the following impairments:

- Edema
- Joint contracture
- Impaired aerobic capacity
- Impaired gait pattern
- Impaired integument
- Residual limb pain
- Impaired sensation
- Muscle weakness

Functional limitations may include the following:

- Decreased community access
- Inability to perform ADLs

Please refer to the *Guide*[1] for a complete list of possible impairments and functional limitations. As you work through this case, think about which of these the patient is experiencing.

Vocabulary List

Gangrenous	Auscultation
Sepsis	Hepatosplenomegaly
Doppler	Cellulitis
Murmur	

PHYSICIAN'S HISTORY AND PHYSICAL

PATIENT NAME: Bonnie K. Martin
ADMIT DATE: September 2, 2010
BIRTH DATE: August 18, 1944
SEX: Female
ROOM/BED: 326-01
MEDICAL RECORD #: 12345678
CHIEF COMPLAINT: LLE nonhealing wound; **sepsis**
ATTENDING: Dr. Sharon Williams, MD

HISTORY OF PRESENT ILLNESS: This 66-year-old woman is being admitted for left transtibial amputation. She has diabetes and has not controlled her blood glucose levels well over the years. Vascular studies of the LLE show ABI of 0.75, and arterial **Doppler** studies show marked arterial obstruction below the knee not amenable to intervention. She had her left foot amputated at the forefoot but continued with problems related to wound healing and now presents with signs of sepsis. She has been on a regimen of multiple antibiotics and has been having diarrhea the past 2 weeks. She complains of severe pain in the LLE, and pain management has been difficult. She has been NWB on the left for some time to promote wound healing. She has been informed of the benefits as well as the potential risks of this procedure, including blood clot, cardiac arrest, stroke, and death, but still chooses to proceed. She anticipates the need for rehabilitation before D/C home.

PAST MEDICAL HISTORY: The patient's medical history includes the following: obesity, HTN, dyslipidemia, DM II with peripheral neuropathy and retinopathy, GERD, and DJD bilateral knees, hips, and spine.

PAST SURGICAL HISTORY: Left foot amputation; cholecystectomy

ALLERGIES: Ibuprofen, hydrocodone

MEDICATIONS: rosuvastatin 20 mg daily
diltiazem CR 180 mg daily
ranitidine 150 mg twice daily
Voltaren 50 mg twice daily
Lantus basal insulin 78 units daily at bedtime and NovoLog sliding scale before main meal of the day; has been using 34 units daily
Extra strength Tylenol 500 mg 1 to 2 tablets every 4 hours PRN for pain

FAMILY HISTORY: Mother died of heart disease; father died of lung cancer and had diabetes; children both have diabetes and are obese.

SOCIAL HISTORY: The patient smokes two packs of cigarettes per day and drinks a beer a day. She lives with a significant other who has his own health problems and smokes; he is unable to assist the patient upon D/C. Two grown children from a prior marriage live nearby, and she has three grandchildren.

REVIEW OF SYSTEMS: See HPI; otherwise negative

PHYSICAL EXAMINATION:

VITAL SIGNS: Temperature 39°C, pulse 74 BPM, respiratory rate 20 respirations per minute, blood pressure 130/84 mm Hg, O_2 saturation 98% on 2 LPM. BMI of 32.9 with height 122 cm and weight 49 kg.

GENERAL: She feels lethargic and generally poor but no acute pain or distress.

SKIN: Cool to touch in distal extremities; surgical wound left foot with drainage; 2-cm diameter grade 3 ulceration above lateral malleolus with associated surrounding redness and swelling in entire lower leg.

HEENT: Unremarkable

SPINE: Kyphotic

CARDIAC: Regular rate and rhythm; grade 2/6 systolic **murmur**

LUNGS: Clear to **auscultation**

ABDOMEN: Bowel sounds present, nontender, nondistended. No **hepatosplenomegaly.**

EXTREMITIES: Left forefoot amputation; BLE edema present 2+.

NEUROLOGICAL: Alert and oriented. Cranial nerves intact.

LABORATORY DATA: Hg A_{1C} 8.6; creatinine 2.1; WBC 42,000 with 40% bandemia

IMAGING STUDIES: ABI 0.75 on LLE last year; RLE currently 1.0

ASSESSMENT: Nonhealing surgical wound of left foot (with prior forefoot amputation) with a new nonhealing wound with **cellulitis** now on mid-leg and laboratory studies supporting ongoing sepsis.

PLAN: The plan is to admit her to the surgical floor for left transtibial amputation and monitor her blood sugars. Physiatry, physical therapy, occupational therapy, and social work consults are planned, along with discharge planning. To quit smoking, the patient opts to use a nicotine patch while hospitalized.

SEEING THE DIAGNOSIS IN ACTION 8-1

Patients need limb amputations for a variety of reasons, and physical therapy can play a large role in their satisfactory rehabilitation. Often, patients must address not only the physical concerns but also the emotional challenges related to the loss of the limb. In addition to exercises and functional mobility training, the patient generally needs a significant amount of education on the care of the residual limb and the prosthesis. Early physical therapy in the hospital and subacute settings often will include wound care and special wrapping procedures to promote optimal shaping of the residual limb in preparation for a prosthesis.

When a patient is discharged from outpatient physical therapy after having a lower extremity amputation, he or she may continue to need support from the physical therapy team as well as the prosthetist, who can help with any adjustments needed as the patient changes. A home exercise program is important to help these patients achieve and maintain their goals.

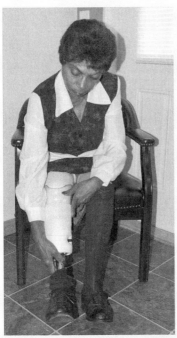

Figure 8-1 This patient with right transtibial amputation dons her prosthesis in preparation for ambulation.

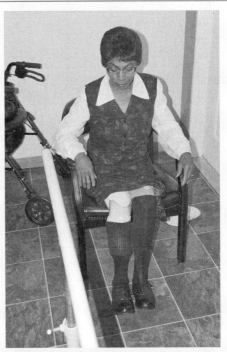

Figure 8-3 Preparing for a sit to stand procedure, the patient can learn appropriate adjustments that may still need to be made before standing.

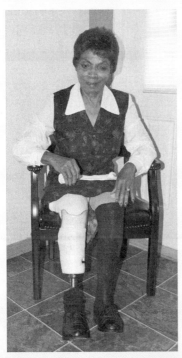

Figure 8-2 After adjusting her prosthesis, she is ready for standing and gait training.

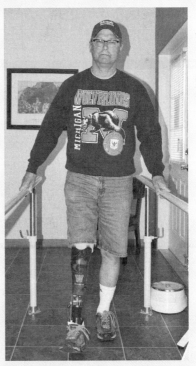

Figure 8-4 The initial gait-training sessions are generally performed in parallel bars for added stability for the patient. Here, another patient demonstrates a pre-gait activity in the parallel bars.

continued

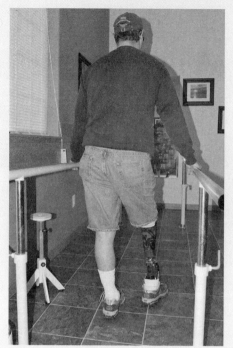

Figure 8-5 Here, the patient continues gait training in the parallel bars.

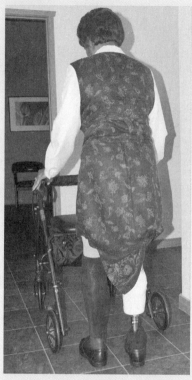

Figure 8-7 Here, the patient continues gait training with the four-wheeled walker. Some patients may find that a front-wheeled walker or standard walker provides better support while learning to ambulate with a prosthesis.

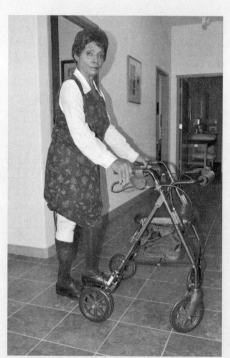

Figure 8-6 Once the patient is able, gait training can be progressed to using a four-wheeled walker.

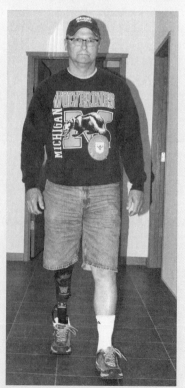

Figure 8-8 Here, the patient has progressed to gait training without an assistive device.

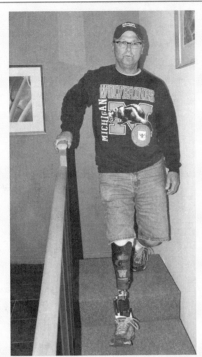

Figure 8-9 Stair training with a patient who is using a prosthesis is similar to training other patients.

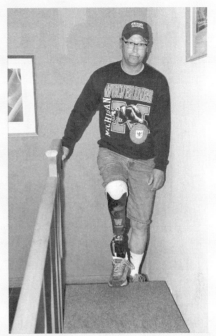

Figure 8-10 Patients with a prosthesis may need to use additional supportive devices and practice longer on steps with bilateral rails than other patients but typically should be able to accomplish the goal of independent stair climbing.

REVIEWING THE MEDICAL HISTORY

1. What do you already know about diabetes and lower extremity amputations?

_____

_____

_____

_____

_____

2. Review the vocabulary list and physician's notes. Look up the meanings of any terms you do not understand in a medical dictionary or other text.

_____

_____

_____

_____

_____

_____

3. Review the diagnoses in the past medical history using a medical or pathology text, Internet resource, or other available resource.

_____

_____

_____

_____

_____

4. Which diagnoses in the past medical history would be significant and potentially affect the patient's response to the physical therapy interventions?

_____

_____

_____

_____

_____

continued

REVIEWING THE MEDICAL HISTORY *continued*

5. List the purpose and potential side effects of each of the medications the patient is taking.

_____

_____

_____

_____

_____

_____

_____

6. Describe what each laboratory result measures and list considerations for physical therapy if the results for this patient were *not* in the normal range.

_____

_____

_____

_____

_____

_____

Acute Care Physical Therapy Initial Evaluation
Patient History

NAME	Bonnie Martin			hips, spine, left foot amputation; cholecystectomy
ROOM # & BED	B326-01			
MEDICAL RECORD #	12345678		SURGERY	Left transtibial amputation
ATTENDING PHYSICIAN	Dr. Williams		SURGERY DATE	09/02/2010
CHIEF COMPLAINT	Nonhealing wound		PRECAUTIONS	Contact precautions; C-diff
AGE	66		WEIGHT-BEARING STATUS	WBAT RLE; NWB LLE
DATE OF BIRTH	08/18/1944			
SEX	Female		LIVING SITUATION	Mobile home
PRIMARY LANGUAGE	English		PRIOR LEVEL OF FUNCTION	Independent with ambulation and all other ADLs with no fall risk before left foot amputation; NWB and using FWW after left foot amputation
ISOLATION	Yes; C-diff			
HEIGHT (CM)	122			
WEIGHT (KG)	49			
MEDICATION ALLERGIES	Ibuprofen; hydrocodone		ASSISTANCE AVAILABLE	None
FOOD ALLERGIES	None		STAIRS TO ENTER HOME	6
INITIATED BY	Donna Smith, PT		RAIL(S) ON STAIRS	One side
DATE	09/03/2010		ASSISTIVE DEVICE USED PRIOR	FWW past 4 weeks since foot amputation
TIME	14:13			
TREATING DIANOSIS	Decreased mobility S/P left transtibial amputation		EQUIPMENT PATIENT HAS	FWW
ONSET DATE	09/02/2010		DRIVING PRIOR TO ADMIT	Yes
PERTINENT MEDICAL HISTORY	Per H & P: obesity, HTN, dyslipidemia, DM II with peripheral neuropathy and retinopathy, GERD, DJD bilateral knees,		OCCUPATION/LIFE ROLE	Retired caregiver; cares for boyfriend who is not healthy

Systems Review

HEARING	Intact	ACTIVITY RESPIRATORY RATE (respirations per minute)	22
VISION	Intact		
SPEECH	Normal		
PAIN SCALE	VPS	ACTIVITY BLOOD PRESSURE (mm Hg)	142/83
PAIN LEVEL	5		
PAIN LOCATION	LLE	ACTIVITY SpO$_2$	98% on 2 LPM
PAIN TYPE	Surgical	POSTACTIVITY HEART RATE (BPM)	84
PAIN INTERVENTION	Notified RN		
RESTING HEART RATE (BPM)	72	POSTACTIVITY RESPIRATORY RATE (respirations per minute)	21
RESTING RESPIRATORY RATE (respirations per minute)	18	POSTACTIVITY BLOOD PRESSURE (mm Hg)	140/80
		POSTACTIVITY SpO$_2$	97% on 2 LPM
RESTING BLOOD PRESSURE (mm Hg)	138/82	LEVEL OF CONSCIOUSNESS	Alert
RESTING SpO$_2$	98% on 2 LPM; 88% on room air	ORIENTATION	x 4
ACTIVITY HEART RATE (BPM)	86	SHORT-TERM MEMORY	Intact

Tests and Measures

ROM NECK/TRUNK	WFL	SKIN INTEGRITY	LLE residual limb with sutures and dressing; dressing and ACE wrap in place
ROM BUE	WNL		
ROM RLE	PROM knee flexion 8 to 125 degrees; ankle plantarflexion 55 degrees; dorsiflexion 0, hip flexion to 95 degrees (limited by obesity), and extension 5 degrees from neutral	BED MOBILITY	Mod. A to roll; total assist to scoot up in bed, but with trapeze Mod. A
		SUPINE TO SIT/SIT TO SUPINE	Mod. A with head of bed elevated
ROM LLE	PROM knee flexion 15 to 80 degrees; hip flexion to 95 degrees (limited by obesity) and extension 5 degrees from neutral	SIT TO STAND/STAND TO SIT	Unable after several attempts in parallel bars
		TRANSFERS	Mod. A slide board toward right side
BUE STRENGTH	WNL	SITTING BALANCE	Good; edge of bed
RLE STRENGTH	Hip flexion, knee extension 3+/5; ankle dorsiflexion/plantarflexion 4/5, eversion/inversion 3+/5	STANDING BALANCE	Unable
		GAIT	Unable
		STAIRS	Unable
LLE STRENGTH	Hip flexion, knee extension 3+/5	SITTING TOLERANCE	5 minutes edge of bed
SENSATION	Absent light touch and temperature sensation BLE below mid-thigh; proprioception intact bilateral hips and knees but impaired in right ankle and foot	DIABETIC FOOT TESTING	Right foot with dry skin, hammertoes, absent protective sensation using monofilament testing
EDEMA CIRCUMFERENCE	2 cm below distal patella: left 47 cm, right 45.5 cm Mid-patella: left 51 cm, right 49 cm 10 cm above patella: left 55 cm, right 54 cm		

continued

Acute Care Physical Therapy Initial Evaluation *continued*
Evaluation

DIAGNOSIS	Musculoskeletal, pattern J, and integumentary, pattern C		her to progress toward goals of independent self-care and eventual ambulation on prosthesis. Her boyfriend present during evaluation and emotionally supportive but unable to assist with care at D/C or cook his own meals. He is currently getting help from neighbors for meals.
PROGNOSIS	Good. Patient is S/P left transtibial amputation due to sepsis LLE with residual pain, edema, decreased strength, and ROM, all limiting her ability to return home and take care of herself. She needs skilled physical therapy services to enable		

Plan of Care

PATIENT'S GOALS	Home ASAP		Therapeutic activities Family training PRN
DISCHARGE GOALS	1. Bed mobility and transfers: Min. A 2. Gait: Mod. A 10 feet in parallel bars 3. Home exercise program: Min. A	FREQUENCY	BID
		PATIENT EDUCATION TOPIC(S)	Activity; LLE positioning in bed to prevent skin breakdown and contractures; call for help with transfers for safety
TIME TO ACHIEVE GOALS	By time of discharge		
PATIENT/FAMILY UNDERSTAND/AGREES WITH GOALS	Patient/significant other: yes	TAUGHT BY	PT
		WHO WAS TAUGHT	Patient/significant other
INTERVENTIONS	Bed mobility training Transfer training Balance training Gait training Home program Therapeutic exercise	METHOD OF INSTRUCTION	Verbal/demonstration
		EVALUATION OF LEARNING	Needs reinforcement

Acute Care Nursing Note

09/03/2010   1:19 PM

The patient has been resting quietly, although she reports pain at 10/10 in her LLE. IV Dilaudid has been given with good effect. She is unable to move in bed and agrees to use a trapeze to assist. Foley is draining dark amber urine. She experiences nausea and dizziness with dangle at edge of bed; she is returned to supine with assist and head of bed elevated. She is asking for ice cream but does not want the diabetic type. She is on ADA diet, and the need for controlling blood sugars has been explained to her. She complains of having to quit smoking due to being in the hospital and that the patch is not working well; she still wants to smoke. She will be referred to a dietitian for patient education. Diarrhea is positive for C-diff; contact precautions are in place. Her dressing is clean, dry, and intact. Patient education is planned for joint contracture prevention measures including use of no pillow under LLE and need for prone position several times per day. She has attempted prone position but is unable to tolerate it longer than 15 minutes. The patient states she is willing to try again tomorrow. Patient instructed to lie prone several times per day to prevent contractures.

Acute Care Social Work Note

09/03/2010   2:52 PM

The patient is S/P left transtibial amputation and has Medicaid insurance coverage; she is also on disability. She has lived with her boyfriend, who is also ill, for the past 3 years; she reports that he is alcoholic and does have anger problems. She does not admit to any abuse. The plan is for D/C to inpatient rehabilitation, and a bed will be available per the admissions coordinator there. The patient will need long-term social work follow-up regarding financial concerns and need for assistance through local agencies for support for herself and her boyfriend. She does have two grown daughters in the area: one works full-time and is unable to provide support beyond visits in the evenings, and the other is on disability herself with lupus.

Acute Care Occupational Therapy Summary

09/03/2010   5:23 PM

The patient is S/P left transtibial amputation with onset of C-diff. She is alert, oriented x 4. Foley is in place. Surgical pain at 5/10 is interfering with mobility. Currently she requires Mod. A to roll and sit up in bed and to transfer via slide board to right side. At a bench commode, the patient requires Max. A for clothing management and hygiene. In bed, the patient requires Max. A for lower body care and Min. A for upper body dressing, setup for grooming, and self-feeding. However, with C-diff. present, bedpan use is recommended until diarrhea and mobility have improved. Small (about 1 cm), round burn marks noted on the patient's buttocks during toileting activities; the patient is unaware of the origin. She will benefit from skilled occupational therapy services to address the above problems. D/C to inpatient rehabilitation unit recommended.

ACUTE CARE CRITICAL THINKING QUESTIONS

After reviewing the acute care physical therapy initial evaluation and other discipline notes, address the following:

1. What are the patient's impairments? Functional limitations? Is there a disability?

2. Find assessments of gait, strength, ROM, and balance if available from the initial evaluation and list.

   a. How could each potentially be used to assess function and demonstrate progress toward goals or show the patient's response to physical therapy interventions?

   b. What would be the most important items to document for this patient?

3. After reviewing the POC, describe a possible next treatment session.

   a. List the activities/exercises and your rationale for the order of treatment activities that you selected.

4. What subjective information will you gather during your session to help in your treatment of this patient and why?

5. What tests or measures will you use to assess the patient's progress and response to treatment?

continued

ACUTE CARE CRITICAL THINKING QUESTIONS *continued*

6. What subjective or objective information that you gather during the treatment might cause you to alter your treatment for this patient and why?

_____

_____

7. How would you document your treatment in the SOAP or Patient/Client Management format?

_____

_____

_____

_____

8. If the treatment goes as expected, what will you do for the next treatment?

_____

_____

9. How would you expect this patient to progress over time?

_____

_____

10. If the patient does not progress as expected, what might be some reasons for a lack of progress?

_____

_____

11. What signs or symptoms, if observed or reported by the patient, would cause you to hold treatment and check with the nursing staff, primary PT, or MD?

_____

_____

12. Are there any cultural, socioeconomic, or ethical issues presented in this case that might affect your interventions or communication with this patient? If so, how?

_____

_____

_____

13. Re-review this case. Are there any coexisting medical diagnoses that might affect how this patient responds to physical therapy? If so, what are they, and how might they cause the patient to respond to physical therapy differently than you expected?

_____

_____

_____

_____

14. After reviewing the other disciplines' notes regarding this patient, is there any other information that will help you to plan your treatment sessions?

_____

_____

_____

_____

15. Compare your responses on this case with those of your classmates or instructors. What, if anything, would you change and why?

_____

_____

_____

_____

Medical Update

09/07/2010

Upon D/C from the acute setting 09/07/10, the patient is S/P left transtibial amputation. Laboratory results include WBC 18,000 with 15% bandemia. Her medication remains the same except for the following: discontinued Voltaren, added Flagyl 500 mg every 6 hours for a total of 14 days (began on 9/3), added Lyrica 50 mg three times daily for neuropathy pain, and added aspirin 81 mg. The plan is to monitor blood sugars and CBC and to begin inpatient rehabilitation.

Inpatient Rehabilitation Physical Therapy Initial Evaluation

NAME	Bonnie Martin	SURGERY	Left transtibial amputation
ROOM # & BED	B306-01	SURGERY DATE	09/02/2010
MEDICAL RECORD #	12345678	PRECAUTIONS	Contact precautions; C-diff
ATTENDING PHYSICIAN	Dr. Gordon	WEIGHT-BEARING STATUS	WBAT RLE; NWB LLE
CHIEF COMPLAINT	S/P left transtibial amputation		
AGE	66	LIVING SITUATION	Mobile home
DATE OF BIRTH	08/18/1944	PRIOR LEVEL OF FUNCTION	Independent with ambulation and all other ADLs with no fall risk
SEX	Female		
PRIMARY LANGUAGE	English	ASSISTANCE AVAILABLE	Friends currently providing meals but unable to help long-term
ISOLATION	Yes; C-diff		
HEIGHT (CM)	122	STAIRS TO ENTER HOME	6
WEIGHT (KG)	49	RAIL(S) ON STAIRS	One side
MEDICATION ALLERGIES	Ibuprofen; hydrocodone	ASSISTIVE DEVICE USED PRIOR	FWW last 4 weeks since foot amputation
FOOD ALLERGIES	None		
INITIATED BY	Roger Lee, PT	EQUIPMENT PATIENT HAS	FWW
DATE	09/07/2010		
TIME	11:42	DRIVING PRIOR TO ADMIT	Yes
TREATING DIAGNOSIS	Decreased mobility S/P left transtibial amputation		
		OCCUPATION/LIFE ROLE	Retired caregiver; cares for boyfriend who has COPD and other multiple medical issues as well as alcoholism, per patient
ONSET DATE	09/02/2010		
PERTINENT MEDICAL HISTORY	Per H & P: obesity, HTN, dyslipidemia, DM II with peripheral neuropathy and retinopathy, GERD, DJD bilateral knees, hips, spine, prior left foot amputation; cholecystectomy		

Systems Review

HEARING	Intact	ACTIVITY RESPIRATORY RATE (respirations per minute)	20
VISION	Intact		
SPEECH	Normal		
PAIN SCALE	VPS	ACTIVITY BLOOD PRESSURE (mm Hg)	140/78
PAIN LEVEL	7		
PAIN LOCATION	LLE	ACTIVITY SpO$_2$	98% on 1 LPM
PAIN TYPE	Surgical, ache	POSTACTIVITY HEART RATE (BPM)	76
PAIN INTERVENTION	Notified RN		
RESTING HEART RATE (BPM)	70	POSTACTIVITY RESPIRATORY RATE (respirations per minute)	19
RESTING RESPIRATORY RATE (respirations per minute)	18		
		POSTACTIVITY BLOOD PRESSURE (mm Hg)	137/76
RESTING BLOOD PRESSURE (mm Hg)	136/78	POSTACTIVITY SpO$_2$	98% on 1 LPM
		LEVEL OF CONSCIOUSNESS	Alert
RESTING SpO$_2$	98% on 1 LPM; 89% on room air	ORIENTATION	x 4
ACTIVITY HEART RATE (BPM)	78	SHORT-TERM MEMORY	Intact

continued

Inpatient Rehabilitation Physical Therapy Initial Evaluation *continued*

Tests and Measures

ROM NECK/TRUNK	WFL	SKIN INTEGRITY AND RESIDUAL LIMB	Sutures and dressing with ACE wraps
ROM BUE	WNL	BED MOBILITY	Min. A to roll; Max. A to scoot up in bed, but with trapeze Min. A
ROM RLE	PROM knee flexion 5 to 125 degrees; ankle plantarflexion 55 degrees; dorsiflexion 0; hip flexion to 95 degrees (limited by obesity) and extension 5 degrees from neutral	SUPINE TO SIT/SIT TO SUPINE	Mod. A
		SIT TO STAND/ STAND TO SIT	Max. A in parallel bars
ROM LLE	PROM knee flexion 10 to 95 degrees; hip flexion to 95 degrees (limited by obesity) and extension 5 degrees from neutral	TRANSFERS	Mod. A slide board toward right side; Max. A stand pivot with FWW
BUE STRENGTH	WNL	SITTING BALANCE	Normal; edge of bed
RLE STRENGTH	Hip flexion, knee extension 3+/5; ankle dorsiflexion/plantarflexion 4/5, eversion/inversion 3+/5	STANDING BALANCE	Poor with FWW
		GAIT	2 steps in parallel bars, hopping on RLE Mod. A
LLE STRENGTH	Hip flexion, knee extension 3+/5	STAIRS	Unable
SENSATION	Absent light-touch and temperature sensation BLE below mid-thigh; intact proprioception bilateral hips and knees but impaired right ankle and foot	SITTING TOLERANCE	15 minutes edge of bed; 3 hours in chair
		DIABETIC FOOT TESTING	Right foot with dry skin, hammertoes, absent protective sensation
EDEMA CIRCUMFERENCE	2 cm below distal patella: left 46.5 cm; right 45.5 cm Mid-patella: left 51 cm, right 49.5 cm 10 cm above patella: left 54.5 cm, right 54 cm		

Evaluation

DIAGNOSIS	Musculoskeletal, pattern J, and integumentary, pattern C		ambulation on prosthesis. She demonstrates good motivation; however, multiple medical concerns and DM II will likely slow healing. Financial concerns may be a factor for long-term follow-up care, along with household help until she is more able. She will need a wheelchair and FWW for discharge, as well as other equipment per occupational therapy recommendations.
PROGNOSIS	Good. The patient is S/P left transtibial amputation due to sepsis LLE with residual pain, edema, decreased strength, and ROM, all limiting her ability to return home and take care of herself. She needs skilled physical therapy services to enable her to progress toward goals of independent self-care and eventual		

Plan of Care

PATIENT'S GOALS	Walk again with prosthesis		5. Diabetic foot care: Mod. I
DISCHARGE GOALS	1. Bed mobility and transfers: Mod. I		6. Amputee care: Mod. I
	2. Car transfers: supervised	TIME TO ACHIEVE GOALS	By time of discharge
	3. Gait: Min. A x 50 ft. with FWW for household distance	PATIENT/FAMILY UNDERSTAND/AGREES WITH GOALS	Patient yes
	4. Home exercise program: supervised		

INTERVENTIONS	Bed mobility training		Therapeutic activities
	Transfer training		Family training PRN
	Balance training		Diabetic foot education
	Gait training		Amputee care education
	Home program	FREQUENCY	BID
	Therapeutic exercise		

BOX 8-1 | Physical Therapy Specialty: Diabetes Education

The PTA can play a significant role in educating patients with diabetes regarding the care of their bodies. The physical therapy POC often includes this specific training, and communication with the primary PT is important to ensure that all appropriate education is provided. Depending on the patient's needs, diabetes education may include daily foot checks and foot care, such as use of lotion for dry skin and daily cleansing of the skin to prevent infections. It usually includes assessment of and recommendation for appropriate footwear and often includes special diabetes shoes. It is important to teach, as well as to document the teaching, regarding the effects of exercise on patients with diabetes. Patients eventually will be discharged from physical therapy and need to have the knowledge and skills to effectively monitor themselves while exercising. Educating patients in these areas typically involves providing both verbal and written information, having discussions with the patients to ensure understanding, and giving demonstrations and return demonstrations of specific skills, such as the use of a small mirror to see the plantar surfaces of feet. In addition to the education that physical therapy typically provides, nursing and nutritionist or dietitian staff educate patients regarding the use of insulin, smoking cessation programs, and food or meal planning to help manage the diabetes. Working together, the healthcare team can help many patients avoid further complications of diabetes and promote a lifestyle that will help them attain a higher quality of life. More information on diabetes education can be found at the American Association of Diabetes Educators website (http://www.diabeteseducator.org) and at the American Diabetes Association website (http://www.diabetes.org).

Inpatient Rehabilitation Nursing Note

09/07/2010   12:12 PM

The patient is requesting pain pills every 4 hours to manage LLE pain; she describes phantom pain as well. She is continent of bladder but continues with diarrhea intermittently related to C-diff and is incontinent of bowel about once per day. She does not always want to wait for nursing staff to supervise for transfers and is impulsive at times. A bed and chair alarm is in use. Her boyfriend is present at all times, requesting meals also for himself from the cafeteria. No other family is present. The patient is hoping to D/C home in a couple of weeks. She eats independently and is on an ADA diet.

Inpatient Rehabilitation Social Work Summary

09/09/2010   10:39 AM

A team conference was held today. The MD reports that the patient's wound is healing well and that the residual limb appears to be taking good shape for eventual prosthesis. Blood sugars are being monitored. The MD is requesting a rehabilitation psychologist consult for possible depression, but patient denies being depressed. Nursing staff report patient impulsivity and lack of safety awareness but that she is continent of bladder, is gaining more control of her bowel, and otherwise is participating well in the program and that the dietitian is planning to work with the patient for diabetes education regarding meal planning. The PT reports good progress so far with functional mobility training and exercise program and is encouraging the patient to stick with the program because it will entail long-term rehabilitation. The OT reports that the patient needs Mod. A for ADLs and will work toward appropriate equipment and home evaluation before D/C. The OT will plan for family training with the boyfriend before D/C in about 2 weeks. The patient requests smoking privileges, but the staff are unable to comply because of hospital policies. We discussed a day pass after some initial training with the boyfriend in about a week.

BOX 8-2 | Health-Care Team Member Role: Nutritionist and Dietitian

Nutritionists and dietitians work with other team members to ensure that patient's nutritional needs are met. They do this through meal planning and preparation as well as individual patient and family counseling. They work in a variety of settings, and they often meet with patients and families in the acute stage of healing and follow up throughout the continuum of care as needed. For more information on the role of these health-care team members and their educational background, see the Bureau of Labor Statistics website at http://www.bls.gov/oco/ocos077.htm.

Inpatient Rehabilitation Occupational Therapy Summary

09/07/2010   1:26 PM

The patient requires Mod. A for lower body dressing, using electric bed, trapeze, and rails to assist with bed mobility during dressing. She requires Mod. A for slide board transfers to right side only using bench commode. She is just beginning to be able to assist with pants by lifting one hip at a time and needs Mod. A. She requires Max. A for toileting hygiene because of diarrhea and setup for upper body care. She needs setup for grooming and oral hygiene from W/C level and for dressing upper body while seated on the bed. Recommendations include home safety evaluation and a ramp to be placed before D/C; specifications have been given to the patient and boyfriend, who states he will take care of the ramp installation before discharge.

INPATIENT REHABILITATION CRITICAL THINKING QUESTIONS

After reviewing the inpatient rehabilitation physical therapy initial evaluation and other discipline notes, address the following:

1. What are the patient's impairments? Functional limitations? Is there a disability?

_____

_____

2. Find assessments of gait, strength, ROM, and balance if available from the initial evaluation and list.

   a. How could each potentially be used to assess function and demonstrate progress toward goals or show the patient's response to physical therapy interventions?

_____

_____

_____

   b. What would be the most important items to document for this patient?

_____

_____

_____

3. After reviewing the POC, describe a possible next treatment session.

   a. List the activities/exercises and your rationale for the order of treatment activities that you selected.

_____

_____

_____

4. What subjective information will you gather during your session to help in your treatment of this patient and why?

_____

_____

_____

5. What tests or measures will you use to assess the patient's progress and response to treatment?

_____

_____

_____

6. What subjective or objective information that you gather during the treatment might cause you to alter your treatment for this patient and why?

_____

_____

7. How would you document your treatment in the SOAP or Patient/Client Management format?

_____

_____

_____

8. If the treatment goes as expected, what will you do for the next treatment?

_____

_____

9. How would you expect this patient to progress over time?

_____

_____

10. If the patient does not progress as expected, what might be some reasons for a lack of progress?

_____

_____

11. What signs or symptoms, if observed or re-ported by the patient, would cause you to hold treatment and check with the nursing staff, primary PT, or MD?

_____

_____

12. Are there any cultural, socioeconomic, or ethical issues presented in this case that might affect your interventions or communication with this patient? If so, how?

_____

_____

_____

13. Re-review this case. Are there any coexisting medical diagnoses that might affect how this patient responds to physical therapy? If so, what are they, and how might they cause the patient to respond to physical therapy differently than you expected?

_____

_____

_____

14. After reviewing the other disciplines' notes regarding this patient, is there any other information that will help you to plan your treatment sessions?

_____

_____

_____

15. Compare your responses on this case with those of your classmates or instructors. What, if anything, would you change and why?

_____

_____

_____

_____

Home Health Physical Therapy Evaluation

NAME	Brenda Martin
DATE	September 22, 2010
DIAGNOSIS	S/P left transtibial amputation
SUBJECTIVE INFORMATION	The patient reports pain at 5/10 and increased swelling in residual limb at times when dangling too long. PMH includes obesity; HTN; dyslipidemia; DM II with peripheral neuropathy and retinopathy; GERD; DJD bilateral knees,

hips, and spine; prior left foot amputation; and cholecystectomy. She continues to report difficulty managing her diabetes and states she feels like it is too late and why bother anymore since she has now lost her leg because of it. She states her boyfriend will not let her spend any money on more healthy choices for food. He is home during evaluation and sitting in other room smoking during the session.

continued

Home Health Physical Therapy Evaluation *continued*

OBJECTIVE INFORMATION	
POSTURE	In standing, hips flexed and forward head and shoulders
GAIT	Hops with FWW about 8 feet in kitchen on linoleum floor, supervised because of decreased balance and risk for fall
BALANCE	Fair with FWW balancing on RLE
STRENGTH	Bilateral hip flexion, knee extension 4–/5; bilateral hip abduction 2+/5, adduction 2+/5; right hamstring 4–/5, left hamstring 3–/5; right ankle dorsiflexion/plantarflexion 4/5, eversion/inversion 4–/5
PROM	RLE: knee flexion 3 to 125 degrees; ankle plantarflexion 60 degrees; dorsiflexion 0; hip flexion to 95 degrees (limited by obesity) and extension 5 degrees from neutral; hip abduction 25 degrees, adduction 10 degrees LLE: knee flexion 5 to 100 degrees; hip flexion to 95 degrees (limited by obesity) and extension 5 degrees from neutral; hip abduction 15 degrees, adduction 7 degrees
CIRCUMFERENCES/ RESIDUAL LIMB SHAPE	2 cm below distal patella: left 46 cm; right 46 cm Mid-patella: left 50 cm, right 50 cm 10 cm above patella: left 54 cm, right 54 cm Residual limb shaping well
SKIN INTEGRITY	LLE residual limb healing scar
SENSATION	Absent light-touch and temperature sensation below mid-thigh BLE; intact proprioception and kinesthesia bilateral hips and knees; impaired in right ankle and foot
DIABETIC FOOT EVALUATION	Hammertoes, callus formation, dry skin, and loss of protective sensation in right foot; when asked what she is doing to take care of her foot, she states she has gotten information from the hospital but does not know where the information is and has not done much. She thinks they told her to put lotion on her foot.
FUNCTIONAL MOBILITY ASSESSMENT	Bed mobility: Min. A, boyfriend assists but has a difficult time himself due to SOB. Stand pivot transfer: Min. A; Mod. I with slide board transfer W/C mobility: inside home Mod. I but does not fit through bathroom door; needs assist to wheel herself up/down ramp and outdoors

	Toilet and shower transfers: Min. A with use of FWW and hopping from bathroom door to toilet then to shower bench.
HOME SAFETY ASSESSMENT	The doorway into the home is 29 inches wide, the hall is 28 inches, the doorway into the bedroom 28 inches, and doorway into the bathroom is 25 inches; a makeshift ramp with a board across the steps is not stable/safe. A bathtub with bench is adequate with handheld shower nozzle; grab bars are not possible because they cannot be placed on wall.
ASSESSMENT	The patient's home is not fully accessible or safe. Recommend a full ramp and provided specifications. Also, W/C does not fit through the bathroom door, so that she has to hop with the FWW into there to use the shower. She otherwise uses a bedside commode in the bedroom. Recommend a shower aide and an occupational therapy consult to address toileting, bathing, toilet, and shower transfers. The safety judgment and awareness of both patient and her boyfriend are questionable. She does wish to proceed with getting a LLE prosthesis and walking with it eventually but does not show motivation to care for herself and manage the diabetes. RN consulted about possible depression; the RN will contact the MD regarding a trial of medication if needed. The patient will benefit from therapy services to address the following goals:
STG (2 weeks)	1. Decrease pain in residual limb to 3/10 to allow patient to perform home exercise program consistently. 2. Increase PROM bilateral hip extension to neutral, ankle dorsiflexion to 5 degrees, knee extension to full, all to improve ambulation in environment. 3. Increase bilateral hip abduction and adduction to 3+/5 and remainder of BLE muscle groups by half grade each to improve ambulation in environment.
LTG	Mod. I with all transfers and functional mobility in home including car transfers and floor transfers.
PLAN	Functional mobility training, pre-gait activities, strengthening and ROM exercise; contact prosthetist for prosthesis assessment. Two times per week for 4 weeks.

BOX 8-3 | Health-Care Team Member Role: Prosthetist and Orthotist

Prosthetists and orthotists work with patients in a wide variety of settings to provide specialized equipment in the form of orthoses and prostheses to assist patients in meeting their mobility goals. Their work involves evaluating the patient, making the brace or prosthesis, and custom-fitting it to the patient. Sometimes, they fabricate or recommend a brace and help to fit it to the patient without need for extensive follow-up. Other times, they follow a patient over months or longer to ensure optimal fit and function over time. Especially in the case of a prosthesis, the patient's needs may change over time as a result of changing circumferences of the residual limb related to weight gain/loss, edema changes, and muscle atrophy/hypertrophy. For these and other reasons, it is important to maintain a positive working relationship with the prosthetist and to keep him or her involved in the care of the patient. For more information, please see the website of the American Academy of Orthotists and Prosthetists at http://www.oandp.org and their career page at http://www.opcareers.org.

HOME HEALTH CRITICAL THINKING QUESTIONS

After reviewing the home health physical therapy evaluation, address the following:

1. What are the patient's impairments? Functional limitations? Is there a disability?

2. Find assessments of gait, strength, ROM, and balance if available from the initial evaluation and list.

   a. How could each potentially be used to assess function and demonstrate progress toward goals or show the patient's response to physical therapy interventions?

   b. What would be the most important items to document for this patient?

3. After reviewing the POC, describe a possible next treatment session.

   a. List the activities/exercises and your rationale for the order of treatment activities that you selected.

4. What subjective information will you gather during your session to help in your treatment of this patient and why?

5. What tests or measures will you use to assess the patient's progress and response to treatment?

6. What subjective or objective information that you gather during the treatment might cause you to alter your treatment for this patient and why?

7. How would you document your treatment in the SOAP or Patient/Client Management format?

8. If the treatment goes as expected, what will you do for the next treatment?

continued

HOME HEALTH CRITICAL THINKING QUESTIONS *continued*

9. How would you expect this patient to progress over time?

_____

_____

10. If the patient does not progress as expected, what might be some reasons for a lack of progress?

_____

_____

11. What signs or symptoms, if observed or reported by the patient, would cause you to hold treatment and check with the nursing staff, primary PT, or MD?

_____

_____

12. Are there any cultural, socioeconomic, or ethical issues presented in this case that might affect your interventions or communication with this patient? If so, how?

_____

_____

13. Re-review this case. Are there any coexisting medical diagnoses that might affect how this patient responds to physical therapy? If so, what are they, and how might they cause the patient to respond to physical therapy differently than you expected?

_____

_____

14. After reviewing the other disciplines' notes regarding this patient, is there any other information that will help you to plan your treatment sessions?

_____

_____

_____

15. Compare your responses on this case with those of your classmates or instructors. What, if anything, would you change and why?

_____

_____

_____

Outpatient Physical Therapy Evaluation

NAME	Brenda Martin
DATE	October 24, 2010
DIAGNOSIS	S/P left transtibial amputation
SUBJECTIVE INFORMATION	The patient reports occasional pain at 2/10 and minimal swelling in residual limb at times. PMH includes obesity; HTN; dyslipidemia; DM II with peripheral neuropathy and retinopathy; GERD; DJD bilateral knees, hips, spine; prior left foot amputation; and cholecystectomy. She reports that a trial of antidepressant medication is helping her cope with the realities of a lost limb. She is also getting help through a support group. She hopes to make some positive changes in her lifestyle and lose some weight in the process to prevent losing her other leg or worse. While her boyfriend was out having a smoke, she stated that she is

thinking of asking him to move out because he is "not very nice at times." However, she is not sure how she will survive because he does work some and helps support them both.

OBJECTIVE INFORMATION	
POSTURE	In standing, hips flexed and forward head and shoulders
GAIT	Hops on RLE with FWW 30 feet Mod. I
BALANCE	Fair with FWW
STRENGTH	Bilateral hip flexion, knee extension 4–/5; bilateral hip abduction 3–/5, adduction 3–/5, extension 3–/5; right hamstring 4/5, left hamstring 3/5; right ankle dorsiflexion/plantarflexion 4/5, eversion/inversion 4/5

PROM	RLE: knee flexion 0 to 125 degrees; ankle plantarflexion 60 degrees, dorsiflexion 3 degrees; hip flexion to 95 degrees (limited by obesity) and extension to neutral; hip abduction 25 degrees, adduction 15 degrees LLE: knee flexion 0 to 115 degrees; hip flexion to 95 degrees (limited by obesity) and extension to neutral; hip abduction 20 degrees, adduction 15 degrees	**ASSESSMENT**	
		STG (2 weeks)	1. Decrease pain in LLE to 0/10 to allow full participation in therapy program. 2. Increase bilateral hip extension to 5 degrees, right ankle dorsiflexion to 10 degrees, and remainder of LLE PROM to equal RLE, all to improve posture and gait. 3. Increase BLE strength to 4/5 in all muscle groups to decrease potential of gait deviations and allow her to use left prosthesis for gait. 4. Patient independent with use of shrinker and temporary prosthesis including donning/doffing safely.
CIRCUMFERENCES/ RESIDUAL LIMB SHAPE	2 cm below distal patella: left 46 cm; right 46 cm Mid-patella: left 50 cm, right 50 cm 10 cm above patella: left 54 cm, right 54 cm Residual limb shaping well		
		LTG	Mod. I with home exercise program; gait with temporary prosthesis 100 feet Mod. I with FWW.
SKIN INTEGRITY	LLE residual limb healing scar		
SENSATION	Absent light-touch and temperature sensation below mid-thigh BLE; intact proprioception and kinesthesia bilateral hips and knees but impaired right ankle and foot	PLAN	Pre-gait and gait training, progression of strengthening and stretching exercise program; progression of cardiovascular exercise program and development of home exercise program; education regarding use of shrinker and temporary prosthesis including donning/doffing. Training is planned for three times per week for 4 weeks, with reassessment for further training depending on progress with prosthesis.
DIABETIC FOOT EVALUATION	Hammertoes, callus formation, dry skin and loss of protective sensation R foot; demonstrates ability to check R foot for pressure areas, check shoe for potential pressure issues, and use lotion for dry skin to prevent cracks. Has new diabetic shoe with adequate room in toe box to prevent pressure due to hammertoes.		
FUNCTIONAL MOBILITY ASSESSMENT ON MAT	Bed mobility: Mod. I Stand pivot transfer: Mod. I with FWW W/C mobility: inside therapy office and outdoors on pavement Mod. I		

OUTPATIENT CRITICAL THINKING QUESTIONS

After reviewing the outpatient physical therapy evaluation, address the following:

1. What are the patient's impairments? Functional limitations? Is there a disability?

_____

_____

_____

_____

_____

_____

2. Find assessments of gait, strength, ROM, and balance if available from the initial evaluation and list.

   a. How could each potentially be used to assess function and demonstrate progress toward goals or show the patient's response to physical therapy interventions?

_____

_____

_____

continued

OUTPATIENT CRITICAL THINKING QUESTIONS *continued*

b. What would be the most important items to document for this patient?

_____

_____

_____

3. After reviewing the POC, describe a possible next treatment session.

a. List the activities/exercises and your rationale for the order of treatment activities that you selected.

_____

_____

_____

4. What subjective information will you gather during your session to help in your treatment of this patient and why?

_____

_____

5. What tests or measures will you use to assess the patient's progress and response to treatment?

_____

_____

6. What subjective or objective information that you gather during the treatment might cause you to alter your treatment for this patient and why?

_____

_____

7. How would you document your treatment in the SOAP or Patient/Client Management format?

_____

_____

_____

_____

8. If the treatment goes as expected, what will you do for the next treatment?

_____

_____

9. How would you expect this patient to progress over time?

_____

_____

10. If the patient does not progress as expected, what might be some reasons for a lack of progress?

_____

_____

11. What signs or symptoms, if observed or reported by the patient, would cause you to hold treatment and check with the nursing staff, primary PT, or MD?

_____

_____

12. Are there any cultural, socioeconomic, or ethical issues presented in this case that might affect your interventions or communication with this patient? If so, how?

_____

_____

13. Re-review this case. Are there any coexisting medical diagnoses that might affect how this patient responds to physical therapy? If so, what are they, and how might they cause the patient to respond to physical therapy differently than you expected?

_____

_____

14. After reviewing the other disciplines' notes regarding this patient, is there any other information that will help you to plan your treatment sessions?

_____

_____

_____

15. Compare your responses on this case with those of your classmates or instructors. What, if anything, would you change and why?

_____

_____

CONTINUUM OF CARE CRITICAL THINKING QUESTIONS

After reviewing the continuum of care for this patient, consider the following:

1. How did the patient's problems change over the weeks after her surgery?

_____

_____

_____

_____

_____

2. How did this affect the goals and the interventions that the PT included in the POC?

_____

_____

_____

_____

3. How were the same interventions modified over time to progress the patient according to her changing needs?

_____

_____

_____

_____

_____

4. What are some potential community resources that this patient might like to participate in and how would these help her to maintain and improve her physical fitness?

_____

_____

_____

_____

IMPLICATIONS OF PATHOLOGY FOR THE PTA[2]

1. What signs and symptoms of hypoglycemia and hyperglycemia should the PTA be aware of when working with a patient who has diabetes?

_____

_____

_____

_____

_____

2. What signs and symptoms of ketoacidosis should the PTA be aware of when working with a patient who has diabetes?

_____

_____

_____

_____

_____

3. What potential complications should the PTA be watching for in a patient with diabetes who is exercising?

_____

_____

_____

_____

_____

4. How would exercise in the water compare with that on land in a patient with diabetes in regard to insulin regulation?

_____

_____

_____

_____

_____

continued

IMPLICATIONS OF PATHOLOGY FOR THE PTA[2] *continued*

5. What are the risks associated with using modalities with patients with diabetes?

_____

_____

_____

_____

_____

_____

_____

_____

_____

6. What should the PTA be aware of when working with patients with the following?
- Type 1 diabetes
- Transfemoral amputation
- BLE amputation
- UE amputation
- Finger or toe amputation

_____

_____

_____

_____

_____

References

1. American Physical Therapy Association: Guide to Physical Therapist Practice, Second Edition. Alexandria, VA: Author, 2001.

2. Goodman CC, Boissonnault FG, Fuller KS: Pathology: Implications for the Physical Therapist, Second Edition. Philadelphia: Saunders, 2003.

Todd Norton: A Patient With Traumatic Brain Injury

 Preferred Practice Pattern: Neuromuscular, Pattern I, Then Pattern D

CHAPTER OUTLINE

Introducing Todd Norton

Todd Norton is 13 years old and sustained a traumatic brain injury during a skateboarding versus car accident. According to the APTA's *Guide to Physical Therapy Practice* (the *Guide*), he could have the following impairments in the acute phase of his rehabilitation when under pattern I:

- Impaired arousal
- Impaired motor function
- Impaired ROM
- Impaired sensory integrity
- Lack of response to stimuli

After he transitions into pattern D, he might have the following impairments:

- Impaired affect
- Impaired arousal, attention, and cognition
- Impaired communication
- Impaired balance

Functional limitations may include the following:

- Difficulty negotiating terrains
- Difficulty planning movements
- Frequent falls
- Inability to keep up with peers or perform work

Please refer to the *Guide*[1] for a complete list of possible impairments and functional limitations. As you work through this case, think about which of these the patient is experiencing.

Vocabulary List

Obtunded	Cyanosis
Glasgow Coma Scale	Babinski
Normocephalic	Rancho scale
Lymphadenopathy	Hemianopsia
Thyromegaly	Dysarthria
Auscultation	Ataxic, ataxia
Hepatosplenomegaly	Trendelenburg

PHYSICIAN'S HISTORY AND PHYSICAL

PATIENT NAME: Todd R. Norton
ADMIT DATE: July 9, 2010
BIRTH DATE: June 14, 1997
SEX: Male
ROOM/BED: 334-01
MEDICAL RECORD #: 12345678

CHIEF COMPLAINT: Traumatic brain injury

ATTENDING: Dr. Melvin Peterson, MD

HISTORY OF PRESENT ILLNESS: This 13-year-old boy was skateboarding, fell when hit by a car, and hit his head, losing consciousness within an hour. He was attended in the field by EMS, who provided oxygen and IV fluid support and monitored vital signs while en route to the emergency department. CT shows subdural hemorrhage in the frontal and left parietal lobes. He is now **obtunded** and responding minimally to stimuli. His **Glasgow Coma Scale** score is 8. His mother and stepfather are present at his bedside.

PAST MEDICAL HISTORY: None

PAST SURGICAL HISTORY: Tonsillectomy

ALLERGIES: Seasonal allergies

MEDICATIONS: Claritin daily during spring and summer months

FAMILY HISTORY: Mother has thyroid disease; father has HTN

SOCIAL HISTORY: The patient lives with his mother and stepfather and two full siblings, ages 4 and 9. He attends middle school, entering 8th grade next year. Other than skateboarding, he enjoys playing basketball and football.

REVIEW OF SYSTEMS: See HPI; otherwise negative

PHYSICAL EXAMINATION:

VITAL SIGNS: Temperature 36.6°C, pulse 95 BPM, respiratory rate 27 respirations per minute, blood pressure 105/60 mm Hg, O_2 saturation 98% on 2 LPM.

GENERAL: Obtunded; moving head to pain and voice stimuli. Grimaces with passive motion to upper extremities but does not attempt to communicate or respond to questions or follow directions.

SKIN: Pale; abrasions on face and arms.

HEENT: **Normocephalic.** Pupils unequal and left eye unreactive. Unable to track visually. Oropharynx unremarkable; using suction to manage secretions.

NECK: Supple without obvious **lymphadenopathy** or **thyromegaly.** Axillary region without obvious lymphadenopathy.

CARDIAC: Unremarkable

LUNGS: Clear to **auscultation**

ABDOMEN: Bowel sounds present, nontender, nondistended. No **hepatosplenomegaly.**

EXTREMITIES: 2+ peripheral pulses without **cyanosis** or edema. No evidence of fractures or dislocation.

NEUROLOGICAL: Mildly increased tone throughout especially right extremities. Reflexes 1+ diffusely. Positive **Babinski** right side. Appears hemiparetic on the right side, but unable to assess fully, as well as sensation, because of his inability to effectively communicate.

LABORATORY DATA: Normal PT/PTT

IMAGING STUDIES: CT axial view demonstrates a hyperdense crescenteric collection adjacent to the inner table over right frontal and parietal lobes.

ASSESSMENT: Left frontal and parietal subdural hematoma S/P traumatic brain injury with right hemiparesis; still in coma-like state, obtunded with minimal response to stimuli.

PLAN: The patient will be admitted to ICU with an immediate neurosurgical consult. Physiatry, physical therapy, occupational therapy, speech therapy, and medical social work consults are needed.

SEEING THE DIAGNOSIS IN ACTION 9-1

Head injuries are either closed or open, but both cause damage to the brain. The effects of a head injury can be wide and varied from a mild concussion to a massive injury resulting in severely impaired mobility in the patient. In the acute setting, physical therapy focuses on functional activities and beginning strengthening, while often working within potential restraints because of the patient's medical instability. As the patient progresses through the typical stages of healing, he or she may exhibit a wide variety of challenges related to cognition, memory, and emotional instability. These factors must be considered when working with any patient with a head injury and may affect overall progress toward functional goals. The following photos show a young patient who actually suffered a CVA but presents as a typical patient with head trauma. He is performing exercises in an outpatient setting.

As with all patients, but especially those with any type of head trauma, the team members will need to work together closely to facilitate an optimal recovery. No two patients are alike, and each must be continually observed for changes in behavior, communication, and cognition as well as physical function. The PTA can provide valuable information to the primary PT to help monitor progress within the POC.

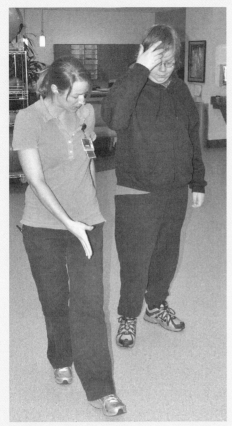

Figure 9-1 Here, a patient receives instruction for balance exercises from the PT.

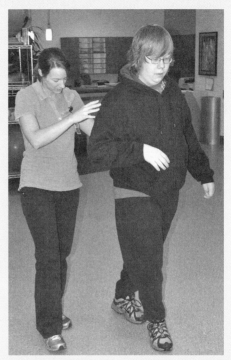

Figure 9-3 A patient with a head injury might perform tandem walking as an activity to improve balance, especially during ambulation.

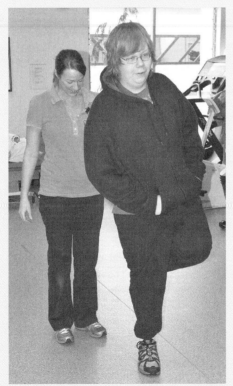

Figure 9-2 A patient performing unilateral stance balance exercise.

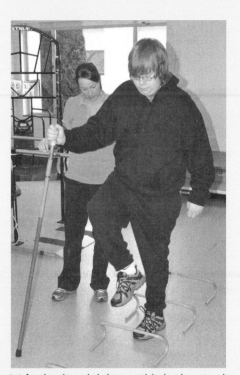

Figure 9-4 Another dynamic balance activity involves stepping over obstacles.

continued

SEEING THE DIAGNOSIS IN ACTION 9-1 *continued*

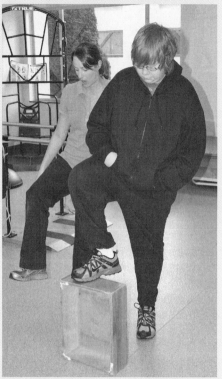

Figure 9-5 Balance exercises are an important part of a physical therapy plan for most patients with a head injury.

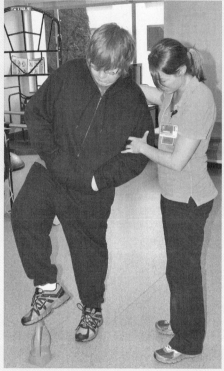

Figure 9-6 Balance and other exercises will typically be included in a home exercise program for these patients.

REVIEWING THE MEDICAL HISTORY

1. What do you already know about traumatic brain injuries?

_____

_____

_____

_____

_____

2. Review the vocabulary list and physician's notes. Look up the meanings of any terms you do not understand in a medical dictionary or other text.

_____

_____

_____

_____

3. Review the diagnoses in the past medical history using a medical or pathology text, Internet resource, or other available resource.

_____

_____

_____

_____

_____

4. Which diagnoses in the past medical history would be significant and potentially affect the patient's response to the physical therapy interventions?

_____

_____

_____

_____

5. List the purpose and potential side effects of each of the medications the patient is taking.

_____

_____

_____

_____

_____

_____

6. Describe what each laboratory result measures and list considerations for physical therapy if the results for this patient were *not* in the normal range.

_____

_____

_____

_____

_____

Acute Care Physical Therapy Initial Evaluation
Patient History

NAME	Todd Norton	SURGERY	Craniotomy
ROOM # & BED	B334-01	SURGERY DATE	07/09/2010
MEDICAL RECORD #	12345678	PRECAUTIONS	Head of bed elevated
ATTENDING PHYSICIAN	Dr. Peterson	WEIGHT-BEARING STATUS	WBAT
CHIEF COMPLAINT	Traumatic brain injury		
AGE	13	LIVING SITUATION	Home
DATE OF BIRTH	06/14/1997	PRIOR LEVEL OF FUNCTION	Independent at home and school
SEX	Male		
PRIMARY LANGUAGE	English	ASSISTANCE AVAILABLE	Family; mother works part-time
ISOLATION	No	STAIRS TO ENTER HOME	12
HEIGHT (CM)	175	RAIL(S) ON STAIRS	One side
WEIGHT (KG)	61	ASSISTIVE DEVICE USED PRIOR	None
MEDICATION ALLERGIES	NKDA		
FOOD ALLERGIES	None	EQUIPMENT PATIENT HAS	None
INITIATED BY	Donna Smith, PT		
DATE	07/10/2010	DRIVING PRIOR TO ADMIT	No
TIME	15:45		
TREATING DIAGNOSIS	Decreased mobility S/P TBI	OCCUPATION/LIFE ROLE	Going into 8th grade; participates in basketball, football, skateboarding
ONSET DATE	07/09/2010		
PERTINENT MEDICAL HISTORY	Per H & P: tonsillectomy		

Systems Review

HEARING	Unable to assess	PAIN TYPE	Unable to assess
VISION	Unable to assess	PAIN INTERVENTION	Limited motion in assessment
SPEECH	Does not attempt to verbalize/communicate	RESTING HEART RATE (BPM)	94
PAIN SCALE	Nonverbal	RESTING RESPIRATORY RATE (respirations per minute)	28
PAIN LEVEL	Grimaces		
PAIN LOCATION	With UE PROM		

continued

Acute Care Physical Therapy Initial Evaluation *continued*
Systems Review

RESTING BLOOD PRESSURE (mm Hg)	106/58	POSTACTIVITY RESPIRATORY RATE (respirations per minute)	26
RESTING SpO$_2$	100% on 2 LPM	POSTACTIVITY BLOOD PRESSURE (mm Hg)	108/60
ACTIVITY HEART RATE (BPM)	99	POSTACTIVITY SpO$_2$	99% on 2 LPM
ACTIVITY RESPIRATORY RATE (respirations per minute)	30	LEVEL OF CONSCIOUSNESS	Coma
ACTIVITY BLOOD PRESSURE (mm Hg)	110/61	ORIENTATION	Unable to assess
ACTIVITY SpO$_2$	99% on 2 LPM	SHORT-TERM MEMORY	Unable to assess
POSTACTIVITY HEART RATE (BPM)	95	RANCHO SCALE	Level II

Tests and Measures

ROM NECK/TRUNK	PROM WNL	SUPINE TO SIT/SIT TO SUPINE	Tot. A
ROM BUE	PROM WNL	SIT TO STAND/STAND TO SIT	Unable
ROM BLE	PROM WNL except bilateral ankle dorsiflexion with knees straight 5 degrees from neutral.	TRANSFERS	Tot. A
BUE STRENGTH	Unable to assess	SITTING BALANCE	Poor
BLE STRENGTH	Unable to assess	STANDING BALANCE	Unable
SENSATION	Unable to assess	GAIT	Unable
TONE	0 RLE; Modified Ashworth Scale; WNL LLE	STAIRS	Unable
SKIN INTEGRITY	Intact with redness at bilateral heels	SITTING TOLERANCE	30 seconds edge of bed
BED MOBILITY	Tot. A		

Evaluation

DIAGNOSIS	Neuromuscular, pattern I
PROGNOSIS	Fair; pending medical stability. The patient is a 13-year-old who suffered a closed head injury when he was hit by a car while skateboarding. He is only minimally responsive, but his parents report that he is a little more responsive today than yesterday. The mother works part-time, and stepfather works full-time in construction. Two younger siblings are both in day care while the parents work, with the youngest starting kindergarten in the fall. The grandmother is coming to

help out at home for a while. The biological father is apparently not in contact with the children. The patient will benefit from skilled therapy services to teach the family appropriate and helpful ways to interact with him and to maintain ROM while he is unable to move his own extremities. These services will progress as his medical condition stabilizes and hopefully he comes out of the coma. He is a good candidate to consider inpatient rehabilitation at D/C.

Plan of Care

PATIENT'S GOALS	Family's goal is to take him home.			Therapeutic exercise
DISCHARGE GOALS	1. Bed mobility and transfers: Mod. A			Therapeutic activities
	2. Gait: TBD			Family training
	3. Home exercise program: Mod. A by		FREQUENCY	BID
	family to maintain PROM		PATIENT EDUCATION TOPIC(S)	Activity: stimulation; calf stretches
TIME TO ACHIEVE GOALS	By time of discharge			
PATIENT/FAMILY UNDERSTAND/AGREES WITH GOALS	Family yes		TAUGHT BY	PT
			WHO WAS TAUGHT	Mother
INTERVENTIONS	Bed mobility training		METHOD OF INSTRUCTION	Verbal/demonstration
	Transfer training			
	Balance training		EVALUATION OF LEARNING	Needs reinforcement
	Gait training			
	Home program			

Acute Care Nursing Note

07/11/2010   3:13 PM

The patient opens his eyes to verbal and tactile stimuli and groans with apparent pain with UE PROM consistent with Glasgow Coma Scale 8. The pupils are equal and reactive to light. The parents and siblings visit often, and the patient demonstrates increasing alertness for about half an hour at these times and then becomes tired and sleeps several hours. Vital signs are stable. Foley catheter is draining dark amber urine.

Acute Care Social Work Note

07/12/2010   2:36 PM

The patient is S/P TBI. He is more alert each day and making progress in therapies. I met with his parents regarding D/C plan, and they hope for inpatient rehabilitation when he is ready for D/C from acute setting. The plan is to move him to floor from ICU tomorrow and will follow up and assist with D/C planning.

Medical Update

07/13/2010

The patient received emergent craniotomy to evacuate hematoma. The head of the bed was elevated to reduce intracranial pressures; he is being monitored for vital signs. Medications after surgery include dexamethasone IV 8 mg, which will then be continued at 4 mg IM every 4 hours for 2 to 4 days. On postoperative day 2, he is awakening from coma and moving left extremities. On postoperative day 4, he is able to begin oral feedings, and Decadron has been changed to 4 mg orally daily.

Acute Care Occupational Therapy Summary

07/13/2010   1:11 PM

The patient is S/P TBI 7/9/10. Occupational therapy evaluation was completed today. Foley was just removed. **Rancho scale** level III to IV. He has just started oral feedings and medications. He is oriented to self and family and follows one-step concrete instructions with 25% accuracy. He responds best to hand-over-hand guidance when initiating unfamiliar tasks and is able to automatically initiate self-feeding and light grooming with just minimal cues for safety and technique. He currently displays right visual deficit noted during testing, but no neglect observed. He is able to perform full AROM of BUE with grossly 3+/5 strength and mild flexor tone in R biceps. He demonstrates slowed but adequate fine and gross motor coordination for functional tasks. He requires Mod. A for low pivot transfer to toilet and Min. A for sitting balance. He needs Mod. A overall for upper body self-care but Max. A for lower body. He demonstrates moderate to severely impaired cognition in sequencing, attention to task, and motor planning. He will require the services of occupational therapy to address deficits and train family with his ADL needs.

BOX 9-1 | Health-Care Team Member Role: Speech Language Pathologist

Speech language pathologists, or speech therapists, like other rehabilitation team members, work in a variety of settings, from acute to outpatient, and also in schools. They work with patients who have both expressive and comprehensive language problems. They also assess and provide appropriate interventions for patients who have swallowing problems and work closely with nurses regarding those needs. Because they are trained extensively in cognitive assessments and interventions, they may work closely with occupational therapists to help patients with cognitive and behavior deficits. Often, PTAs may notice improved speech in patients after or during postural re-education or other movement therapy with patients. Working closely with speech therapy staff will help the PTA understand how to approach difficult patients in terms of their behaviors or cognitive deficits. For more information, see the American Speech-Language-Hearing Association website at http://www.asha.org.

Acute Care Speech Language Pathology Summary

07/14/2010   1:15 PM

The patient has been making progress toward speech therapy goals. He has progressed to dysphagia thick diet and nectar thick liquids. He needs supervision when feeding himself. His speech continues to be dysarthritic, but his intelligibility improves daily. He is also working on improving rate of articulation. He works hard at therapy sessions. His family is involved and asking questions about how to help him. They have been provided education regarding appropriate stimulation and the need for a calm environment because he tends to get distracted easily and has difficulty focusing.

ACUTE CARE CRITICAL THINKING QUESTIONS

After reviewing the acute care physical therapy initial evaluation and other discipline notes, address the following:

1. What are the patient's impairments? Functional limitations? Is there a disability?

_____

_____

_____

_____

_____

2. Find assessments of gait, strength, ROM, and balance if available from the initial evaluation and list.

   a. How could each potentially be used to assess function and demonstrate progress toward goals or show the patient's response to physical therapy interventions?

   _____

   _____

   _____

b. What would be the most important items to document for this patient?

_____

_____

_____

3. After reviewing the POC, describe a possible next treatment session.

   a. List the activities/exercises and your rationale for the order of treatment activities that you selected.

_____

_____

_____

4. What subjective information will you gather during your session to help in your treatment of this patient and why?

_____

_____

5. What tests or measures will you use to assess the patient's progress and response to treatment?

_____

_____

6. What subjective or objective information that you gather during the treatment might cause you to alter your treatment for this patient and why?

_____

_____

7. How would you document your treatment in the SOAP or Patient/Client Management format?

_____

_____

_____

_____

8. If the treatment goes as expected, what will you do for the next treatment?

_____

_____

9. How would you expect this patient to progress over time?

_____

_____

10. If the patient does not progress as expected, what might be some reasons for a lack of progress?

_____

_____

11. What signs or symptoms, if observed or reported by the patient, would cause you to hold treatment and check with the nursing staff, primary PT, or MD?

_____

_____

12. Are there any cultural, socioeconomic, or ethical issues presented in this case that might affect your interventions or communication with this patient? If so, how?

_____

_____

13. Re-review this case. Are there any coexisting medical diagnoses that might affect how this patient responds to physical therapy? If so, what are they, and how might they cause the patient to respond to physical therapy differently than you expected?

_____

_____

14. After reviewing the other disciplines' notes regarding this patient, is there any other information that will help you to plan your treatment sessions?

_____

_____

15. Compare your responses on this case with those of your classmates or instructors. What, if anything, would you change and why?

_____

_____

Medical Update

07/16/2010

Upon discharge from the acute setting on July 16, 2010, the patient is S/P craniotomy for subdural hematoma. His medications include Decadron 4 mg daily and Tylenol 325 mg 1 to 2 tablets every 4 to 6 hours PRN for headache. The plan is for inpatient rehabilitation.

Inpatient Rehabilitation Physical Therapy Initial Evaluation

Patient History

NAME	Todd Norton	SURGERY	Craniotomy
ROOM # & BED	B362-2	SURGERY DATE	07/09/2010
MEDICAL RECORD #	12345678	PRECAUTIONS	Head of bed elevated; aspiration precautions; fall risk
ATTENDING PHYSICIAN	Dr. Gordon		
CHIEF COMPLAINT	Traumatic brain injury	WEIGHT-BEARING STATUS	WBAT
AGE	13		
DATE OF BIRTH	06/14/1997	LIVING SITUATION	Home
SEX	Male	PRIOR LEVEL OF FUNCTION	Independent at home and school
PRIMARY LANGUAGE	English	ASSISTANCE AVAILABLE	Family; mother works part-time. Grandmother has been here to help with family while patient in hospital.
ISOLATION	No		
HEIGHT (CM)	175		
WEIGHT (KG)	58	STAIRS TO ENTER HOME	12
MEDICATION ALLERGIES	NKDA	RAIL(S) ON STAIRS	One side
FOOD ALLERGIES	None	ASSISTIVE DEVICE USED PRIOR	None
INITIATED BY	Roger Lee, PT		
DATE	07/16/2010	EQUIPMENT PATIENT HAS	None
TIME	11:25		
TREATING DIAGNOSIS	Decreased mobility S/P TBI	DRIVING PRIOR TO ADMIT	Not applicable
ONSET DATE	07/09/2010		
PERTINENT MEDICAL HISTORY	Per H & P: tonsillectomy	OCCUPATION/LIFE ROLE	Going into 8th grade; participates in basketball, football, skateboarding, youth group at church

Systems Review

HEARING	Intact	RESTING RESPIRATORY RATE (respirations per minute)	25
VISION	Right hemianopsia		
SPEECH	Dysarthria and able to understand about 25% of time; other times incoherent and inappropriate	RESTING BLOOD PRESSURE (mm Hg)	104/56
PAIN SCALE	VPS	RESTING SpO$_2$	100% on 1 LPM
PAIN LEVEL	4	ACTIVITY HEART RATE (BPM)	100
PAIN LOCATION	Neck		
PAIN TYPE	Ache	ACTIVITY RESPIRATORY RATE (respirations per minute)	27
PAIN INTERVENTION	Alerted RN		
RESTING HEART RATE (BPM)	92	ACTIVITY BLOOD PRESSURE (mm Hg)	110/60

ACTIVITY SpO$_2$	99% on 2 LPM	LEVEL OF CONSCIOUSNESS	Alert but drowsy
POSTACTIVITY HEART RATE (BPM)	96	ORIENTATION	To self, place; not time or situation
POSTACTIVITY RESPIRATORY RATE (respirations per minute)	26	SHORT-TERM MEMORY	No short-term memory. Impaired with no selective attention to environment and able to focus on general environment about 30 seconds at a time.
POSTACTIVITY BLOOD PRESSURE (mm Hg)	106/58	RANCHO SCALE	Level IV
POSTACTIVITY SpO$_2$	100% on 1 LPM		

Tests and Measures

ROM NECK/TRUNK	PROM WNL	BED MOBILILTY	Min. A to roll; Mod. A to scoot up in bed
ROM BUE	PROM WNL	SUPINE TO SIT/SIT TO SUPINE	Mod. A to sit; Min. A to return to supine
ROM BLE	PROM WNL except bilateral ankle dorsiflexion with knees straight to neutral.	SIT TO STAND/STAND TO SIT	Mod. A
BUE STRENGTH	3+/5 shoulder, elbow, wrist, hand	TRANSFERS	Mod. A; low pivot
BLE STRENGTH	Hip flexors, quadriceps, ankle plantarflexion, eversion, inversion all able to move against gravity but with increased tone with resistance, ankle dorsiflexion able to achieve partial range with gravity eliminated RLE; all of above 4–/5 LLE	SITTING BALANCE	Fair
		STANDING BALANCE	Poor with bars
		GAIT	Mod. A in parallel bars x 6 feet; scissor gait pattern with shorter stance time on RLE and shorter step length on LLE; ataxic; right foot drop
SENSATION	Light touch intact BLE; proprioception impaired right ankle, toes	STAIRS	Unable
TONE	2+ RLE, especially hip adductors and ankle plantarflexors on Modified Ashworth Scale	SITTING TOLERANCE	10 minutes edge of bed
		WHEELCHAIR MOBILITY	Min. A forward, backward, turning each direction
SKIN INTEGRITY	Intact		

Evaluation

DIAGNOSIS	Neuromuscular, pattern D
PROGNOSIS	Good. The patient is a 13-year-old who suffered a closed head injury when he fell while skateboarding. He progressed from coma-like status to being alert and partially oriented. He follows one-step directions about 25% of time because of decreased attention. He has balance, strength, coordination, and motor control deficits evident throughout evaluation. Increased tone also limits functional mobility. Will consult with the MD about whether additional medication may be tried to decrease tone and allow greater functional progress. The mother works part-time, and stepfather works full-time

in construction. Two younger siblings are being cared for by the maternal grandmother, who came to help. He will benefit from skilled therapy services to progress functional mobility. He should be able to D/C home with grandmother and parental support and assistance. He will likely need home health and then outpatient physical therapy to follow up long term, as well as speech and occupational therapy to address communication, behavior, and cognitive impairments. He will need a rental W/C, FWW, and likely a custom AFO for RLE to improve gait and safety.

continued

Inpatient Rehabilitation Physical Therapy Initial Evaluation *continued*

Plan of Care

PATIENT'S GOALS	Skateboarding again	INTERVENTIONS	Bed mobility training
DISCHARGE GOALS	1. Bed mobility and transfers: supervision		Transfer training
	2. Car and floor transfers: Min. A		Balance training
	3. Gait: Min. A x 50 feet with FWW		Gait training
	4. Wheelchair mobility: Mod. I indoors; supervised outdoors and in community		Wheelchair mobility training
	5. Home exercise program: Min. A		Home program
	6. Family ability to assist: independent with all care needed for D/C home		Therapeutic exercise
			Therapeutic activities
			Family training
TIME TO ACHIEVE GOALS	By time of discharge	FREQUENCY	BID
PATIENT/FAMILY UNDERSTAND/AGREES WITH GOALS	Family yes		

Inpatient Rehabilitation Nursing Note

07/16/2010   1:19 PM

The patient needs Mod. A to transfer and loses balance easily but does not use call light and moves impulsively. A 1:1 sitter is used during the night, and family members are taking turns watching him during the daytime hours. Foley is removed; the patient is incontinent of urine about twice per day. The patient seems to prefer that a nurse assist him with toileting needs rather than have family help because of his embarrassment. He demonstrates some agitation at times during meals and therapies. It is recommended that he have only one family member at a time for supervision and only one additional visitor per day. He plans to have visits from school friends some days.

Inpatient Rehabilitation Social Work Summary

07/19/2010   10:55 AM

A team conference was held today. The MD reports that the latest laboratory results are negative for UTI, which was suspected. He recommends short treatment sessions and low stimulation areas be used for therapy as well as meals. He provided a short summary of expectations for recovery for the family to support the TBI family packet of information already provided. He explained to the family and patient the benefit of trial of a new medication to help control emerging tone and how this can help him make better functional progress. The MD is considering a trial of muscle relaxant for this purpose but explained to the staff and family the need to report any excessive fatigue or drowsiness with the new medication. The PT reports that the patient needs three 30-minute sessions rather than the typical two 45-minute sessions per day to reduce agitation and improve participation. The OT is providing a 45-minute session in AM for self-care activity training. Speech therapy is also providing 45 minutes per day for speech and swallowing training. Both OT and SLP are focusing on cognitive development. All disciplines are incorporating cognitive strategies to improve attention and motor planning during therapeutic activities. The recreational therapist is meeting with the patient and providing quiet games to play with his brother and sister. A rehabilitation psychologist will meet with the patient and family regarding coping and moods. The patient is requesting help to contact his biological father. The mother states outside of the meeting that the father has not had contact with the children for 4 years and that she does not wish to contact him. The rehabilitation psychologist will follow up with patient during counseling sessions. Family training is planned for 8/17 and 8/18 before D/C home on 8/20.

Inpatient Rehabilitation Occupational Therapy Summary

07/20/2010   4:22 PM

The patient is making progress toward occupational therapy goals. He continues to need supervision to Min. A for most ADLs. Primary deficits continue to be balance during standing activities, such as dressing and grooming, and cognition. He compensates automatically for right **hemianopsia.** He exhibits poor safety judgment and motor planning, is impulsive, and is beginning to show signs of aggression, consistent with Rancho level IV. His short attention span requires a quiet environment and repetition of cues for learning. He will likely need home health and then outpatient occupational therapy services for further rehabilitation after D/C to focus on return to school and leisure activities.

Inpatient Rehabilitation Speech Language Pathology Summary

07/22/2010   3:09 PM

The patient continues to have **dysarthria** and therefore is still on mechanical soft diet and nectar thick liquids. Speech therapy is focused on enunciation of words and rate of articulation. Familiar and simple games are being taught to improve memory and concentration. He is able to work only in nondistracting environments. He continues to be unable to complete new learning exercises. After D/C, he will need continued speech therapy in home health and outpatient settings to focus on speech, swallowing, and cognitive impairments.

INPATIENT REHABILITATION CRITICAL THINKING QUESTIONS

After reviewing the inpatient rehabilitation physical therapy initial evaluation and other discipline notes, address the following:

1. What are the patient's impairments? Functional limitations? Is there a disability?

2. Find assessments of gait, strength, ROM, and balance if available from the initial evaluation and list.

   a. How could each potentially be used to assess function and demonstrate progress toward goals or show the patient's response to physical therapy interventions?

   b. What would be the most important items to document for this patient?

3. After reviewing the POC, describe a possible next treatment session.

   a. List the activities/exercises and your rationale for the order of treatment activities that you selected.

4. What subjective information will you gather during your session to help in your treatment of this patient and why?

5. What tests or measures will you use to assess the patient's progress and response to treatment?

6. What subjective or objective information that you gather during the treatment might cause you to alter your treatment for this patient and why?

continued

INPATIENT REHABILITATION CRITICAL THINKING QUESTIONS *continued*

7. How would you document your treatment in the SOAP or Patient/Client Management format?

_____

_____

_____

_____

8. If the treatment goes as expected, what will you do for the next treatment?

_____

_____

9. How would you expect this patient to progress over time?

_____

_____

10. If the patient does not progress as expected, what might be some reasons for a lack of progress?

_____

_____

11. What signs or symptoms, if observed or reported by the patient, would cause you to hold treatment and check with the nursing staff, primary PT, or MD?

_____

_____

12. Are there any cultural, socioeconomic, or ethical issues presented in this case that might affect your interventions or communication with this patient? If so, how?

_____

_____

13. Re-review this case. Are there any coexisting medical diagnoses that might affect how this patient responds to physical therapy? If so, what are they, and how might they cause the patient to respond to physical therapy differently than you expected?

_____

_____

14. After reviewing the other disciplines' notes regarding this patient, is there any other information that will help you to plan your treatment sessions?

_____

_____

_____

15. Compare your responses on this case with those of your classmates or instructors. What, if anything, would you change and why?

_____

_____

BOX 9-2 | Physical Therapy Specialty: Home Health

Many PTs make home health their specialty. PTAs are also widely utilized in home health. Because therapists and assistants work primarily alone in patients' homes, it is usually recommended that new graduates from either physical therapy or physical therapist assistant programs receive mentoring from other therapists in an acute or subacute setting before working in the home health setting. It is often more challenging in the home setting than in other settings to maintain good communication among the PT and PTA, other clinical team members, and office staff. Home health care can be both rewarding and challenging because of the ability to see patients in their homes, interact closely with the family, and see first hand the barriers that patients encounter at home. For insurance to pay for home health services, the patient must be considered "homebound," which means that the patient has physical difficulty getting to an outpatient facility. Thus, home health therapists and assistants often don't work with patients very long; as patients recover and progress in their rehabilitation, they move on to an outpatient setting. The APTA has a Home Health Section, and more information can be found at their website (see http://www.homehealthsection.org).

Home Health Physical Therapy Evaluation

NAME	Todd Norton
DATE	August 21, 2010
DIAGNOSIS	S/P TBI with right-sided weakness
SUBJECTIVE INFORMATION	The patient is 13 years old and planning to enter 8th grade in the fall. He suffered TBI in a skateboarding vs. car accident on July 9, 2010. He was just discharged from an inpatient rehabilitation unit where family were involved in his care. His grandmother is available to assist with care at home while both parents work, the mother part-time. The patient states he hopes to find his biological father because he thinks his dad will help him get better care. He is angry that his parents are continuing to work while he needs so much help at home. He wants to get back to school in the fall, and they are talking about having him take a year out instead. That will put him a year behind his friends. He doesn't think he is "that bad" and thinks he is pretty close to normal now. He does not report any pain. His mother states that the patient continues to deny he has any problems but that he is clearly unable to focus well enough to return to school. She also states that he is still impulsive and unable to walk alone because of poor balance.
OBJECTIVE INFORMATION	
COGNITION, COMMUNICATION, AND VISION	Rancho level V; follows one or two simple steps about 75% of time; able to focus on activity for about 5 minutes in nondistracting environment. He demonstrates aggression when frustrated and is easily frustrated. He needs a calm, quiet approach and simple directions to participate in therapy sessions. He has right visual hemianopsia.
POSTURE	Leans to the left in standing and sitting; in standing, right knee hyperextended
GAIT	Scissor-like gait 25 feet with FWW and right AFO, Min. A; decreased stance time on right; right **Trendelenburg;** mildly **ataxic.** Unable to negotiate steps.
BALANCE	BERG 29/56; high risk for falls
STRENGTH	Takes moderate resistance without increased tone RLE, except hip abductors take no resistance and ankle dorsiflexors only able to achieve full range with gravity eliminated; 4/5 LLE
PROM	WFL except right ankle plantarflexion 60 degrees; dorsiflexion 0
WHEELCHAIR MOBILITY	Mod. I in house using manual W/C on carpets and wood flooring 50 feet; supervised for safety because he tends to get out of chair alone to try walking and has fallen twice since he got home from hospital according to mother. Needs Mod. A to manage up ramp into home and Min. A to negotiate down ramp.
TONE	3+ right hip adductors and ankle plantarflexors; WNL LLE
SENSATION	Impaired proprioception right foot and great toe; otherwise, intact light touch and proprioception
FUNCTIONAL MOBILITY ASSESSMENT	Bed mobility Mod. I Transfers low pivot supervised Car transfers Min. A Mother, stepfather, and grandmother all demonstrate ability to safely assist with transfers. His 9-year-old brother helps supervise him and plays with him.
HOME SAFETY ASSESSMENT	His family has a temporary ramp placed at the front entrance. Doors and halls all accommodate W/C. The bathroom is accessible, and the patient is using a shower bench with a handheld shower in walk-in shower. He has FWW for gait training and hopes to be out of the W/C by the time school starts. His bed is a twin bed with a rail on one side and a wall on the other.
ASSESSMENT	The patient is S/P TBI and continues to deal with emotional aspects of coping with his injuries and deficits. He clearly has made functional physical progress, but his ambulation is not where he or his family would like it to be. During a session today, the patient demonstrated decreased tolerance to stress and some unpredictable behaviors, such as aggression and cursing, with the therapist and family members. He would benefit from continued counseling and follow-up with a rehabilitation psychologist as outpatient. Message also left with the MD stating that the patient demonstrates signs of depression.

continued

Home Health Physical Therapy Evaluation *continued*

STG (2 weeks)

1. Supervised for home exercise program for upper body strengthening to improve W/C mobility up ramp and outdoors.
2. Supervised for home exercise program for strengthening BLE for improved gait.
3. Increase right hip abduction strength to decrease Trendelenburg gait deviation.
4. Increase right ankle plantarflexion to 65 degrees and dorsiflexion to 5 degrees passively to improve gait.
5. Increase BERG balance score to 36/56.

LTG

Independent with W/C mobility outdoors including ramp, transfers. Supervised gait with FWW, 50 feet.

PLAN

The plan includes development of a home exercise program for upper body and lower body strengthening, BLE stretching especially for gastrocnemius, and further balance training, along with functional mobility training, gait training, and W/C mobility training. Continued family training is planned to assist with home exercise program and tone reduction techniques. Cognitive strategies outlined by the OT and SLP will be incorporated to facilitate carryover in other aspects of his life.

HOME HEALTH CRITICAL THINKING QUESTIONS

After reviewing the home health physical therapy evaluation, address the following:

1. What are the patient's impairments? Functional limitations? Is there a disability?

_____

_____

2. Find assessments of gait, strength, ROM, and balance if available from the initial evaluation and list.

   a. How could each potentially be used to assess function and demonstrate progress toward goals or show the patient's response to physical therapy interventions?

   _____

   _____

   _____

   b. What would be the most important items to document for this patient?

   _____

   _____

   _____

3. After reviewing the POC, describe a possible next treatment session.

   a. List the activities/exercises and your rationale for the order of treatment activities that you selected.

   _____

   _____

   _____

4. What subjective information will you gather during your session to help in your treatment of this patient and why?

_____

_____

5. What tests or measures will you use to assess the patient's progress and response to treatment?

_____

_____

6. What subjective or objective information that you gather during the treatment might cause you to alter your treatment for this patient and why?

_____

_____

7. How would you document your treatment in the SOAP or Patient/Client Management format?

_____

_____

_____

_____

8. If the treatment goes as expected, what will you do for the next treatment?

_____

_____

_____

9. How would you expect this patient to progress over time?

_____

_____

10. If the patient does not progress as expected, what might be some reasons for a lack of progress?

_____

_____

11. What signs or symptoms, if observed or reported by the patient, would cause you to hold treatment and check with the nursing staff, primary PT, or MD?

_____

_____

12. Are there any cultural, socioeconomic, or ethical issues presented in this case that might affect your interventions or communication with this patient? If so, how?

_____

_____

13. Re-review this case. Are there any coexisting medical diagnoses that might affect how this patient responds to physical therapy? If so, what are they, and how might they cause the patient to respond to physical therapy differently than you expected?

_____

_____

_____

14. After reviewing the other disciplines' notes regarding this patient, is there any other information that will help you to plan your treatment sessions?

_____

_____

_____

15. Compare your responses on this case with those of your classmates or instructors. What, if anything, would you change and why?

_____

_____

Outpatient Physical Therapy Evaluation

NAME	Todd Norton		
DATE	September 14, 2010		
DIAGNOSIS	S/P TBI with mild right-sided weakness and ataxia		

SUBJECTIVE INFORMATION

The patient is 13 years old. He is unable to return to school because of continued cognitive deficits from TBI on 7/9/10, after which he received rehabilitation therapy in the inpatient rehabilitation unit and then home health. He states that he thinks he could handle school, but his parents will not let him go back unless he attends a "special" class, which he does not want to do. Instead, he plans to have a tutor at home and maybe start in the second quarter. The grandmother is living with the family to assist with everything, but she states she will need to return home soon; where she lives out of state with her husband who continues to work. Also, the house is pretty crowded.

OBJECTIVE INFORMATION

COGNITION, COMMUNICATION, AND VISION

Rancho levels VI and VII; communicates in short sentences, alert and oriented but has little memory of TBI and circumstances. Poor judgment affecting safety during ambulation. Continues to have safety risks because of right hemianopsia.

POSTURE

Leans mildly to the left in standing with right knee hyperextended but can correct to midline and unlock knee with mirror and tactile facilitation. Sits unsupported in midline.

GAIT

Scissor-like gait 40 feet with FWW and right AFO, supervised with tactile and verbal cues to maintain control of right knee; decreased stance time on right; mild ataxia improved with two 5-pound weights added to base of FWW. Up and down 2 steps with Min. A and 2 rails using step-to pattern and RLE down first, LLE up first.

continued

Outpatient Physical Therapy Evaluation *continued*

BALANCE	BERG 38/56; high risk for falls		help from a tutor daily and working at home, hoping to keep up with his classmates. His mother states he will likely fall behind and need additional tutoring through the year in the hope that he can catch up by next year.
STRENGTH	Takes moderate resistance RLE, except hip abductors take minimal resistance and ankle dorsiflexors minimal resistance with gravity eliminated, all without increased tone RLE; 4+/5 LLE; moderate resistance RUE; 3+ to 4–/5 LUE.	STG (2 weeks)	1. Increase BLE strength of all muscle groups without increasing tone and PROM WNL to improve ambulation on a variety of surfaces, including stairs. 2. Increase right ankle passive dorsiflexion to 10 degrees to improve gait quality. 3. Decrease gait deviations of right knee hyperextension, scissoring, and ataxia to improve gait speed and quality; and ambulate 75 feet with FWW independently and up and down 12 steps with 1 rail per home situation with supervision. 4. Increase BERG balance test score to 45/56 to improve safety during ambulation.
PROM	WFL except right ankle plantarflexion 60 degrees and dorsiflexion 5 degrees; bilateral hip abduction to 10 degrees with increased tone in right greater than left adductors		
WHEELCHAIR MOBILITY	Mod. I indoors and outdoors on grass and slight inclines and ramp for total distance over 500 feet; supervised for community and crosswalks because of cognitive deficits and decreased safety awareness.		
TONE	2+ in hip adductors and ankle plantarflexors RLE	LTG	Independent ambulation indoors x 100 feet with or without an assistive device. Up and down 12 steps with 1 rail independently. Independent with home exercise program. Supervision only because of cognitive deficits, not physical deficits. Patient able to use tone inhibition techniques to normalize tone during functional activities and exercise program.
SENSATION	Impaired proprioception right foot and great toe; otherwise intact light touch and proprioception BLE and BUE		
FUNCTIONAL MOBILITY ASSESSMENT	Bed mobility Mod. I Transfers low pivot supervised Floor transfers Min. A		
HOME SAFETY ASSESSMENT	Family has a temporary ramp placed at the front entrance. Doors and halls all accommodate W/C. The bathroom is accessible, and the patient sits for showers. He has an FWW for gait training and hopes to be out of the W/C by the time school starts. He sleeps in a twin-sized bed.	PLAN	The plan includes soft tissue and joint mobilization and an exercise program 3 times per week, then reducing to 1 to 2 times per week for up to 12 weeks with focus on return to independent ambulation without an assistive device, if able. The exercise program is to incorporate cardiovascular, strengthening, balance, core stability, flexibility, and proprioceptive exercises using free weights, exercise tubing, PNF techniques, bicycle, and balance equipment such as a therapy ball to enhance balance reactions. It will also incorporate *Wii* and other games to improve participation and overall success. Plan is to teach tone modification techniques for patient to use during exercises and functional mobility tasks. This will be coordinated with the SLP, who is working with him as an outpatient on speech and cognitive deficits, to coordinate care.
FAMILY'S ABILITY TO ASSIST	The mother, stepfather, and grandmother provide assistance with transfers. They need hands-on assistance with gait in order to avoid deviations and promote quality movement patterns. They also need cues to help maintain quality of movement patterns with a home exercise program given by a home health therapist. The patient's 9-year-old brother helps supervise him and plays with him.		
ASSESSMENT	The patient is S/P TBI with residual cognitive deficits as well as impaired mobility. Specifically, he cannot walk independently because of tone abnormalities, muscle weakness, impaired proprioception, and decreased ROM. He also has poor safety awareness. He is working with a school counselor on a plan to return to school but for now is getting		

OUTPATIENT CRITICAL THINKING QUESTIONS

After reviewing the outpatient physical therapy evaluation, address the following:

1. What are the patient's impairments? Functional limitations? Is there a disability?

2. Find assessments of gait, strength, ROM, and balance if available from the initial evaluation and list.

   a. How could each potentially be used to assess function and demonstrate progress toward goals or show the patient's response to physical therapy interventions?

   b. What would be the most important items to document for this patient?

3. After reviewing the POC, describe a possible next treatment session.

   a. List the activities/exercises and your rationale for the order of treatment activities that you selected.

4. What subjective information will you gather during your session to help in your treatment of this patient and why?

5. What tests or measures will you use to assess the patient's progress and response to treatment?

6. What subjective or objective information that you gather during the treatment might cause you to alter your treatment for this patient and why?

7. How would you document your treatment in the SOAP or Patient/Client Management format?

8. If the treatment goes as expected, what will you do for the next treatment?

9. How would you expect this patient to progress over time?

10. If the patient does not progress as expected, what might be some reasons for a lack of progress?

11. What signs or symptoms, if observed or reported by the patient, would cause you to hold treatment and check with the nursing staff, primary PT, or MD?

12. Are there any cultural, socioeconomic, or ethical issues presented in this case that might affect your interventions or communication with this patient? If so, how?

13. Re-review this case. Are there any coexisting medical diagnoses that might affect how this patient responds to physical therapy? If so, what are they, and how might they cause the patient to respond to physical therapy differently than you expected?

continued

OUTPATIENT CRITICAL THINKING QUESTIONS *continued*

14. After reviewing the other disciplines' notes regarding this patient, is there any other information that will help you to plan your treatment sessions?

_____

_____

15. Compare your responses on this case with those of your classmates or instructors. What, if anything, would you change and why?

_____

_____

CONTINUUM OF CARE CRITICAL THINKING QUESTIONS

After reviewing the continuum of care for this patient, consider the following:

1. How did the patient's problems change over the weeks after his surgery?

_____

_____

_____

_____

_____

2. How did this affect the goals and the interventions that the PT included in the POC?

_____

_____

_____

_____

_____

3. How were the same interventions modified over time to progress the patient according to his changing needs?

_____

_____

_____

_____

_____

4. What are some potential community resources that this patient might like to participate in and how would these help him to maintain and improve his physical fitness?

_____

_____

_____

_____

IMPLICATIONS OF PATHOLOGY FOR THE PTA[2]

1. What signs or symptoms might alert the PTA that there may be problems with the cranial nerves in a patient with TBI?

_____

_____

_____

_____

_____

2. What are at least two reasons the head of the bed should be elevated approximately 30 degrees for a patient with TBI in the ICU?

_____

_____

_____

_____

_____

IMPLICATIONS OF PATHOLOGY FOR THE PTA[2]

3. How can the PTA work with the medical team to assist with pulmonary management and problems with respiration, swallowing, and potential skin breakdown during the physical therapy intervention sessions with a TBI patient?

_____

_____

_____

_____

_____

4. What should the PTA be aware of when working with patients with mild concussion?

_____

_____

_____

_____

_____

_____

_____

References

1. American Physical Therapy Association: Guide to Physical Therapist Practice, Second Edition. Alexandria, VA: Author, 2001.

2. Goodman CC, Boissonnault FG, Fuller KS: Pathology: Implications for the Physical Therapist, Second Edition. Philadelphia: Saunders, 2003.

CHAPTER 10

Amy Parker: A Patient With Spinal Cord Injury

Preferred Practice Pattern: Neuromuscular, Pattern H

CHAPTER OUTLINE

Introducing Amy Parker

Amy Parker is a 16-year-old girl who suffered a spinal cord injury due to a fracture at the T9 level. According to the APTA's *Guide to Physical Therapist Practice* (the *Guide*), she could have the following impairments:

- Decreased aerobic capacity
- Impaired ventilation
- Impaired motor function

Functional limitations may include the following:

- Difficulty with accessing community
- Difficulty performing ADLs
- Inability to perform work

Please refer to the *Guide*[1] for a complete list of possible impairments and functional limitations. As you work through this case, think about which of these the patient is experiencing.

Vocabulary List

Normocephalic	Auscultation
Lymphadenopathy	Hepatosplenomegaly
Thyromegaly	Roho cushion

PHYSICIAN'S HISTORY AND PHYSICAL

PATIENT NAME: Amy L. Parker

ADMIT DATE: September 13, 2010

BIRTH DATE: February 8, 1994

SEX: Female

ROOM/BED: 339-01

MEDICAL RECORD #: 12345678

CHIEF COMPLAINT: Numbness and weakness of legs

ATTENDING: Dr. Melvin Peterson, MD

HISTORY OF PRESENT ILLNESS: This 16-year-old female was riding her mountain bike down a steep trail and crashed into a tree. She was wearing a helmet. She did not lose consciousness and does not appear to have any broken bones; however, she could not and still cannot feel her legs or move them. It took emergency services 2 hours to get to her, and then she was transported on a spinal board to the emergency room via helicopter. At this time her vital signs have stabilized, and she is alert and oriented with her father present.

PAST MEDICAL HISTORY: ADHD

Seizure disorder

PAST SURGICAL HISTORY: None

ALLERGIES: Dairy, wheat

MEDICATIONS: Dilantin 300 mg daily
Straterra 40 mg daily

FAMILY HISTORY: Mother died last year of brain cancer; father has depression.

SOCIAL HISTORY: The patient has lived with her father and two brothers since her mother died last year. Her parents were divorced, and the mother had had custody of the three children until her mother's illness prevented her from caring for them. The patient reports that her father drinks too much and is aggressive when he drinks, which is why her parents divorced.

REVIEW OF SYSTEMS: See HPI

PHYSICAL EXAMINATION:

VITAL SIGNS: Temperature 36.2°C, pulse 84 BPM, respiratory rate 21 respirations per minute, blood pressure 110/62 mm Hg, O_2 saturation 98% on 2 LPM.

GENERAL: Alert and oriented, worried about outcome

SKIN: Pale; abrasions on arms, legs, face

HEENT: **Normocephalic.** Pupils equal and reactive. Able to track visually. Oropharynx unremarkable; able to manage secretions.

NECK: Supple without obvious **lymphadenopathy** or **thyromegaly.** Axillary region without obvious lymphadenopathy.

CARDIAC: Unremarkable

LUNGS: Clear to **auscultation**

ABDOMEN: Bowel sounds present, nontender, nondistended. No **hepatosplenomegaly.**

EXTREMITIES: 2+ peripheral pulses, no edema present.

NEUROLOGICAL: Flaccid bilateral lower extremities. Absent bilateral lower extremity reflexes. Absent light-touch and sharp/dull sensation from T9 level down, including S4 to S5. Cranial nerves intact.

LABORATORY DATA: Dilantin level: 11

IMAGING STUDIES: Complete spine series showing comminuted vertebral fracture at T9 level.

ASSESSMENT: T9 ASIA A SCI due to vertebral fracture from fall

PLAN: The plan is to admit the patient to an ICU with neurosurgical consult and MRI of thoracic spine. Methylprednisolone will be started at 1380 mg, followed by infusion of 2484 mg per hour for next 23 hours. Physiatry, physical therapy, occupational therapy, and social work consults will be required.

Medical Update

09/14/2010

Spinal decompression and fusion at T9 were applied on 9/13/10 and are being used now with a TLSO with spinal precautions to avoid rotation. A spinal anesthetic is being used with Versed. Medications include continued Straterra and Dilantin; added Tylenol PRN for neck pain and headaches; and tapering steroids. Follow-up radiographs show hardware in place and T9 stable.

SEEING THE DIAGNOSIS IN ACTION 10-1

A patient with a spinal cord injury must cope with not only the physical effects of the injury but also the emotional aspects of the loss. Spinal cord injuries can be either complete or incomplete, and depending on the level of injury, they can leave a patient without the use of his or her legs or all four extremities. Typically, patients are dependent on a wheelchair for the remainder of their lives but can lead productive lives after a lengthy rehabilitation process.

continued

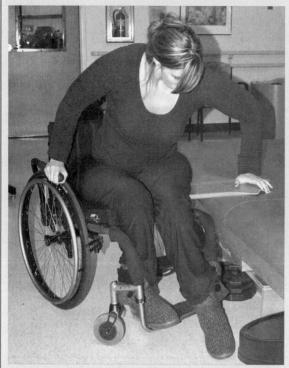

Figure 10-1 In the beginning of the rehabilitation process, patients are often instructed in slide board transfers. Later, they may be able to transfer without the use of a slide board in most situations, using it only for car or toilet transfers as needed.

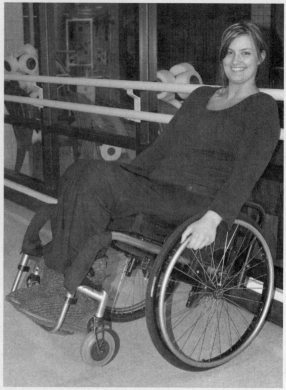

Figure 10-3 Learning to perform wheelies is not only fun but also an important skill to allow patients to negotiate a curb if needed.

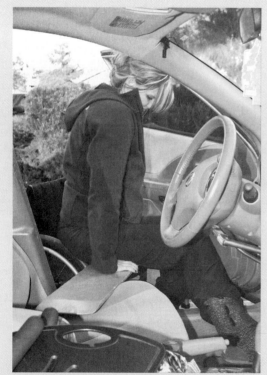

Figure 10-2 Car transfer training is an important part of the training involved in helping a patient reach her full potential. This patient with a thoracic-level injury is now able to drive a car that is modified for her use.

REVIEWING THE MEDICAL HISTORY

1. What do you already know about spinal cord injuries?

_____

_____

_____

_____

2. Review the vocabulary list and physician's notes. Look up the meanings of any terms you don't understand in a medical dictionary or other text.

_____

_____

_____

_____

3. Review the diagnoses in the past medical history using a medical or pathology text, Internet resource, or other available resource.

_____

_____

_____

_____

_____

4. Which diagnoses in the past medical history would be significant and potentially affect the patient's response to the physical therapy interventions?

_____

_____

_____

_____

5. List the purpose and potential side effects for each of the medications the patient is taking.

_____

_____

_____

_____

6. Describe what each laboratory result measures and list considerations for physical therapy if the results for this patient were *not* in the normal range.

_____

_____

_____

_____

_____

BOX 10-1 | Physical Therapy Specialty: Neurology

The physical therapy specialty of neurology focuses on patients with a wide variety of neurological diseases or injuries. Some therapists specialize in one type of neurological problem such as stroke, TBI, or SCI. Others provide services to "neuro" patients in general. Traditionally, and still to some extent, therapists viewed themselves as either "neuro" therapists or "ortho" therapists. Although there are distinct differences between patients with primary dysfunction in one or the other of these broad systems, it is still important to remember that people have both kinds of structures—neurological and musculoskeletal—and that their problems may overlap. For example, patients with TBI may often develop musculoskeletal problems such as shortened or weak muscles and need treatment interventions that are more traditionally used in an orthopedic setting. As in all areas of physical therapy, the PTA should remember that he or she is working with an individual, not a primary diagnosis. For more information on the neurology specialty, see the APTA's Neurology Section website at: http://www.neuropt.org.

Acute Care Physical Therapy Initial Evaluation

Patient History

NAME	Amy Parker	SURGERY	Spinal fusion at T9
ROOM # & BED	B339-01	SURGERY DATE	09/13/2010
MEDICAL RECORD #	12345678	PRECAUTIONS	Spinal, using TLSO at all times Ace wraps and abdominal binder also when up
ATTENDING PHYSICIAN	Dr. Peterson		
CHIEF COMPLAINT	Spinal cord injury		
AGE	16	WEIGHT-BEARING STATUS	WBAT
DATE OF BIRTH	02/08/1994		
SEX	Female	LIVING SITUATION	Home
PRIMARY LANGUAGE	English	PRIOR LEVEL OF FUNCTION	Independent at home and school
ISOLATION	No		
HEIGHT (CM)	163	ASSISTANCE AVAILABLE	Father works full-time in construction; mother deceased. Grandparents unable to assist.
WEIGHT (KG)	54		
MEDICATION ALLERGIES	NKDA		
FOOD ALLERGIES	Dairy, wheat	STAIRS TO ENTER HOME	6
INITIATED BY	Donna Smith, PT	RAIL(S) ON STAIRS	None
DATE	09/15/2010	ASSISTIVE DEVICE USED PRIOR	None
TIME	9:15		
TREATING DIAGNOSIS	Decreased mobility S/P SCI	EQUIPMENT PATIENT HAS	None
ONSET DATE	09/13/2010		
PERTINENT MEDICAL HISTORY	Per H & P: ADHD, seizure disorder	DRIVING PRIOR TO ADMIT	Learner's permit
		OCCUPATION/LIFE ROLE	Just started 11th grade in high school; is a cheerleader

Systems Review

HEARING	WNL	ACTIVITY RESPIRATORY RATE (respirations per minute)	21
VISION	WNL		
SPEECH	WNL		
PAIN SCALE	VPS	ACTIVITY BLOOD PRESSURE (mm Hg)	122/68
PAIN LEVEL	4		
PAIN LOCATION	Neck	ACTIVITY SpO$_2$	99% on 2 LPM
PAIN TYPE	Sore, achy muscles	POSTACTIVITY HEART RATE (BPM)	75
PAIN INTERVENTION	Reported to RN, recommended ice pack		
RESTING HEART RATE (BPM)	72	POSTACTIVITY RESPIRATORY RATE (respirations per minute)	19
RESTING RESPIRATORY RATE (respirations per minute)	18		
		POSTACTIVITY BLOOD PRESSURE (mm Hg)	118/64
RESTING BLOOD PRESSURE (mm Hg)	112/66	POSTACTIVITY SpO$_2$	99% on 2 LPM
RESTING SpO$_2$	99% on 2 LPM	LEVEL OF CONSCIOUSNESS	Alert
ACTIVITY HEART RATE (BPM)	79	ORIENTATION	x 4
		SHORT-TERM MEMORY	Intact

Tests and Measures

ROM NECK/TRUNK	AROM WNL	SIT TO STAND/STAND TO SIT	Unable
ROM BUE	AROM WNL	TRANSFERS	Tot. A with mechanical lift
ROM BLE	PROM WNL except bilateral straight-leg raises to 55 degrees	SITTING BALANCE	Poor
BUE STRENGTH	WNL	STANDING BALANCE	Unable
BLE STRENGTH	Flaccid	GAIT	Unable
SENSATION	Intact above T9 and absent below for light touch and pinprick	STAIRS	Unable
		WHEELCHAIR MOBILITY	Min. A using BUE; fit in recliner W/C to enable her to adjust gradually to upright position
SKIN INTEGRITY	Redness bilateral heels and sacrum		
BED MOBILITY	Tot. A		
SUPINE TO SIT/SIT TO SUPINE	Tot. A	SITTING TOLERANCE	5 seconds edge of bed, then lightheaded and needed to lie down

Evaluation

DIAGNOSIS	Neuromuscular, pattern H
PROGNOSIS	Good. The patient is a 16-year-old high school cheerleader diagnosed with a T9 ASIA A SCI S/P fusion. She has absent light-touch and pinprick sensation below T9 and does not have any voluntary motor control below that level. BLE are flaccid without signs of spasticity. She has decreased hamstring ROM and has not been able to tolerate upright position because of low blood pressure and complaints of dizziness. Her heels are red, and she is at risk for developing pressure ulcers. She states she will walk again and wants to get back to school and her friends as soon as possible. She worries about her two younger brothers at home with their father who drinks too much and

can become aggressive. She states that she usually tries to be the go-between. When asked whether he hits the kids, she said not really but he pushes them around. Overall, she is motivated. She will need ongoing education about her diagnosis and prognosis. Education for the patient, nursing staff, and family will include potential complications, pressure relief and prevention of pressure ulcers, need for ROM, and increasing upright tolerance. Note was posted for staff to keep the patient's heels floated while in bed. She is a good candidate for and will benefit from D/C to inpatient rehabilitation before D/C home for further intensive rehabilitation to facilitate return to highest possible function.

Plan of Care

PATIENT'S GOALS	Walk again, return to high school ASAP		Wheelchair mobility training
DISCHARGE GOALS	1. Bed mobility and transfers: Mod. A		Home program
	2. Wheelchair mobility: independent indoors x 200 feet		Therapeutic exercise
			Therapeutic activities
	3. Sitting tolerance: 1 hour in wheelchair three times daily		Family training
	4. Home exercise program: independent with upper extremity exercises; PROM by family if able to assist	FREQUENCY	BID
		PATIENT EDUCATION TOPIC(S)	Activity: log roll for rolling, use of brace
TIME TO ACHIEVE GOALS	By time of discharge	TAUGHT BY	PT
PATIENT/FAMILY UNDERSTAND/AGREES WITH GOALS	Family yes	WHO WAS TAUGHT	Patient
		METHOD OF INSTRUCTION	Verbal/demonstration
INTERVENTIONS	Bed mobility training	EVALUATION OF LEARNING	Needs reinforcement
	Transfer training		
	Balance training		

Acute Care Nursing Note

09/16/2010   9:30 AM

The patient is alert but tires easily. She is unable to raise her head out of bed because of lightheadedness and refuses to attempt gradual raising of the head. BP drops from 110/65 to 85/50 mm Hg with reclined position and head of bed up to 45 degrees. She was up in her W/C yesterday with the PT for a few minutes and described an "awful headache" afterward. She is using call light regularly and has many needs. One friend and a teacher from high school have visited her. The father came in to visit after work with the two sons. Foley is draining dark amber urine. Log roll is being used for position changes, and a schedule is posted for changing positions every 2 hours. The patient states that she "wishes she was dead" but has made no suicide attempts. MD has been consulted about referral to a psychiatrist for depression and suicidal thoughts. Suction is being used to clear her airway; a respiratory therapist has been in to assist with care.

BOX 10-2 | Health-Care Team Member Role: Respiratory Therapist

The respiratory therapist works closely with physicians, nurses, and other health-care providers, including PTs and PTAs, especially in the acute care setting. They evaluate and treat patients with a wide variety of both acute and chronic respiratory problems. They are also involved in the outpatient setting, typically working with patients/clients who have chronic lung conditions and hope to improve their lung function. Respiratory therapists are able to provide valuable information to the PT or PTA when decisions about use of supplemental oxygen must be made. PTs and PTAs also provide valuable information regarding oxygen saturation and other vital signs in response to activity during physical therapy sessions so that respiratory therapists can make the appropriate recommendation to the physician regarding need for oxygen or other medical treatments in the hospital and also after discharge. For more information, see the American Association for Respiratory Care website at http://www.aarc.org.

Acute Care Social Work Note

09/16/2010   4:43 PM

Discussed with the patient her accident and family situation. She states that she is still very sad about her mother's death a year ago. She and her two brothers had been living with their mother after their parents divorced 4 years ago. She states that her father drinks too much and pushes the kids around. She also reports past sexual abuse by her father before the divorce. When the mother's illness prevented her from caring for the children, they went back to the father. No charges were ever filed. She worries about her brothers because she is not there now to protect them. She does not have many friends because she is in a new high school since moving back with her father. Now, with the recent injury to her spine, she is unsure of what the outcome will be. She admits to suicidal thoughts at times but does not have a plan to carry it out. A psychiatry consult is pending. CPS report has been made because of the patient's report of her home situation.

Acute Care Occupational Therapy Summary

09/16/2010   3:21 PM

The patient's vertigo and lightheadedness related to sitting upright interfere greatly with functional seated ADL tasks. The patient is currently on a Foley catheter and is incontinent of bowel. The OT is to work in conjunction with the PT toward upright sitting ADL tasks. The patient's upper extremity strength is WFL, and she has good gross and fine motor coordination as well as intact cognition. These should allow her to be independent with most or all ADLs once sitting tolerance and functional mobility skills are developed. Discharge to a rehabilitation unit is anticipated. Occupational therapy goals include the following:

1. The patient will tolerate sitting upright in a wheelchair for three meals per day.
2. The patient will sit at the edge of the bed with one arm propping herself for 2 minutes with Mod. A during minimally assisted grooming and upper body dressing.
3. The patient will dry-run transfer between wheelchair and bench commode via slide board with Mod. A.

Patients with spinal cord injuries may need ongoing support and further therapies as their needs change, as they age, and with new life responsibilities. They must constantly adapt their environment in order to be as independent as possible. Some patients with higher-level injuries will need ongoing assistance either part-time or full-time from family members or other caregivers.

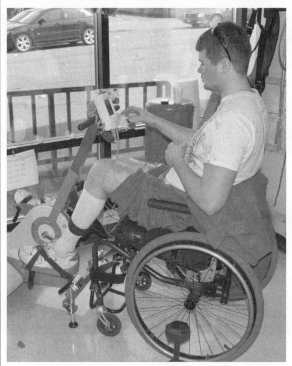

Figure 10-4 Newer interventions for spinal cord injury include the use of functional electrical stimulation.

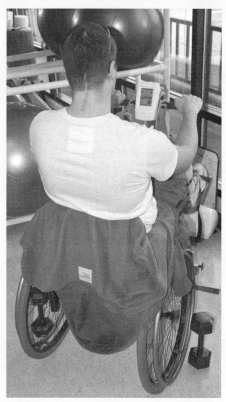

Figure 10-5 In these photos, a patient with spinal cord injury performs exercise on a bike using functional electrical stimulation.

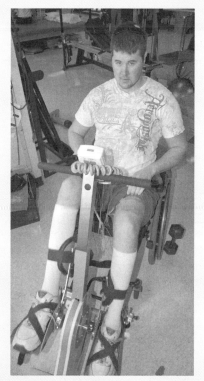

Figure 10-6 The electrical stimulation causes the muscles to contract, moving the pedals on the bike, and helps to maintain a level of muscular fitness when traditional exercise is impossible.

ACUTE CARE CRITICAL THINKING QUESTIONS

After reviewing the acute care physical therapy initial evaluation and other discipline notes, address the following:

1. What are the patient's impairments? Functional limitations? Is there a disability?

_____

_____

2. Find assessments of gait, strength, ROM, and balance if available from the initial evaluation and list.

   a. How could each potentially be used to assess function and demonstrate progress toward goals or show the patient's response to physical therapy interventions?

   _____

   _____

   _____

   b. What would be the most important items to document for this patient?

   _____

   _____

   _____

3. After reviewing the POC, describe a possible next treatment session.

   a. List the activities/exercises and your rationale for the order of treatment activities that you selected.

   _____

   _____

   _____

4. What subjective information will you gather during your session to help in your treatment of this patient and why?

   _____

   _____

5. What tests or measures will you use to assess the patient's progress and response to treatment?

   _____

   _____

6. What subjective or objective information that you gather during the treatment might cause you to alter your treatment for this patient and why?

_____

_____

7. How would you document your treatment in the SOAP or Patient/Client Management format?

_____

_____

_____

_____

8. If the treatment goes as expected, what will you do for the next treatment?

_____

_____

9. How would you expect this patient to progress over time?

_____

_____

_____

10. If the patient does not progress as expected, what might be some reasons for a lack of progress?

_____

_____

11. What signs or symptoms, if observed or reported by the patient, would cause you to hold treatment and check with the nursing staff, primary PT, or MD?

_____

_____

_____

12. Are there any cultural, socioeconomic, or ethical issues presented in this case that might affect your interventions or communication with this patient? If so, how?

_____

_____

13. Re-review this case. Are there any coexisting medical diagnoses that might affect how this patient responds to physical therapy? If so, what are they, and how might they cause the patient to respond to physical therapy differently than you expected?

_____

_____

_____

_____

_____

14. After reviewing the other disciplines' notes regarding this patient, is there any other information that will help you to plan your treatment sessions?

_____

_____

15. Compare your responses on this case with those of your classmates or instructors. What, if anything, would you change and why?

_____

_____

_____

_____

Medical Update _____

_09/22/2010_

Upon discharge from the acute setting on 9/22/10, the patient is S/P T9 fracture, decompression with fusion, and resulting lower extremity paralysis. She is being discharged to inpatient rehabilitation. She is seeing a psychiatrist for depression and suicidal thoughts. She is continuing Strattera and Dilantin as before injury. She is continuing Tylenol PRN for headaches and neck pain. Lexapro 5 mg daily has been added for depression. The plan is to follow up with the surgeon in 1 week and the psychiatrist in the rehabilitation setting. The MSW and psychiatrist are to monitor the home situation and continue assessment regarding the safety of the younger siblings, with possible referral to CPS.

Inpatient Rehabilitation Physical Therapy Evaluation
Patient History

NAME	Amy Parker	TREATING DIAGNOSIS	Decreased mobility S/P SCI
ROOM # & BED	B310-02	ONSET DATE	09/13/2010
MEDICAL RECORD #	12345678	PERTINENT MEDICAL HISTORY	Per H & P: ADHD, seizure disorder
ATTENDING PHYSICIAN	Dr. Gordon, MD		
CHIEF COMPLAINT	Spinal cord injury	SURGERY	Spinal fusion at T9
AGE	16	SURGERY DATE	09/13/2010
DATE OF BIRTH	02/08/1994	PRECAUTIONS	Spinal, using orthosis at all times
SEX	Female	WEIGHT-BEARING STATUS	WBAT
PRIMARY LANGUAGE	English	LIVING SITUATION	Home with father and two younger brothers
ISOLATION	No		
HEIGHT (CM)	163		
WEIGHT (KG)	55	PRIOR LEVEL OF FUNCTION	Independent at home and school
MEDICATION ALLERGIES	NKDA	ASSISTANCE AVAILABLE	Father works full-time in construction; mother deceased. Grandparents unable to assist.
FOOD ALLERGIES	Dairy, wheat		
INITIATED BY	Roger Lee, PT		
DATE	09/23/2010	STAIRS TO ENTER HOME	6
TIME	11:35	RAIL(S) ON STAIRS	None

continued

Inpatient Rehabilitation Physical Therapy Evaluation *continued*

Patient History

ASSISTIVE DEVICE USED PRIOR	None	DRIVING PRIOR TO ADMIT	Learner's permit
EQUIPMENT PATIENT HAS	None	OCCUPATION/LIFE ROLE	Just started 11th grade in high school; is a cheerleader

Systems Review

HEARING	WNL	ACTIVITY RESPIRATORY RATE (respirations per minute)	22
VISION	WNL		
SPEECH	WNL		
PAIN SCALE	VPS	ACTIVITY BLOOD PRESSURE (mm Hg)	90/56
PAIN LEVEL	2	ACTIVITY SpO_2	99% on room air
PAIN LOCATION	Neck	POSTACTIVITY HEART RATE (BPM)	78
PAIN TYPE	Sore, achy muscles		
PAIN INTERVENTION	Notified RN	POSTACTIVITY RESPIRATORY RATE (respirations per minute)	19
RESTING HEART RATE (BPM)	70		
RESTING RESPIRATORY RATE (respirations per minute)	18	POSTACTIVITY BLOOD PRESSURE (mm Hg)	106/60
		POSTACTIVITY SpO_2	99% on room air
RESTING BLOOD PRESSURE (mm Hg)	110/62	LEVEL OF CONSCIOUSNESS	Alert
RESTING SpO_2	99% on room air	ORIENTATION	x 4
ACTIVITY HEART RATE (BPM)	82	SHORT-TERM MEMORY	Intact

Tests and Measures

ROM NECK/TRUNK	AROM WNL	SIT TO STAND/STAND TO SIT	Unable
ROM BUE	AROM WNL		
ROM BLE	PROM WNL	TRANSFERS	Mod. A using slide board
BUE STRENGTH	WNL	SITTING BALANCE	Poor
BLE STRENGTH	Flaccid	STANDING BALANCE	Unable
SENSATION	Intact above T9 and absent below for light touch and pinprick	GAIT	Unable
		STAIRS	Unable
SKIN INTEGRITY	Redness bilateral heels and sacrum	WHEELCHAIR MOBILITY	Supervised using BUE in W/C reclined at 45 degrees
PRESSURE RELEASES	Able to perform pressure releases in chair with moderate assist	SITTING TOLERANCE	1 hour in wheelchair reclined at 45 degrees
BED MOBILITY	Mod. A using log roll		
SUPINE TO SIT/SIT TO SUPINE	Mod. A		

Evaluation

DIAGNOSIS	Neuromuscular, pattern H		to be independent as much as possible. Her father is not present during evaluation and does not answer the phone calls of the PT. The patient will benefit from skilled physical therapy to address functional mobility to achieve independence from a W/C level. She will need a custom W/C assessment and other DME as determined throughout rehabilitation. She will attempt to reach the goal of independent W/C mobility and transfers before D/C in preparation for outpatient therapy to continue. Home health may not be an option, depending on her living situation. MSW is consulting with the patient regarding options and potential assistance available.
PROGNOSIS	Good. The patient is motivated, although she appears to be lacking in family support. She is a 16-year-old high school cheerleader who suffered a complete traumatic spinal cord injury from a mountain biking accident during which she was wearing a helmet. She was diagnosed with T9 ASIA A SCI S/P fusion. She has improved sitting tolerance, although still must be reclined to 45 degrees. Thus far in her recovery, she has not developed any pressure ulcers but continues to have intermittent redness on her sacrum and bilateral heels. She states that she hopes that she can live with a friend after hospitalization and will need		

Plan of Care

PATIENT'S GOALS	States she would like to walk again	TIME TO ACHIEVE GOALS	By time of discharge
DISCHARGE GOALS	1. Bed mobility and transfers: Mod. I	PATIENT/FAMILY UNDERSTAND/AGREES WITH GOALS	Patient yes
	2. Wheelchair mobility: independent indoors and outdoors x 1000 feet, including community settings and in crosswalks	INTERVENTIONS	Bed mobility training Transfer training Balance training Wheelchair mobility training Home program Therapeutic exercise Therapeutic activities Family training
	3. Sitting tolerance: 4 hours 3 times per day		
	4. Patient will be able to perform adequate pressure releases in chair to prevent pressure ulcers.		
	5. Home exercise program: independent with upper extremity exercises; assist with BLE exercises but unclear who will provide assist	FREQUENCY	BID

Inpatient Rehabilitation Nursing Note

09/25/2010   11:19 AM

The patient complains of pain in her neck at 3/10 and legs with any movement at 7/10. She has spasms at night in her legs. Tylenol has been given to her with good relief. She was offered an ice pack for her neck but declined. She is eating about 50% of her meals and drinking water, juice, and soda. Her urine output is good. She needs a suppository in the AM for bowel movements. Her stool is formed.

Inpatient Rehabilitation Social Work Summary

09/27/2010   9:34 AM

A team conference was held today. The patient's father was present and yelled at staff when asked questions about the home environment. He left after the MD report. The MD reports that the patient's vital signs and laboratory results look good, but he is concerned about the patient's living situation and depression. The MD encourages the patient to work with a rehabilitation psychologist and the rest of team to have the best possible outcome. The RN reports that the patient is beginning a bowel program and is appropriately using her call light. No concerns were brought up. The PT reports addressing bed mobility and transfers, which are limited somewhat by patient's inability to achieve an upright position. Currently, the patient can tolerate the head of the bed up to about 30 degrees. Pain and spasms with PROM of BLE are another limitation. The OT reports the same limitations. When the patient is able to sit upright, she can be more functional and independent with dressing and grooming. The team will begin to address these skills even in the reclined position. The rehabilitation psychologist reports that, based on yesterday's assessment, the patient will be starting new medication for depression. This will not take effect for a few days to weeks, and he encouraged the patient to talk to staff and any others who are available for counseling. A definite challenge is the lack of social and emotional support in the life of this patient. It was discussed that the hospital will be contacting CPS regarding the younger siblings as well as the patient. The situation is serious because the patient at this time does not have an adequate living situation for D/C, which is planned for approximately 10/28/10.

BOX 10-3 | Health-Care Team Member Role: Rehabilitation Psychologist

The rehabilitation psychologist typically works in an acute rehabilitation hospital or unit and also sees patients in the outpatient setting. He or she typically evaluates patients in the inpatient setting who are especially at risk for developing mood disorders such as depression or anxiety or otherwise need help coping emotionally with the great changes in life due to the accident or disease process. Psychologists work closely with the other team members to help the patient and family cope with the changes. As the patient progresses through the rehabilitation process, his or her needs for emotional support will change. The psychologist or counselor will often continue to see the patient as an outpatient until he or she can cope well enough to either be discharged from this service or be able to follow with a school or work counselor and thus integrate into the community network of resources. The counselor or psychologist may also be involved in developing a plan for the patient to return to school or work activities, perhaps assisting the patient in pursuing alternate work if he or she cannot return to the prior work setting. For more information on rehabilitation psychology, see the American Psychological Association website for rehabilitation psychology at http://www.apa.org/about/division/div22.aspx.

Inpatient Rehabilitation Occupational Therapy Summary

09/24/2010   9:45 AM

The patient is alert, oriented, aware of the situation, and voicing feelings of depression exacerbated by poor sitting tolerance. BLE spasm and vertigo still interfere with sitting. At this point, the patient is most capable and focused on tasks when in a semi-reclined position. Occupational therapy is planned to work toward supine and then upright seated ADL tasks to provide opportunities for independence and improved sense of self. Her prognosis is good once upright sitting tolerance is achieved. Poor social support affects discharge planning. She may need continued occupational therapy as an outpatient once discharged to address any residual deficits in dressing, bathing, and home environment modifications.

Discharge Goals for Occupational Therapy

1. The patient will improve sitting balance to SBA to be able to dress her upper body on the edge of the bed at Mod. I level.
2. The patient will dress her lower body from bed with SBA.
3. The patient will transfer via slide board to commode independently for toileting or bathing. She will successfully lift her hips off the seat with SBA while receiving full assist for clothing management and hygiene.
4. The patient will bathe at the commode bench with SBA overall using long-handled sponge and shower hose.
5. The patient will independently direct caregivers in safely managing her functional mobility and ADLs, including bowel and Foley care.

INPATIENT REHABILITATION CRITICAL THINKING QUESTIONS

After reviewing the inpatient rehabilitation physical therapy initial evaluation and other discipline notes, address the following:

1. What are the patient's impairments? Functional limitations? Is there a disability?

_____

_____

2. Find assessments of gait, strength, ROM, and balance if available from the initial evaluation and list.

   a. How could each potentially be used to assess function and demonstrate progress toward goals or show the patient's response to physical therapy interventions?

   _____

   _____

   _____

   b. What would be the most important items to document for this patient?

   _____

   _____

   _____

3. After reviewing the POC, describe a possible next treatment session.

   a. List the activities/exercises and your rationale for the order of treatment activities that you selected.

   _____

   _____

   _____

4. What subjective information will you gather during your session to help in your treatment of this patient and why?

   _____

   _____

5. What tests or measures will you use to assess the patient's progress and response to treatment?

   _____

   _____

   _____

6. What subjective or objective information that you gather during the treatment might cause you to alter your treatment for this patient and why?

   _____

   _____

7. How would you document your treatment in the SOAP or Patient/Client Management format?

   _____

   _____

   _____

   _____

8. If the treatment goes as expected, what will you do for the next treatment?

   _____

   _____

9. How would you expect this patient to progress over time?

   _____

   _____

10. If the patient does not progress as expected, what might be some reasons for a lack of progress?

   _____

   _____

11. What signs or symptoms, if observed or reported by the patient, would cause you to hold treatment and check with the nursing staff, primary PT, or MD?

   _____

   _____

   _____

12. Are there any cultural, socioeconomic, or ethical issues presented in this case that might affect your interventions or communication with this patient? If so, how?

   _____

   _____

   _____

continued

INPATIENT REHABILITATION CRITICAL THINKING QUESTIONS *continued*

13. Re-review this case. Are there any coexisting medical diagnoses that might affect how this patient responds to physical therapy? If so, what are they, and how might they cause the patient to respond to physical therapy differently than you expected?

_____

_____

_____

_____

_____

14. After reviewing the other disciplines' notes regarding this patient, is there any other information that will help you to plan your treatment sessions?

_____

_____

15. Compare your responses on this case with those of your classmates or instructors. What, if anything, would you change and why?

_____

_____

_____

Outpatient Physical Therapy Evaluation

NAME	Amy Parker
DATE	November 6, 2010
DIAGNOSIS	T9 complete spinal cord injury
SUBJECTIVE INFORMATION	The patient is 16 years old and S/P SCI almost 2 months ago. She is now living with an older woman who "adopted" her from her church. This woman is providing meals and laundry care, and a caregiver provides assistance with Foley care, bowel program, and skin care. She has a hospital bed with trapeze. The patient is still not having regular bowel movements, needing suppositories regularly. She had one UTI after being discharged from the hospital and is still on antibiotics for that. She states she feels overwhelmed by everything that has happened and depressed that her friends do not come to see her more often. She notes that she thinks her father is likely too hard on her little brothers, and she does not know what to do about it. She does not want to go back to the psychologist but may because of her depressive feelings. She reports increased pain in her legs now, especially with stretching of calf muscles, that goes up to 8/10. Her new W/C should arrive in about 2 weeks. She is using public specialized transportation for appointments. She is accompanied today by the woman in whose house she now lives (Doris). At home, she has a hospital bed with trapeze, bed rails, and loops to assist with bed mobility as well as a bench commode for bathtub and toilet use. Doris states that she has had several foster children in the past but that CPS is looking for a permanent placement for the patient because she is unable to provide the type of care needed long term. She also reports that the patient's two younger siblings are in foster care at this time.
OBJECTIVE INFORMATION	
WHEELCHAIR POSITIONING/MOBILITY	The patient sits in a temporary manual W/C with **Roho cushion,** and has adequate posture, although she tends to lean to either side. She propels the W/C using BUE inside clinic and outdoors on the sidewalk, including safe negotiation of a crosswalk and busy street.
TRANSFERS	Supervised with slide board between W/C and mat table
SITTING BALANCE/ENDURANCE ON MAT	Fair. The patient sits on edge of a mat table with upper body support and supervision for 10 minutes before fatiguing; long sits for 5 minutes with supervision because of impaired balance reactions
ROLLING ON MAT	Log roll to either direction with standby assist
SUPINE TO SIT AND SIT TO SUPINE ON MAT	Min. A

STRENGTH	BUE WNL; 0/5 BLE
PROM	Bilateral ankle dorsiflexion 5 degrees from neutral; bilateral SLR to 75 degrees. All other LE PROM WNL.
TONE	Increased tone in bilateral ankle plantarflexors and hamstrings, hip adductors
SKIN INTEGRITY	Grade 1 pressure ulcer on sacrum 1.0 cm x 0.75 cm
SENSATION	Absent below T9 for light touch and pinprick
ASSESSMENT	The patient demonstrates impaired sitting balance and endurance as well as difficulty with rolling and supine-to-sit and sit-to-supine movement; she still needs standby assist for slide board transfers. She is at risk for developing ankle plantarflexion contractures and has hamstring tightness. She continues to be at risk for skin breakdown with a grade 1 pressure ulcer on sacrum. Her social support system is minimal.
STG (2 weeks)	1. Increase bilateral SLR to 75 degrees to allow improved safety with transfers. 2. Increase bilateral ankle dorsiflexion to neutral to promote improved positioning in W/C and prevent skin breakdown.
LTG	1. Independent with bed mobility 2. Safe, independent sitting balance on edge of mat table during transfers and bed mobility tasks in order for her to return to highest possible function in home setting. 3. Supervised car transfers to allow her access to transportation in private vehicle to and from medical and social appointments. 4. Patient is independent with pressure releases and is able to maintain skin integrity on sacrum and other at-risk areas.
PLAN	The following exercises will be performed three times per week for 6 weeks: stretching techniques for BLE, functional mobility training and sitting balance activities, and car transfers. The plan includes a trial of functional electrical stimulation BLE for increased motor control. Patient education will be provided on pressure releases and assessment of wheelchair cushion to prevent further skin breakdown.

OUTPATIENT CRITICAL THINKING QUESTIONS

After reviewing the outpatient physical therapy evaluation, address the following:

1. What are the patient's impairments? Functional limitations? Is there a disability?

_____

_____

2. Find assessments of gait, strength, ROM, and balance if available from the initial evaluation and list.

   a. How could each potentially be used to assess function and demonstrate progress toward goals or show the patient's response to physical therapy interventions?

   _____

   _____

   _____

b. What would be the most important items to document for this patient?

_____

_____

_____

_____

3. After reviewing the POC, describe a possible next treatment session.

   a. List the activities/exercises and your rationale for the order of treatment activities that you selected.

   _____

   _____

   _____

   _____

continued

OUTPATIENT CRITICAL THINKING QUESTIONS *continued*

4. What subjective information will you gather during your session to help in your treatment of this patient and why?

_____

_____

5. What tests or measures will you use to assess the patient's progress and response to treatment?

_____

_____

6. What subjective or objective information that you gather during the treatment might cause you to alter your treatment for this patient and why?

_____

_____

7. How would you document your treatment in the SOAP or Patient/Client Management format?

_____

_____

8. If the treatment goes as expected, what will you do for the next treatment?

_____

_____

9. How would you expect this patient to progress over time?

_____

_____

10. If the patient does not progress as expected, what might be some reasons for a lack of progress?

_____

_____

11. What signs or symptoms, if observed or reported by the patient, would cause you to hold treatment and check with the nursing staff, primary PT, or MD?

_____

_____

12. Are there any cultural, socioeconomic, or ethical issues presented in this case that might affect your interventions or communication with this patient? If so, how?

_____

_____

13. Re-review this case. Are there any coexisting medical diagnoses that might affect how this patient responds to physical therapy? If so, what are they, and how might they cause the patient to respond to physical therapy differently than you expected?

_____

_____

14. After reviewing the other disciplines' notes regarding this patient, is there any other information that will help you to plan your treatment sessions?

_____

_____

15. Compare your responses on this case with those of your classmates or instructors. What, if anything, would you change and why?

_____

_____

CONTINUUM OF CARE CRITICAL THINKING QUESTIONS

After reviewing the continuum of care for this patient, consider the following:

1. How did the patient's problems change over the weeks after her surgery?

_____

_____

_____

_____

_____

2. How did this affect the goals and the interventions that the PT included in the POC?

_____

_____

_____

_____

_____

_____

3. How were the same interventions modified over time to progress the patient according to her changing needs?

_____

_____

_____

_____

4. What are some potential community resources that this patient might like to participate in and how would these help her to maintain and improve her physical fitness?

_____

_____

_____

_____

_____

IMPLICATIONS OF PATHOLOGY FOR THE PTA[2]

1. What are the signs and symptoms of orthostatic hypotension and autonomic dysreflexia and why are these potentially life-threatening to the patient with SCI?

_____

_____

_____

_____

_____

2. How should the PTA monitor the patient with SCI in order to prevent a negative outcome with orthostatic hypotension and autonomic dysreflexia?

_____

_____

_____

_____

_____

3. How can the PTA work with the health-care team to prevent pressure ulcers, contractures, thromboembolism, and respiratory problems with a patient with SCI?

_____

_____

_____

_____

_____

_____

_____

_____

_____

_____

_____

continued

IMPLICATIONS OF PATHOLOGY FOR THE PTA[2] *continued*

4. What is heterotopic ossification and how can this condition affect physical therapy interventions?

_____

_____

_____

_____

_____

_____

_____

_____

5. What should the PTA be aware of when working with patients with the following?
- Quadriplegia from traumatic SCI
- Central cord syndrome
- Posterior cord syndrome
- Brown-Sequard syndrome
- Anterior cord syndrome

_____

_____

_____

_____

References

1. American Physical Therapy Association: Guide to Physical Therapist Practice, Second Edition. Alexandria, VA: Author, 2001.

2. Goodman CC, Boissonnault FG, Fuller KS: Pathology: Implications for the Physical Therapist, Second Edition. Philadelphia: Saunders, 2003.

CHAPTER 11

Mrs. Ramos: A Patient With Cerebrovascular Accident

 Preferred Practice Pattern: Neuromuscular, Pattern D

CHAPTER OUTLINE

Introducing Mrs. Ramos

Mrs. Ramos is a 64-year-old woman who just suffered a cerebrovascular accident. She has had a left ischemic CVA with right hemiparesis. According to the APTA's *Guide to Physical Therapist Practice* (the *Guide*), she could have the following impairments:

- Difficulty planning movements, positioning
- Frequent falls
- Impaired affect, arousal, attention, cognition, communication
- Impaired motor function and balance

Functional limitations may include difficulty negotiating terrains and performing ADLs. Please refer to the *Guide*[1] for a complete list of possible impairments and functional limitations. As you work through this case, observe which of these the patient is experiencing.

Vocabulary List

Murmur	Rhonchi
Auscultation	Hepatosplenomegaly
Wheezes	Upward toe signs
Rales	

PHYSICIAN'S HISTORY AND PHYSICAL

PATIENT NAME: Dionisia A. Ramos
ADMIT DATE: January 16, 2010
BIRTH DATE: 03/07/1945
SEX: Female
ROOM/BED: 445-02
MEDICAL RECORD #: 12345678
CHIEF COMPLAINT: Right-sided weakness
ATTENDING: Dr. Anne Proffit, MD

HISTORY OF PRESENT ILLNESS: This 64-year-old woman was brought by ambulance to the emergency department with complaint of right extremity weakness and difficulty speaking. Apparently, earlier in the day, her right side went numb and weak, and she collapsed to the floor. Her speech was confused, and her family then called 9-1-1. At this time, she is comfortable in bed, with her husband and son at her side. She does not speak English, and her son translates information for her. Her husband also speaks limited English. Their primary language is Filipino.

PAST MEDICAL HISTORY: The patient has not received regular medical care, but her son states she has heart problems and probably diabetes, with possible hypertension.

He also states she has osteoporosis. Records here show that she was brought to the emergency department 2 years ago with a myocardial infarction. She was discharged to home with family at that time. She does not appear to have had any prior fractures.

PAST SURGICAL HISTORY: Cesarean section x 2, appendectomy

ALLERGIES: NKDA

MEDICATIONS: Not currently taking any medications

FAMILY HISTORY: The son states he is not aware of the health problems of family members other than that he himself has HTN and his brother has diabetes. The patient's husband also does not see a doctor regularly and is not aware of any problems.

SOCIAL HISTORY: The patient is married and lives with her husband and son and his wife and children in a three-bedroom apartment. She had been working in the laundry department of a local nursing home.

REVIEW OF SYSTEMS: See HPI

PHYSICAL EXAMINATION:

VITAL SIGNS: Temperature 36°C, pulse 80 BPM, respiratory rate 19 respirations per minute, blood pressure 155/84 mm Hg, O$_2$ saturation 98% on room air.

GENERAL: Patient resting comfortably in bed

SKIN: Pale but otherwise normal overall, with slight redness bilateral heels

HEENT: Speech is slurred

NECK: No evidence of stiffness, holds her head toward the left side

CARDIAC: Normal rate and rhythm without **murmur**

LUNGS: Clear to **auscultation**; no **wheezes, rales,** or **rhonchi**

ABDOMEN: Bowel sounds present, nontender, nondistended. No **hepatosplenomegaly.**

EXTREMITIES: RUE and RLE are flaccid without active movement

NEUROLOGICAL: Flaccid right side with absent reflexes right side, appears to have absent or at least diminished sensation as well on the right side. Right-sided facial droop. **Upward toe signs** on right. Cranial nerves intact.

LABORATORY DATA: Fasting blood sugar 210; hematocrit 45; hemoglobin 15; creatinine 1.4 PT/INR: 1.1

IMAGING STUDIES: CT shows no evidence of intracranial bleeding.

ASSESSMENT: Right hemiparesis with probable thrombotic event

PLAN: The plan includes MRA after 24 to 48 hours and tube feedings via a nasogastric tube. Physiatry, physical therapy, occupational therapy, and speech therapy consults, as well as social work for discharge planning, are planned.

SEEING THE DIAGNOSIS IN ACTION 11-1

Patients with CVA can have mild, moderate, or severe effects, depending on how extensive the damage is to the brain. Treatment interventions typically focus on functional training and use a wide variety of techniques to facilitate more normalized movement patterns. Because of the nature of many CVAs, one side of the body is left weak or paralyzed. If the patient is able to move that side of the body, it often is with poor movement patterns. With repetition of use, a patient can relearn functional activities and learn to use more normalized patterns; however, with severe injuries, the patient may never fully recover.

Coping with the loss becomes part of the patient's rehabilitation, and the PT/PTA team will need to consider this when planning to work with patients who have had a CVA.

After discharge from outpatient physical therapy, the patient with CVA must continue to live with the residual effects of the CVA. Patients may return to their prior level of function but usually have some residual problems. They may need follow-up therapy after several months or even intermittently over the years after a CVA in order to progress the home exercise program and instruct the family if needed.

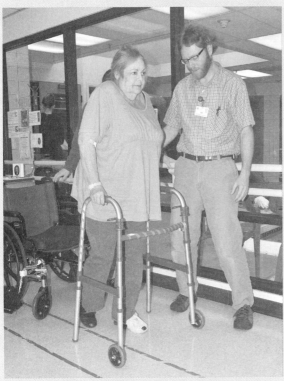

Figure 11-1 When a patient is ready for gait training, it may begin with the use of one rail on the side the patient still has use. Mirrors can give the patient feedback regarding alignment and posture. Here, a patient with CVA has progressed to gait training with a FWW.

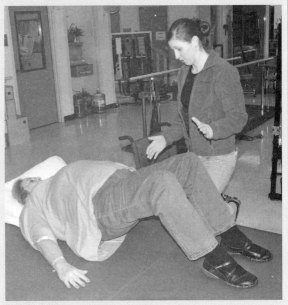

Figure 11-3 Bridging exercises to increase hip strength and stability can be an important part of a patient's exercise routine and provide for weight-bearing through the lower extremities, which facilitates improved motor control.

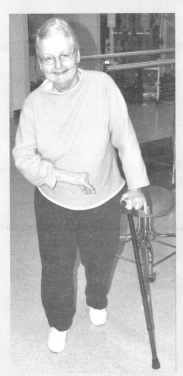

Figure 11-2 When appropriate, many patients progress to gait training with cane and perhaps later to no device at all. Often, assistive devices are recommended to patients even though they can walk without them, in order to improve gait quality and reduce deviations.

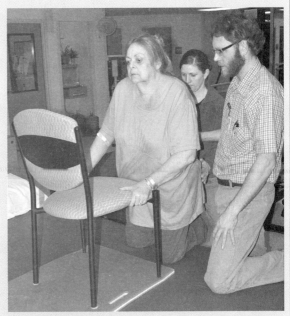

Figure 11-4 A kneeling activity can be useful to increase trunk stability and balance while providing some weight-bearing for improved motor control.

continued

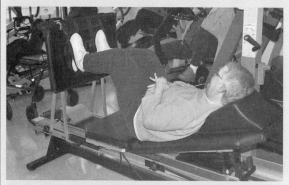

Figure 11-5 Another example of a weight-bearing or closed-chain activity includes squats to improve functional strength of the lower extremity.

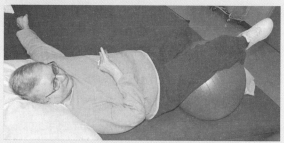

Figure 11-6 Therapy balls, this one used for a RLE exercise, can be useful for many problems. They provide a dynamic surface to work on balance and coordination while also addressing strength and ROM.

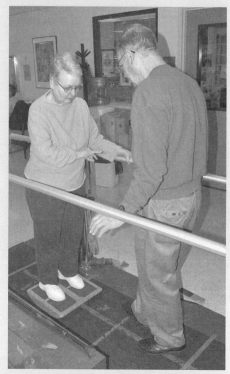

Figure 11-8 Here, he assists the patient with balance exercises.

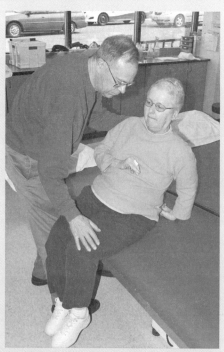

Figure 11-7 Often, family members must be trained in how to best assist the patient with functional activities and the exercise program. Here, the patient's husband assists her with a transfer.

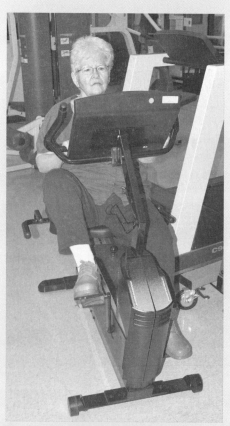

Figure 11-9 To reduce the risk for recurrent CVA, the patient may be instructed in a general exercise program. Here, the patient uses a recumbent bike to increase cardiovascular conditioning.

REVIEWING THE MEDICAL HISTORY

1. What do you already know about cerebrovascular accidents?

_____

_____

_____

_____

_____

_____

2. Review the vocabulary list and physician's notes. Look up the meanings of any terms you do not understand in a medical dictionary or other text.

_____

_____

_____

_____

_____

3. Review the diagnoses in the past medical history using a medical or pathology text, Internet resource, or other available resource.

_____

_____

_____

_____

_____

4. Which diagnoses in the past medical history would be significant and potentially affect the patient's response to the physical therapy interventions?

_____

_____

_____

_____

_____

5. List the purpose and potential side effects of each of the medications the patient is taking.

_____

_____

_____

_____

_____

6. Describe what each laboratory result measures and list considerations for physical therapy if the results for this patient were *not* in the normal range.

_____

_____

_____

_____

_____

_____

Acute Care Physical Therapy Initial Evaluation
Patient History

NAME	Dionisia Ramos		PRIMARY LANGUAGE	Filipino; no English
ROOM # & BED	445-02		ISOLATION	No
MEDICAL RECORD #	12345678		HEIGHT (CM)	170
ATTENDING PHYSICIAN	Dr. Anne Proffit, MD		WEIGHT (KG)	64
CHIEF COMPLAINT	Weakness		MEDICATION ALLERGIES	NKDA
AGE	64		FOOD ALLERGIES	None
DATE OF BIRTH	03/07/1945		INITIATED BY	Donna Smith, PT
SEX	Female		DATE	01/17/2010

continued

Acute Care Physical Therapy Initial Evaluation

Patient History

TIME	10:18	ASSISTANCE AVAILABLE	Two sons are in the area but both work. A daughter-in-law can help some but has two small children to care for. Her husband works nights and sleeps days.
TREATING DIAGNOSIS	Decreased mobility S/P left CVA with right hemiparesis		
ONSET DATE	01/16/2010	STAIRS TO ENTER HOME	Three steps into ground-floor apartment
PERTINENT MEDICAL HISTORY	Per H & P: possible DM II, cesarean section x 2, appendectomy, MI, osteoporosis	RAIL(S) ON STAIRS	One side
		ASSISTIVE DEVICE USED PRIOR	None
PRECAUTIONS	Fall risk, osteoporosis, nasogastric tube	EQUIPMENT PATIENT HAS	None
WEIGHT-BEARING STATUS	WBAT		
LIVING SITUATION	Home	DRIVING PRIOR TO ADMIT	No
PRIOR LEVEL OF FUNCTION	Independent with ambulation, ADLs, and IADLs without an assistive device	OCCUPATION/LIFE ROLE	Works in a laundry department at local SNF

Systems Review

HEARING	Intact	ACTIVITY RESPIRATORY RATE (respirations per minute)	24
VISION	Intact per family before CVA, unable to assess because of aphasia		
SPEECH	Patient appears both receptive and expressive aphasic	ACTIVITY BLOOD PRESSURE (mm Hg)	145/84
PAIN SCALE	Nonverbal adult	ACTIVITY SpO$_2$	98% on room air
PAIN LEVEL	Grimaces with PROM of right extremities	POSTACTIVITY HEART RATE (BPM)	88
PAIN LOCATION	RUE, RLE	POSTACTIVITY RESPIRATORY RATE (respirations per minute)	22
PAIN TYPE	Unable to assess		
PAIN INTERVENTION	Notified RN		
RESTING HEART RATE (BPM)	86	POSTACTIVITY BLOOD PRESSURE (mm Hg)	140/80
RESTING RESPIRATORY RATE (respirations per minute)	20	POSTACTIVITY SpO$_2$	99% on room air
		LEVEL OF CONSCIOUSNESS	Drowsy
RESTING BLOOD PRESSURE (mm Hg)	138/80	ORIENTATION	Unable to assess because of aphasia
RESTING SpO$_2$	97% on room air	SHORT-TERM MEMORY	Unable to assess because of aphasia
ACTIVITY HEART RATE (BPM)	95		

Tests and Measures

ROM NECK/TRUNK	PROM WNL	LUE STRENGTH	Unable to assess because of aphasia but demonstrates good active movement LUE
ROM BUE	PROM WNL		
ROM BLE	PROM WNL except for bilateral SLR to 60 degrees	RLE STRENGTH	Unable to assess because of aphasia but demonstrates no active movement RLE
RUE STRENGTH	Unable to assess because of aphasia but demonstrates no active movement RUE	LLE STRENGTH	Unable to assess because of aphasia but demonstrates good active movement LLE

SENSATION	Unable to assess because of aphasia	SITTING BALANCE	Poor, Max. A at edge of bed using LUE to support self
BED MOBILITY	Max. A	STANDING BALANCE	Poor; Tot. A of two persons at parallel bars
SUPINE TO SIT/SIT TO SUPINE	Max. A	GAIT	Unable
SIT TO STAND/STAND TO SIT	Max. A	STAIRS	Unable
TRANSFERS	Max. A low pivot transfer	SITTING TOLERANCE	1 minute edge of bed

Evaluation

DIAGNOSIS	Neuromuscular, pattern D
PROGNOSIS	Fair. The patient is S/P left CVA with right hemiparesis, no motor control at this time on right side, global aphasia, mild right neglect, and dependent for basic mobility tasks. During all functional activities, she pushes strongly to the right, leans to the right, and has difficulty unweighting the RLE. She moves her left extremities at will but not to command. Her family is present for evaluation, including her husband and one son. She is Filipino and does not speak English; her husband speaks very little English, and her son interprets today but is unable to be present every therapy session because of his work schedule. The patient has been very active, working full time in a laundry setting and sewing for family at home. She was also active in her local church and caring for her grandchildren at times. The family seems close but is limited financially and cannot afford to take off work to care for her. They will likely need some assistance with caregiver support because she will most likely still need assistance when she goes home, if that is still feasible. She will need SNF or an inpatient rehabilitation setting for continued rehabilitation after this hospital stay.

Plan of Care

PATIENT'S GOALS	The family would like the patient to return home, but they are unsure about how much care she will need and what they can provide.		Home program Therapeutic exercise Therapeutic activities Family training Diabetic foot care education
DISCHARGE GOALS	1. Bed mobility and transfers: Mod. A 2. Gait: TBD if appropriate 3. Home exercise program: Mod. A	FREQUENCY	BID
TIME TO ACHIEVE GOALS	By time of discharge	PATIENT EDUCATION TOPIC(S)	Activity: stimulation to right side; bed rails up for safety
PATIENT/FAMILY UNDERSTAND/AGREES WITH GOALS	Family yes	TAUGHT BY	PT
		WHO WAS TAUGHT	Family
INTERVENTIONS	Bed mobility training Transfer training Balance training Gait training	METHOD OF INSTRUCTION	Verbal/demonstration
		EVALUATION OF LEARNING	Needs reinforcement

Acute Care Nursing Note

01/18/2010   2:00 PM

The patient has an elevated BP to 160/90; there are no new orders, and the patient does not have symptoms. Chest sounds are clear. The patient is receiving tube feedings. Foley is draining dark amber urine. She is incontinent of bowel x 2 today. Family is visiting regularly and bringing their own food from home, attempting to get the patient to eat. Interpreter services are being used for family instruction and communication. The family is instructed that the patient cannot eat anything by mouth yet but is receiving therapeutic feeding with the SLP because of swallowing problems. The family has been educated regarding swallowing difficulties and the risk for aspiration with CVA. The SLP reports that the patient needs a purée diet and honey-thick liquids at this time and only during speech therapy sessions. The patient still grimaces with pain on RUE movement. Medications are being given via tube feedings. The patient attempts to say "no" when she is being repositioned onto her right side. A reddened area has been noted on her sacrum, and barrier cream has been applied. The CNAs have been educated regarding the need for repositioning every 2 hours.

BOX 11-1 | Health-Care Team Member Role: Medical Social Worker

Medical social workers are social workers who specialize in the medical setting versus the educational or community settings. They typically work in a hospital environment and provide a wide variety of services for patients and their families. In many settings, it is the responsibility of the MSW to coordinate the care of the patient from admission to discharge. This includes admissions screening, meeting with the family at the start to provide information about the services available, coordinating team meetings and family education, ordering or providing a list to family for the ordering of needed equipment, and coordinating follow-up therapy or other services after discharge from the hospital. In other settings, the MSW has a part of these responsibilities, with other staff performing the others. The MSW also helps screen patients who may need further assistance in the way of counseling or psychology or psychiatric consults. Finally, the MSW often develops a variety of educational materials used with patients and families in the rehabilitation process. For more information on the MSW and the role of social workers in general, please see the following website: http://www.bls.gov/oco/ocos060.htm.

Acute Care Social Work Note

01/19/2010   4:00 PM

The patient is S/P left CVA with right hemiparesis. The patient is aphasic and unable to communicate verbally at this time; she does nod her head yes or no but is inconsistent. Because she does not speak English, her son provided interpretation. The patient is Filipino and very involved in her church and works in a laundry department at a local SNF. She has young grandchildren that she helps to care for and also is active with sewing and other hobbies. She has lived in the United States about 35 years but has not learned much English. Her husband also speaks very little English. Her son states they are hopeful she can come home, but if she needs rehabilitation, they would like her to go to the SNF where she works because they are sure she will get the best care there, and she knows people there. A call has been placed to this facility, and the patient is placed on a waiting list. The son states that there are financial concerns because the patient does not have private health insurance, only Medicaid. The family has been provided with a list of resources for home care, adult day care, and a Meals on Wheels program and has been informed that the patient will likely require a lengthy rehabilitation stay in the SNF, up to 3 months or longer, before she may be ready for D/C home. The son states his wife has two small children but can provide daytime care and that the patient's husband will provide nighttime care when the patient goes home, if needed. They do not want her to stay long-term in the SNF.

Acute Care Occupational Therapy Summary

01/20/2010   2:20 PM

The patient is aphasic and unable to follow directions consistently but is attempting to follow one-step commands. She has difficulty managing oral secretions. She is currently on a Foley catheter and incontinent of bowel. She demonstrates poor trunk control, pushing to the right. She exhibits flaccid RUE and RLE and pain, with right extremity PROM noted with grimacing. Occupational therapy is focused on trunk control and automatic response to familiar tasks to promote ADL skills and elicit cognitive improvement. She will begin RUE management through positioning and splinting because of onset of minimal edema and ongoing indications of pain. She requires one-person Max. A for bedside sitting, with a second person assisting with positioning and help with dressing and grooming activities. Goals include the following:

1. The patient will sit at bedside with Mod. A for balance during left-handed functional task for 5 to 10 minutes.
2. The patient will wash her face with Min. A in seated position.
3. The patient will tolerate right resting hand splint for 4 hours twice per day with the assistance of trained staff and family with donning and doffing of splint.

Acute Care Speech Therapy Summary

01/21/2010   12:30 PM

The patient is making progress with swallowing. She is able to safely handle puréed foods and honey-thick liquids. She is still unable to tolerate full meals and continues to receive supplemental nutrition through the feeding tube. The patient's husband, son, and daughter-in-law were taught safe methods of assisting the patient with eating foods with these consistencies. Feeding directions are posted at the patient's bedside. Family education included stimulation techniques to encourage vocalization, and these directions are also posted at the bedside. Speech evaluation also demonstrates primarily unintelligible utterances because of the patient's aphasia. The patient continues to attempt saying "yes" and "no" and occasionally produces a word. The family reports that these Filipino words are often mixed up or incorrect. The patient is beginning to be able to point to objects and pictures on command with about 70% accuracy for a short period of time. Further work on language and swallowing in a SNF setting after D/C is recommended.

ACUTE CARE CRITICAL THINKING QUESTIONS

After reviewing the acute care physical therapy initial evaluation and other discipline notes, address the following:

1. What are the patient's impairments? Functional limitations? Is there a disability?

_____

_____

2. Find assessments of gait, strength, ROM, and balance if available from the initial evaluation and list.

   a. How could each potentially be used to assess function and demonstrate progress toward goals or show the patient's response to physical therapy interventions?

   _____

   _____

   _____

b. What would be the most important items to document for this patient?

_____

_____

_____

3. After reviewing the POC, describe a possible next treatment session.

   a. List the activities/exercises and your rationale for the order of treatment activities that you selected.

   _____

   _____

   _____

   _____

continued

ACUTE CARE CRITICAL THINKING QUESTIONS *continued*

4. What subjective information will you gather during your session to help in your treatment of this patient and why?

_____

_____

5. What tests or measures will you use to assess the patient's progress and response to treatment?

_____

_____

6. What subjective or objective information that you gather during the treatment might cause you to alter your treatment for this patient and why?

_____

_____

7. How would you document your treatment in the SOAP or Patient/Client Management format?

_____

_____

_____

_____

8. If the treatment goes as expected, what will you do for the next treatment?

_____

_____

9. How would you expect this patient to progress over time?

_____

_____

10. If the patient does not progress as expected, what might be some reasons for a lack of progress?

_____

_____

11. What signs or symptoms, if observed or reported by the patient, would cause you to hold treatment and check with the nursing staff, primary PT, or MD?

_____

_____

12. Are there any cultural, socioeconomic, or ethical issues presented in this case that might affect your interventions or communication with this patient? If so, how?

_____

_____

13. Re-review this case. Are there any coexisting medical diagnoses that might affect how this patient responds to physical therapy? If so, what are they, and how might they cause the patient to respond to physical therapy differently than you expected?

_____

_____

14. After reviewing the other disciplines' notes regarding this patient, is there any other information that will help you to plan your treatment sessions?

_____

_____

15. Compare your responses on this case with those of your classmates or instructors. What, if anything, would you change and why?

_____

_____

Medical Update

01/21/2010

Upon discharge from the acute setting on 1/21/10, the patient is S/P left middle cerebral artery occlusive CVA with right hemiparesis. Her blood pressure is 172/98 mm Hg; an ECG shows normal sinus rhythm. Transesophageal echocardiogram shows no atrial thrombus. MRA shows occlusion of left middle cerebral artery. Updated laboratory results are as follows: total cholesterol is 245, LDL is 160, HDL is 36, and triglycerides are 330; creatinine is 1.6; and Hg A_{1C} is 9.2. Updated medications include added metoprolol 25 mg twice daily, Lipitor 20 mg daily, Lantus 15 mg daily, sliding-scale regular insulin, and aspirin 81 mg daily. The patient is still on tube feedings via PEG tube to supplement oral nutrition.

The plan is to discharge the patient to a SNF. The patient is declining inpatient rehabilitation. She will have a follow-up bone density scan and a neurology follow-up in 2 weeks. She will receive physical, occupational, and speech therapy, as well as social work, later in the SNF setting.

Skilled Nursing Facility Physical Therapy Evaluation

NAME	Dionisia Ramos
SOC DATE	01/22/2010
ONSET DATE	01/16/2010
PRIMARY DIAGNOSIS	Late effects of CVA
TREATMENT DIAGNOSIS	General muscle weakness
PAYOR	Medicaid

SHORT-TERM GOALS (2 weeks)

1. Bed mobility: Patient will transition from supine to sit with Min. A and 50% verbal cues for sequencing to increase level of independence.
2. Transfer: Patient will perform low pivot transfer with Min. A and 50% verbal cues for sequencing to increase level of independence.
3. Sitting balance: Patient will increase her sitting balance to fair to improve her ability to transfer safely.
4. W/C mobility: Patient will use RUE and RLE to propel W/C for 50 feet with Min. A and 50% verbal cues for sequencing.
5. Standing tolerance: Patient will tolerate standing for 2 minutes in parallel bars with Min. A and cues for midline control without a rest break to increase endurance for ambulation in environment.
6. Gait: Patient will ambulate 50 feet with FWW adapted with right hand splint, right AFO, or NDT wrap and Mod. A and cues for right ankle dorsiflexion, knee control, and hip control in order to improve ambulation in her environment.
7. Skin integrity: Stage II decubitus ulcer on sacrum will heal.

OUTCOME (long-term, 12 weeks)

The patient will be independent, with W/C mobility indoors to 300 feet and supervised W/C outdoors for 100 feet on a sidewalk or paved surface. The patient will be independent with ADLs from a W/C level. She will be supervised for a home exercise program. She will require Min. A for car transfers to return home. The family is able to safely assist the patient with all transfers and a home exercise program as well as up and down steps into the apartment. The patient and family can independently manage diabetic foot care, skin checks, and pressure releases. There are no further wounds, and the current decubitus ulcer is healed.

PLAN

97001—PT evaluation
97110—Therapeutic exercise
97116—Gait training
97530—Therapeutic activities
G0283—Electrical stimulation (unattended) to one or more areas, for indications other than wound
G0285—Electrical stimulation (unattended) to one or more areas, for wound healing

continued

Skilled Nursing Facility Physical Therapy Evaluation *continued*

The resident and/or responsible party understands the proposed treatment and the expected benefits and risks that are associated with the plan. The resident and/or responsible party agrees to the treatment as prescribed.	The rehabilitation potential is good. Prognostic indicator: The patient is able to follow one-step directions, is alert and oriented to self and family as well as place, and has good motivation and family support to return home with additional caregiver support.
FREQUENCY/DURATION	6 per week x 12 weeks
CERTIFICATION	N/A
PRIOR HOSPITALIZATION	From 01/16/10 through 01/21/10
PRECAUTIONS	Aspiration risk, fall risk, osteoporosis, cardiac, PEG tube
INITIAL ASSESSMENT (history, medical complications, level of function at start of care, reason for referral)	PLOF: The patient is independent in her home, with three steps and one rail to enter the apartment. She did not use any assistive devices. She has a tub-shower combo in a small bathroom per family. History: Patient is a 64-year-old Filipino woman with left CVA and right hemiparesis. She has good family support and is making progress in her motor control since onset on 1/16/10. She communicates to yes/no questions with head nods or shakes and smiles. She usually does not attempt to speak. She has a PEG tube for feedings. Her PMH includes DM II, HTN, osteoporosis, MI, prior appendectomy, and two cesarean sections. Her husband and son hope to take her home eventually but will need additional caregiver support.
D/C PLANS	The patient will return to home. Family will provide assistance with cooking and cleaning, and an outside caregiver will help with self-care activities. Outpatient follow-up is needed.
ASSESSMENT	Orientation: the patient is alert and oriented x 2.

Cognition: She follows one-step directions but experiences some comprehension breakdown.
Bed mobility: Mod. A
Sitting balance: Poor, pushes to right strongly, needs Mod. A to maintain
Sit to stand with FWW: Mod. A
Standing balance: Poor, pushes to right strongly and Mod. A to Max. A
Low pivot transfer: Mod. A
Gait: Max. A for three steps in parallel bars and W/C follow; leans to the right throughout and has difficulty unweighting RLE during swing phase. Needs assist to lift RLE and in using NDT wrap to facilitate right ankle dorsiflexion.
Endurance: Sits on edge of bed x 10 minutes, in W/C x 45 minutes, stands x 1 minute
SpO_2 before activity: 98% on room air
SpO_2 during activity: 97% on room air
Pain: with PROM to RUE, patient holds right shoulder with left hand and shakes head "no" with any movement.
MMT: left hip flexion 3+/5, quadriceps 3+/5, ankle dorsiflexion and plantarflexion 4/5
RLE not formally tested but exhibits beginning motor control in hip flexion, quadriceps, and ankle dorsiflexion and plantarflexion, all in gravity-eliminated positions and to about 25% of normal ROM.
AROM: WFL on left side, right side limited by weakness
Tone: Decreased RUE and RLE except for increasing tone in right plantarflexors
Sensation: Impaired RLE for light touch
Protective sensation: Impaired bilateral feet
Proprioception: Impaired right ankle, great toe and knee
Skin integrity: Stage II decubitus ulcer on sacrum measured 2.5 x 2.0 cm; wound bed granulating

| FUNCTIONAL STATUS AT SOC | 1. Bed mobility: Patient transitions from supine to sit toward left side with Mod. A and 90% verbal cues for sequencing, tactile facilitation to right hip flexors, and quadriceps and anterior shoulder to initiate roll. She rolls to right side with supervision for verbal cues only.
2. Transfer: The patient is able to perform low pivot transfer with Mod. A and 90% verbal cues for sequencing and tactile facilitation at gluteals for initiation of movement.
3. Sitting balance: Poor; needs tactile facilitation and verbal cues as well as mirror and Mod. A to achieve midline because of strong push toward right side. | 4. W/C mobility: Patient propels W/C using LUE and LLE for 25 feet with Min. A and 90% verbal cues for sequencing.
5. Standing tolerance: Patient stands for 30 seconds in parallel bars without a rest. She needs tactile facilitation to promote activation of left hip abductors and extensors and left quadriceps.
6. Gait: Patient ambulates three steps in parallel bars with NDT wrap to right ankle and Max. A to achieve right knee and hip control and right lower extremity unweighting for swing phase.
7. Skin integrity: Stage II decubitus ulcer on sacrum measured 2.5 x 2.0 cm; wound bed granulating. |

BOX 11-2 | Physical Therapy Specialty: Osteoporosis

Although the treatment of osteoporosis is not considered a true specialty, it is one of those pathologies that does require the PTA to consider several factors specific to the disease process. These include certain precautions, appropriate interventions that not only help in the short-term but also help prevent future complications, as well as appropriate exercise programs for the general population with osteoporosis. PTAs can be involved in all of these areas, from direct intervention to wellness and prevention education, as delegated by the PT. Many clinical settings include protocols to be used with patients who have osteoporosis as well as exercise classes to enhance the well-being and quality of life of these patients. For more information on osteoporosis and its treatment, see the National Osteoporosis Foundation website at http://www.nof.org.

Skilled Nursing Facility Nursing Note

01/21/2010   3:21 PM

The patient is able to verbalize "yes" and "no," but answers are inconsistently correct. She cries out when she needs something and points or gestures to communicate to staff what she needs with limited success. A PEG tube is in place for feedings. The Foley is draining amber urine. She is incontinent of bowel and is using Depends. She is toileting in the AM after daily suppository on the commode to prevent feces contamination of urinary tract. A stage II decubitus ulcer on sacrum measured 2.4 x 1.8 cm and stage I on left heel measured 0.6 x 1.1 cm. Allevyn dressing has been applied to the sacrum. The patient's heels are floated with foam boots and repositioned every 2 hours, with pressure taken off the sacrum using pillows. PT has provided a Roho cushion for the W/C. Physical therapy with modalities is being used for enhanced wound healing. She requires two-person assist for transfers and bed baths only so far. The family is present at all times, taking shifts to be with the patient. At times, the nursing staff asks the family to leave to give more space when providing care. There is no respiratory distress, and the patient's breath sounds are clear.

Skilled Nursing Facility Social Work Summary

01/23/2010   4:42 PM

A care conference was held today. The patient's son Tom interpreted between the team and the family. The nursing staff report that wounds appear to be healing, getting smaller in size. Pressure relief is very important. The Roho cushion on the W/C is helping the sacral wound. The PT reports that the patient is making progress and working on sitting balance, transfers, and motor control activities to strengthen RLE. Occupational therapy will address self-feeding, grooming, upper body dressing, RUE management for patient positioning, and along with nursing, a bowel program to achieve regular bowel movements. Speech therapy is addressing improved swallowing function. The patient is now able to manage dysphagia, mechanical textures, and nectar-thick liquids. She is still on PEG feedings because she is only eating about 20% of a meal. A communication board has been developed, and the team and family are encouraged to use it, asking the patient to point to pictures of things she needs or would like to express, such as pain, drink, food, change pants, TV, etc. She should also be encouraged to say the words next to the pictures. Her son, Tom, will provide Filipino words with correct pronunciations to include on the board.

Skilled Nursing Facility Occupational Therapy Summary

01/24/2010   10:45 AM

The patient is working toward a pre-ADL goal of independent trunk control and dressing in supported sitting position; she currently requires Mod. A. She demonstrates apraxia with grooming and dressing and is unable to orient clothing, needing hand-over-hand Mod. A. She is able to self-feed with minimal cues and supervision for safety. She is receiving low pivot transfer training to bedside commode with Max. A and second-person assist with clothing. Foley catheter is still present. Nursing staff is providing a suppository and then occupational therapy about 30 minutes later for transfer training, sitting balance activity on a commode; the patient usually achieves a BM. The patient has ongoing pain indications in RUE with one-finger subluxation. The OT introduced a sling for transfer purposes only and half lap tray for support in the W/C. Family members are typically present and observe all activities, with verbal education provided by the OT when the son is present to interpret. The son and daughter-in-law are trained in UE self-ROM exercises and in hand splint purpose and wearing schedule. Long-term goals for discharge include the following:

1. The patient will perform functional transfers with Min. A by trained family member who will protect RUE during transfers.
2. The patient will follow RUE ROM, positioning, and splinting program with assist of trained family members.
3. The patient will sit at bedside independently during self-care tasks for up to 15 minutes assisted by trained family members.
4. With environmental modifications and family education, the patient will have safe D/C to home.

   Outpatient physical therapy is to address residual RUE deficits after discharge because outpatient occupational therapy is unavailable.

Skilled Nursing Facility Speech Language Pathology Summary

01/25/2010   3:29 PM

Filipino words are now included on the communication board, and education has been provided to the PT, OT, and nursing staff to facilitate improved communication with the patient using these words with the pictures. The patient is able to answer yes or no correctly about 75% of the time. Expressive aphasia continues to make speech attempts mostly unintelligible. The patient is eating a mechanical soft diet with ground meats and nectar-thick liquids. The daughter-in-law is trained and able to safely provide these to the patient while following posted techniques. She is still receiving supplemental feeding via PEG tube. She is eating about 25% of meals. Outpatient speech therapy services are recommended so that the patient will continue to improve speech, communication, swallowing, and cognition.

SKILLED NURSING FACILITY CRITICAL THINKING QUESTIONS

After reviewing the SNF physical therapy initial evaluation and other discipline notes, address the following:

1. What are the patient's impairments? Functional limitations? Is there a disability?

_____

_____

2. Find assessments of gait, strength, ROM, and balance if available from the initial evaluation and list.

   a. How could each potentially be used to assess function and demonstrate progress toward goals or show the patient's response to physical therapy interventions?

   _____

   _____

   _____

   b. What would be the most important items to document for this patient?

   _____

   _____

   _____

3. After reviewing the POC, describe a possible next treatment session.

   a. List the activities/exercises and your rationale for the order of treatment activities that you selected.

   _____

   _____

   _____

4. What subjective information will you gather during your session to help in your treatment of this patient and why?

   _____

   _____

5. What tests or measures will you use to assess the patient's progress and response to treatment?

   _____

   _____

6. What subjective or objective information that you gather during the treatment might cause you to alter your treatment for this patient and why?

_____

_____

7. How would you document your treatment in the SOAP or Patient/Client Management format?

_____

_____

_____

_____

8. If the treatment goes as expected, what will you do for the next treatment?

_____

_____

9. How would you expect this patient to progress over time?

_____

_____

10. If the patient does not progress as expected, what might be some reasons for a lack of progress?

_____

_____

11. If the patient's decubitus ulcer progressed to a stage III, what changes would you expect to observe in the wound?

_____

_____

_____

12. What signs or symptoms, if observed or reported by the patient, would cause you to hold treatment and check with the nursing staff, primary PT, or MD?

_____

_____

_____

continued

SKILLED NURSING FACILITY CRITICAL THINKING QUESTIONS *continued*

13. Are there any cultural, socioeconomic, or ethical issues presented in this case that might affect your interventions or communication with this patient? If so, how?

_____

_____

_____

14. Re-review this case. Are there any coexisting medical diagnoses that might affect how this patient responds to physical therapy? If so what are they, and how might they cause the patient to respond to physical therapy differently than you expected?

_____

_____

_____

15. After reviewing the other disciplines' notes regarding this patient, is there any other information that will help you to plan your treatment sessions?

_____

_____

_____

_____

16. Compare your responses on this case with those of your classmates or instructors. What, if anything, would you change and why?

_____

_____

_____

_____

Outpatient Physical Therapy Evaluation

NAME	Dionisia Ramos
DATE	April 18, 2010
DIAGNOSIS	S/P left CVA with right hemiparesis
SUBJECTIVE INFORMATION	The patient can communicate through interpretation by her son; in her language, she can speak a few words but uses gestures and pictures on communication board primarily. She has pain in her right shoulder and uses a sling at all times to protect it from jarring; she is unable to rate on pain scale because of aphasia. The family has the help of a caregiver through a special program for low-income patients in the AM and PM for help with dressing, meals, and bathing. Between those times, the daughter-in-law provides supervision and assistance with transfers and lunch meal while she also cares for her two young children. She and the patient's husband are also home at night providing assist to the bedside commode at night as needed. The son and husband basically carry her up and down the three steps into the apartment when she goes to medical appointments. They declined home health, wanting to begin outpatient therapy right away instead. The son states that the family and patient goals are to get the right shoulder better and walk independently, including up and down the three steps into apartment. They realize she may not be able to return to work. They are trying to get her disability pay.
OBJECTIVE INFORMATION	
POSTURE	Sits and stands with slight lean to the right of midline; holds head turned toward the left
GAIT	Ambulates 40 feet with FWW with modified support for right wrist and Mod. A, tactile facilitation to engage right gluteus medius and maximus, quadriceps, and hamstring; right AFO and verbal cues for heel strike and weight shift. Left step length shorter than right with decreased stance time on right. Up and down one step with rail on left side both ways and Max. A.

BALANCE	Tinetti balance score: 16/28 for high risk for falling Sitting balance: Fair	STG (2 weeks)	1. Ambulates 60 feet with Min. A and modified FWW, right AFO. 2. Ascend/descend one step with rail on both sides Mod. A. 3. Family able to safely and effectively assist patient with supine or sitting ROM, stretching, and strengthening exercises using written home exercise program.
SITTING AND STANDING TOLERANCE	Sits on mat table without support for 5 minutes; stands with bar on left for 8 minutes		
STRENGTH	LUE and LLE WNL; RLE not formally tested but exhibits fair motor control of hip flexion, quadriceps, and ankle dorsiflexors and plantarflexors. Beginning motor control of hip abduction, extension, ankle eversion, and inversion. Right elbow flexion and extension, wrist flexion and extension beginning motor control.	LTG	1. Ambulates 100 feet on even surfaces with right AFO and modified FWW with supervision; equal step lengths and verbal cues for weight shifting and heel strike. 2. Ambulates up and down three steps with one rail on left side ascending with Min. A and family able to assist. 3. Supervised for home exercise program for RUE and RLE ROM, strengthening; sitting and standing balance. 4. Reduced right shoulder subluxation and minimal pain that allows AAROM to 130 degrees flexion and abduction and 45 degrees external rotation.
PROM	WNL BUE and BLE except for right SLR 65 degrees and right ankle dorsiflexion to neutral; right shoulder flexion and abduction to 110 degrees, external rotation 10 degrees with pain at end range.		
PALPATION	Tenderness to palpation of right supraspinatus with 1 finger width of subluxation		
SENSATION	Impaired light-touch RLE and proprioception for right ankle, great toe, and knee	PLAN	Functional electrical stimulation to right shoulder for subluxation and pain; motor control activities; therapeutic exercise; gait training; balance training; cardiovascular exercise program; and development of home exercise program. Three times per week x 4 weeks.
VITAL SIGNS	BP 122/78 mm Hg; HR 76 bpm; SpO$_2$ 99% on room air		
ASSESSMENT			

OUTPATIENT CRITICAL THINKING QUESTIONS

After reviewing the outpatient physical therapy evaluation, address the following:

1. What are the patient's impairments? Functional limitations? Is there a disability?

_____

_____

2. Find assessments of gait, strength, ROM, and balance if available from the initial evaluation and list.

a. How could each potentially be used to assess function and demonstrate progress toward goals or show the patient's response to physical therapy interventions?

_____

_____

b. What would be the most important items to document for this patient?

_____

_____

_____

_____

3. After reviewing the POC, describe a possible next treatment session.

a. List the activities/exercises and your rationale for the order of treatment activities that you selected.

_____

_____

_____

continued

OUTPATIENT CRITICAL THINKING QUESTIONS *continued*

4. What subjective information will you gather during your session to help in your treatment of this patient and why?

_____

_____

5. What tests or measures will you use to assess the patient's progress and response to treatment?

_____

_____

6. What subjective or objective information that you gather during the treatment might cause you to alter your treatment for this patient and why?

_____

_____

7. How would you document your treatment in the SOAP or Patient/Client Management format?

_____

_____

_____

_____

8. If the treatment goes as expected, what will you do for the next treatment?

_____

_____

_____

9. How would you expect this patient to progress over time?

_____

_____

10. If the patient does not progress as expected, what might be some reasons for a lack of progress?

_____

_____

11. What signs or symptoms, if observed or reported by the patient, would cause you to hold treatment and check with the nursing staff, primary PT, or MD?

_____

_____

12. Are there any cultural, socioeconomic, or ethical issues presented in this case that might affect your interventions or communication with this patient? If so, how?

_____

_____

_____

13. Re-review this case. Are there any coexisting medical diagnoses that might affect how this patient responds to physical therapy? If so, what are they, and how might they cause the patient to respond to physical therapy differently than you expected?

_____

_____

_____

14. After reviewing the other disciplines' notes regarding this patient, is there any other information that will help you to plan your treatment sessions?

_____

_____

_____

15. Compare your responses on this case with those of your classmates or instructors. What, if anything, would you change and why?

_____

_____

_____

CONTINUUM OF CARE CRITICAL THINKING QUESTIONS

After reviewing the continuum of care for this patient, consider the following:

1. How did the patient's problems change over the months after her CVA?

_____

_____

_____

_____

_____

2. How did this affect the goals and the interventions that the PT included in the POC?

_____

_____

_____

_____

_____

_____

3. How were the same interventions modified over time to progress the patient according to her changing needs?

_____

_____

_____

_____

_____

4. What are some potential community resources that this patient might like to participate in and how would these help her to maintain and improve her physical fitness?

_____

_____

_____

_____

_____

IMPLICATIONS OF PATHOLOGY FOR THE PTA[2]

1. List the signs and symptoms of the following potential complications for a patient with CVA and the appropriate response of the PTA:
   • Angina or myocardial infarction
   • Peripheral vascular disease
   • Deep vein thrombosis
   • Aspiration
   • Development of pressure ulcers
   • Development of contractures
   • Shoulder subluxation on hemiparetic side

_____

_____

_____

_____

_____

_____

2. What precautions should the PTA take when working with patients who have osteoporosis?

_____

_____

_____

_____

_____

3. What additional physical therapy interventions can be used to help facilitate wound healing for decubitus ulcers at stages II through IV or when other, more conservative interventions have not helped?

_____

_____

_____

_____

continued

IMPLICATIONS OF PATHOLOGY FOR THE PTA[2] *continued*

4. What are the common clinical manifestations in a patient who has had a right-sided CVA as opposed to a left-sided CVA?

_____
_____
_____
_____
_____
_____
_____
_____
_____
_____
_____
_____
_____
_____
_____
_____
_____
_____
_____
_____
_____
_____

5. How might the following sensorimotor, cognitive, and perceptual deficits commonly observed after a CVA affect physical therapy interventions?
- One-sided neglect
- Visual disturbances such as homonymous hemianopsia
- Aphasia (comprehensive and expressive)
- Apraxia and motor planning deficiencies
- Attention deficits
- Disorientation
- Short-term memory loss
- Loss of judgment and safety awareness
- Ataxia
- Dysarthria
- Poor coordination
- Language difficulties
- Balance impairment
- Muscle weakness and fatigue
- Altered consciousness

_____
_____
_____
_____
_____
_____
_____
_____
_____
_____
_____

References

1. American Physical Therapy Association: Guide to Physical Therapist Practice, Second Edition. Alexandria, VA: Author, 2001.

2. Goodman CC, Boissonnault FG, Fuller KS: Pathology: Implications for the Physical Therapist, Second Edition. Philadelphia: Saunders, 2003.

chapter 12

Mr. Jones: A Patient With Parkinson Disease and Hip Fracture

Preferred Practice Pattern: Neuromuscular, Pattern E, and Musculoskeletal, Pattern I

CHAPTER OUTLINE

Introducing Mr. Jones

Mr. Jones is an 83-year-old man who has Parkinson disease and just fell at home and fractured his hip. According to the APTA's *Guide to Physical Therapist Practice* (the *Guide*), he could have the following impairments:

- Decreased coordination
- Impaired endurance, arousal, attention, and cognition
- Impaired motor function, sensory integrity, and balance
- Limited ROM
- Muscle weakness
- Pain

Functional limitations may include the following:

- Difficulty negotiating different terrains and community environments
- Frequent falls
- Progressive loss of function
- Limited independence in ADLs

Please refer to the *Guide*[1] for a complete list of possible impairments and functional limitations. As you work through this case, think about which of these the patient is experiencing.

Vocabulary List

Orthopnea	Rhonchi
Auscultation	Hepatosplenomegaly
Wheeze	Physiatry
Rales	Trendelenburg

PHYSICIAN'S HISTORY AND PHYSICAL

PATIENT NAME: Alfred M. Jones
ADMIT DATE: January 2, 2010
BIRTH DATE: July 23, 1926
SEX: Male
ROOM/BED: 327-01
MEDICAL RECORD #: 12345678
CHIEF COMPLAINT: Ground-level fall
ATTENDING: Dr. Charles Hinkley, MD

HISTORY OF PRESENT ILLNESS: This is an 83-year-old male with a past medical history of Parkinson disease, HTN, DM II, peripheral neuropathy, obesity, osteoarthritis with chronic pain, and pneumonia 1 year ago. He presents with a ground-level fall. The patient states that he tripped while coming down the stairs in his home and fell onto his right hip at the bottom of the stairs. He reports no loss of consciousness and that his wife called 9-1-1 when he could not get up. He now complains of right shoulder and right hip pain. He denies any chest pain, palpitations, shortness of breath, or lightheadedness before the fall. He also denies any fever, cough, **orthopnea,** lower extremity edema, abdominal pain, nausea, or vomiting. He does have constipation.

PAST MEDICAL HISTORY: The patient's medical history is significant for Parkinson disease, HTN, hyperlipidemia, DM type II, peripheral neuropathy, osteoarthritis, mild obesity, and aspiration pneumonia 1 year ago.

PAST SURGICAL HISTORY: Left total knee replacement 5 years ago with good results; tonsillectomy

ALLERGIES: None

MEDICATIONS: Sinemet 10 mg carbidopa/100 mg levodopa PO three times daily
Colace 100 mg PO twice daily
lisinopril 5 mg PO daily
Lipitor 40 mg PO daily
hydrocodone 5 mg/325 mg acetaminophen PO daily PRN
Glucophage 500 mg PO twice daily

FAMILY HISTORY: Reviewed and noncontributory

SOCIAL HISTORY: The patient is married with three grown children and five grandchildren. He denies smoking and drinks about 1 beer per day.

REVIEW OF SYSTEMS: See HPI; otherwise negative

PHYSICAL EXAMINATION:

VITAL SIGNS: Temperature 36.5°C, pulse 84 BPM, respiratory rate 17 respirations per minute, blood pressure 115/62 mm Hg, O_2 saturation 98% on 2 liters.

GENERAL: Uncomfortable, with right shoulder and right hip pain

SKIN: Warm and dry without rash or jaundice. Bruising at right shoulder and face.

HEENT: Unremarkable

NECK: Tenderness to palpation at base of the neck; able to flex neck

CARDIAC: Regular rate and rhythm

LUNGS: Clear to **auscultation** bilaterally without **wheeze, rales,** or **rhonchi.**

ABDOMEN: Bowel sounds present, nontender, nondistended. No **hepatosplenomegaly.**

EXTREMITIES: Tenderness to palpation of right rotator cuff. Right hip is flexed; patient is unable to move his right leg. Left leg is normal.

NEUROLOGICAL: Alert and oriented. Moving his left extremities well, right shoulder slowly due to pain. Cranial nerves intact.

LABORATORY DATA: Hematocrit 34, which is stable. Platelets 148,000. Troponin is negative.
Hg A_{1C} 7

IMAGING STUDIES: CT of head—right occipital scalp hematoma. CT of cervical spine—negative. Right shoulder x-ray negative. Right hip x-ray—intertrochanteric fracture of the right femur.

ASSESSMENT:
1. Right intertrochanteric hip fracture
2. Right shoulder and head contusions

PLAN: The plan is to admit the patient to the surgical floor with an orthopedic consult for right hip surgical repair. Pain control will be provided, and the patient's current medications will be continued. **Physiatry,** physical therapy, occupational therapy, and social work consults will be provided.

SEEING THE DIAGNOSIS IN ACTION 12-1

Parkinson disease is a progressive disease that often has minimal effects in the beginning. Patients may need education on an effective exercise program designed to maintain balance, strength, and flexibility and can often live a number of years until the disease progresses to the point they need more help. The later effects of Parkinson disease can be devastating, causing a great deal of difficulty with ADLs and IADLs. Patients often fall frequently and suffer fractures and other problems related to the falls. In the end, respiratory or other dysfunction often leads to death.

When the patient has been diagnosed with Parkinson disease, he or she may not receive physical therapy right away. As the patient's needs change, physical therapy will be indicated at various points along the progression of the disease and in a variety of settings along the continuum of care. The physical therapy POC will be based on the patient's needs at the time and will be dependent on the patient's current stage of progression. Toward the later stages, family and other caregivers will require training in order to provide care in the most effective way.

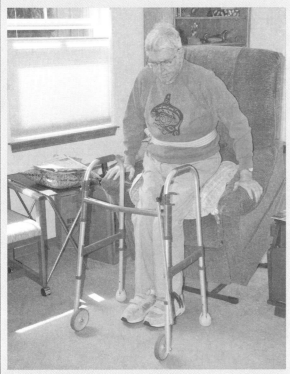

Figure 12-1 Because of the progressive nature of the disease and the inability to restore normal function at later stages, patients with Parkinson disease may need to learn compensatory strategies. Here, a patient uses a lift chair for sit to stand at the FWW.

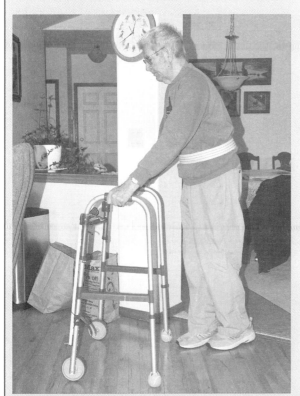

Figure 12-2 To reduce fall risk, patients with Parkinson disease may benefit from using a FWW.

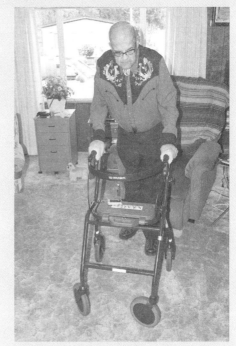

Figure 12-3 This patient uses a 4WW for ambulation to help decrease "freezing" episodes during the activity.

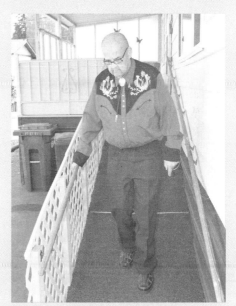

Figure 12-4 Patients learn how to safely ambulate on a variety of surfaces in order to safely negotiate all home and community settings. Here, the patient is practicing at home as in a home health setting.

continued

SEEING THE DIAGNOSIS IN ACTION 12-1 *continued*

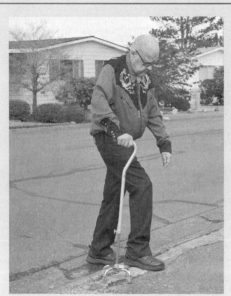

Figure 12-5 Some patients with Parkinson disease are able to safely use a cane for ambulation some or all of the time. Here, the patient performs gait training on a curb using a cane.

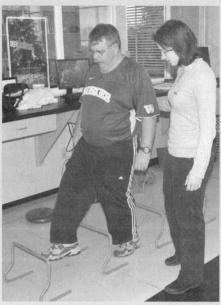

Figure 12-7 In addition to the many functional mobility tasks the patient with Parkinson disease must learn, the PT/PTA team must also include a home exercise program designed to help the patient maintain and improve function where possible. This patient performs a balance activity by stepping over obstacles. Balance is affected by a variety of factors such as strength, flexibility, and vision and sensory changes. An effective program will address all areas that are problems for the particular patient.

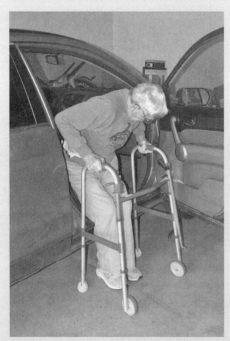

Figure 12-6 Another skill many patients must learn to perform safely is car transfers. Here, a patient demonstrates his car transfer technique. This patient is still able to drive, but as the disease progresses, he will likely stop driving because of safety concerns.

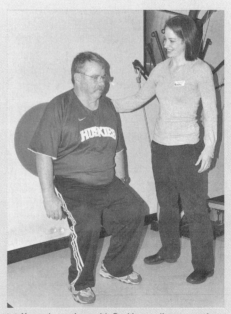

Figure 12-8 Here, the patient with Parkinson disease performs a squat exercise using a therapy ball. This exercise promotes improved function for sit to stand and other weight-bearing activities, such as ambulation. It is commonly included (with or without the therapy ball) in a home exercise program for patients with Parkinson disease.

REVIEWING THE MEDICAL HISTORY

1. What do you already know about Parkinson disease? About hip fractures?

_____
_____
_____
_____
_____

2. Review the vocabulary list and physician's notes. Look up the meanings of any terms you do not understand in a medical dictionary or other text.

3. Review the diagnoses in the past medical history using a medical or pathology text, Internet resource, or other available resource.

4. Which diagnoses in the past medical history would be significant and potentially affect the patient's response to the physical therapy interventions?

_____
_____
_____
_____
_____

5. List the purpose and potential side effects of each of the medications the patient is taking.

_____
_____
_____
_____
_____
_____
_____
_____

6. Describe what each laboratory result measures and list considerations for physical therapy if the results for this patient were _not_ in the normal range.

_____
_____
_____
_____
_____
_____
_____

Acute Care Physical Therapy Initial Evaluation
Patient History

NAME	Alfred Jones	INITIATED BY	Donna Smith, PT
ROOM # & BED	B327-01	DATE	01/03/2010
MEDICAL RECORD #	12345678	TIME	14:52
ATTENDING PHYSICIAN	Dr. Hinkley	TREATING DIAGNOSIS	Decreased mobility S/P ORIF with intermedullary screw secondary to right intertrochanteric fracture sustained in ground-level fall in home
CHIEF COMPLAINTS	Right hip fracture		
AGE	83		
DATE OF BIRTH	07/23/1926	ONSET DATE	01/02/2010
SEX	Male	PERTINENT MEDICAL HISTORY	Per H & P: significant for PD x 3 years, HTN, DM II, peripheral neuropathy, osteoarthritis, mild obesity, and aspiration pneumonia 1 year ago
PRIMARY LANGUAGE	English		
ISOLATION	No		
HEIGHT (CM)	170		
WEIGHT (KG)	102	SURGERY	ORIF right hip
MEDICATION ALLERGIES	NKDA	SURGERY DATE	01/02/2010
FOOD ALLERGIES	None		

continued

Acute Care Physical Therapy Initial Evaluation *continued*

Patient History

PRECAUTIONS	Fall risk, risk for skin breakdown with overlay mattress in use on bed	STAIRS TO ENTER HOME	Two plus one flight of stairs in home to upstairs bedrooms with two rails
WEIGHT-BEARING STATUS	TTWB RLE	RAIL(S) ON STAIRS	One side on outdoor steps
LIVING SITUATION	Home	ASSISTIVE DEVICE USED PRIOR	Cane
PRIOR LEVEL OF FUNCTION	Independent with ambulation using cane and had history of five or six falls in past year, per wife his gait has been deteriorating	EQUIPMENT PATIENT HAS	Cane and FWW
		DRIVING PRIOR TO ADMIT	No
ASSISTANCE AVAILABLE	Spouse for meals and household cleaning, she is unable to do any lifting due to back problems; she is 82 years old but able to care for herself	OCCUPATION/LIFE ROLE	Retired high school math teacher

Systems Review

HEARING	Intact	ACTIVITY RESPIRATORY RATE (respirations per minute)	24
VISION	Intact, wears glasses		
SPEECH	Impaired swallowing with prior speech therapy	ACTIVITY BLOOD PRESSURE (mm Hg)	123/74
PAIN SCALE	VPS	ACTIVITY SpO$_2$	97% on 1 LPM supplemental O$_2$
PAIN LEVEL	4	POSTACTIVITY HEART RATE (BPM)	84
PAIN LOCATION	RLE		
PAIN TYPE	Surgical	POSTACTIVITY RESPIRATORY RATE (respirations per minute)	20
PAIN INTERVENTION	Notified RN and was medicated before mobility assessments		
RESTING HEART RATE (BPM)	80	POSTACTIVITY BLOOD PRESSURE (mm Hg)	122/70
RESTING RESPIRATORY RATE (respirations per minute)	19	POSTACTIVITY SpO$_2$	97% on 1 LPM supplemental O$_2$
		LEVEL OF CONSCIOUSNESS	Alert
RESTING BLOOD PRESSURE (mm Hg)	118/72	ORIENTATION	x 4
RESTING SpO$_2$	98% on 1 LPM supplemental O$_2$; 90% on room air	SHORT-TERM MEMORY	Impaired; unable to remember TTWB status at end of evaluation after verbal education with demonstration by PT
ACTIVITY HEART RATE (BPM)	85		

Tests and Measures

ROM NECK/TRUNK	Impaired; general rigidity with trunk rotation about 50% of normal, neck rotation about 20 degrees bilaterally	ROM RLE	WNL except as noted; supine, right hip flex to 90 degrees, extension to 5 degrees from neutral, abduction to 20 degrees; knee extension lacks 20 degrees; ankle dorsiflexion to neutral
ROM RUE	WNL except as noted; PROM shoulder flexion to 60 degrees, abduction to 55 degrees		
		ROM LLE	WNL except as noted; hip extension lacks 5 degrees from neutral; knee extension lacks 20 degrees; ankle dorsiflexion to neutral
ROM LUE	WNL except as noted; PROM shoulder flexion to 90 degrees, abduction to 90 degrees		

RUE STRENGTH	2+/5		SIT TO STAND/STAND TO SIT	Max. A
LUE STRENGTH	3–/5			
RLE STRENGTH	Ankle dorsiflexion/plantarflexion 4–/5, supine hip and knee flexion to about 90 degrees hip flexion with assistance of therapist		TRANSFERS	Tot. A stand pivot with TTWB RLE, using FWW; second person needed to stand by for safety, to manage RLE and also assist with IV
LLE STRENGTH	3–/5		SITTING BALANCE	Good; edge of bed using BUE to support self
SENSATION	Intact for light-touch sensation except for lack of protective sensation in all areas of plantar surfaces of feet, proprioception intact except for impaired in bilateral great toes and ankles		STANDING BALANCE	Poor; needs moderate assist with FWW
			GAIT	Unable
			STAIRS	Unable
BED MOBILITY	Tot. A of 1 person		SITTING TOLERANCE	10 minutes edge of bed
SUPINE TO SIT/SIT TO SUPINE	Max. A			

Evaluation

DIAGNOSIS	Neuromuscular, pattern E, and musculoskeletal, pattern I
PROGNOSIS	Good. The patient is S/P right hip fracture and ORIF after falling at the bottom of the stairs in his home where he lives independently with his wife of 61 years. She is in good health but has some back problems and is 81 years old and unable to assist him with any lifting. She can handle cooking, cleaning, etc. Two grown children live in the area but work full time and are unable to help at home after discharge. Because of complications, especially of diabetes and Parkinson disease, the patient will experience a slow but gradual return to his prior level of function. He does have the motivation and wants to work toward a return to his home. He states eventually he will have to live in a "home" but hopes to postpone that as long as possible. He has been participating in a group exercise class for Parkinson patients and had been ambulating with a cane, although not for distances greater than household distances (about 100 feet). He states he is interested in trying a pool program because he heard it was good for people with Parkinson. He has recently started

taking Sinemet for his PD symptoms of bradykinesia, rigidity, and balance problems. The patient will be evaluated for transfer to an inpatient rehabilitation setting at D/C for transitioning to home setting. If he is unable to tolerate the intensive therapies, he will need a 6- to 12-week ECF stay to achieve at least a supervised level of ADLs so that his wife can provide care as he continues to recover. The patient will also benefit from a speech therapy consult because of slowness of speech and swallowing problems that may have worsened with this hospitalization; a consult has been requested. As a result of complications of PD and neuropathies related to diabetes, the patient will likely have a slower-than-normal return to functional level and slow healing of this recent hip fracture because of delayed wound healing secondary to diabetes; he has a supportive wife and children who live in the area and also appears to be motivated for rehabilitation. He has good potential to eventually reach his goal of returning home but will likely need additional inpatient rehabilitation after this acute stay.

Plan of Care

PATIENT'S GOALS	The goal is for him to go home, but he agrees he may need additional rehabilitation before going home; he would also like to be able to return to his group exercise classes for people with PD at the local YMCA.	DISCHARGE GOALS	1. Bed mobility and transfers: Mod. A of two persons 2. Gait: Mod. A of two persons, 10 ft with FWW 3. Home exercise program: Min. A

continued

Acute Care Physical Therapy Initial Evaluation *continued*
Plan of Care

TIME TO ACHIEVE GOALS	By time of discharge	FREQUENCY	BID
PATIENT/FAMILY UNDERSTAND/AGREES WITH GOALS	Patient/Spouse yes	PATIENT EDUCATION TOPIC(S)	Activity; RLE TTWB status; call for help with transfers for safety
INTERVENTIONS	Bed mobility training	TAUGHT BY	PT
	Transfer training	WHO WAS TAUGHT	Patient, spouse
	Balance training	METHOD OF INSTRUCTION	Verbal/demonstration
	Gait training		
	Home program	EVALUATION OF LEARNING	Needs reinforcement
	Therapeutic exercise		
	Therapeutic activities		
	Family training PRN		
	Diabetic foot care education		

Acute Care Nursing Note

01/03/2010   5:00 PM

The patient reports pain at 7/10 after a physical therapy session earlier in the afternoon; he is being given two Percocet tablets with good effect. Oxygen saturation is in the 85% to 88% range on room air, so continuous monitoring is in place. The orders are to maintain above 93% oxygen saturation. The patient is on 2 LPM supplemental O_2 via nasal cannula. Foley is draining amber urine. The suture line is approximated, and the dressing is clean, dry, and intact. He complains of constipation, which is relieved with a suppository. He gets up on a bedside commode with two-person assist. He is eating about 50% of meals. His wife and family are visiting. The patient plans to D/C to ECF.

Acute Care Social Work Note

01/04/2010   5:55 PM

The patient has Parkinson disease and was admitted for hip fracture. The patient and his wife state they wish to have the patient D/C to ECF because wife is unable to care for him. He would prefer to go to one near his home so will be placed on a hotlist for Country Gardens and Healing Touch Convalescent Centers for the next available bed. The patient is on Medicare with Blue Cross supplemental and would qualify for an ECF stay. No other social work needs have been identified at this time, but follow-up will continue.

BOX 12-1 | Health-Care Team Member Role: Occupational Therapist

OTs and COTAs work in a variety of inpatient and outpatient settings to help patients recover from injury or illness. Their focus is to help patients learn better how to take care of themselves. They may specialize in hand or upper extremity therapy, where PTs work more with lower extremity problems. They also are more specially trained than PTs in general to assess and provide treatment for patients with cognitive dysfunction. They work closely with speech language pathologists in that area as well as with feeding concerns. OTs may also work in settings providing consultation for return to work. For more information on the occupational therapy profession, see the following website: http://www.aota.org.

Acute Care Occupational Therapy Summary

01/03/2010   2:55 PM

Patient is an 83-year-old male who presents with right hip fracture and ORIF. PMH includes Parkinson disease and DM II. He is alert and oriented to self and place. He is unable to recall TTWB precautions, nor can he follow them. His wife states he is unusually confused. He guards RUE use with PROM tolerated to 60 degrees of shoulder flexion. His left shoulder tolerates 90 degrees of flexion. RUE strength is grossly 2+/5 and limited by pain. LUE strength is grossly 3–/5. The patient currently requires Tot. A with lower body dressing, bathing, and toilet use. Commode transfers require Max. A of two persons. He requires Min. A for upper body dressing. He is independent with grooming from W/C level. He is able to feed himself with his right hand, protecting his shoulder, but coughed while eating a meal today. He is motivated to participate in therapies and his own care, but very limited by TTWB precautions, overall weakness, and hip pain. The patient's goal is eventual return to home, but he will need ECF stay for rehabilitation before D/C.

Acute Care Speech Therapy Summary

01/03/2010   10:23 AM

The patient is an 83-year-old male S/P right hip fracture and ORIF with Parkinson disease. He has learned compensatory strategies for swallowing due to poor swallowing and generally does well. He also exhibits diminished vocal intensity during speech evaluation. Nursing staff will supervise while the patient is eating, and the SLP will recommend further services to address both speech and swallowing function in the ECF setting.

ACUTE CARE CRITICAL THINKING QUESTIONS

After reviewing the acute care physical therapy initial evaluation and other discipline notes, address the following:

1. What are the patient's impairments? Functional limitations? Is there a disability?

   _____
   _____

2. Find assessments of gait, strength, ROM, and balance if available from the initial evaluation and list.

   a. How could each potentially be used to assess function and demonstrate progress toward goals or show the patient's response to physical therapy interventions?

   _____
   _____
   _____

   b. What would be the most important items to document for this patient?

   _____
   _____
   _____

3. After reviewing the POC and the treatment principles summarized in Box 12-2, describe a possible next treatment session.

   a. List the activities/exercises and your rationale for the order of treatment activities that you selected.

   _____
   _____
   _____

4. What subjective information will you gather during your session to help in your treatment of this patient and why?

   _____
   _____
   _____
   _____

5. What tests or measures will you use to assess the patient's progress and response to treatment?

   _____
   _____
   _____

continued

ACUTE CARE CRITICAL THINKING QUESTIONS *continued*

6. What subjective or objective information that you gather during the treatment might cause you to alter your treatment for this patient and why?

_____

_____

7. How would you document your treatment in the SOAP or Patient/Client Management format?

_____

_____

_____

_____

8. If the treatment went as expected, what would you do for the next treatment?

_____

_____

9. How would you expect this patient to progress over time?

_____

_____

10. If the patient does not progress as expected, what might be some reasons for a lack of progress?

_____

_____

11. What signs or symptoms, if observed or reported by the patient, would cause you to hold treatment and check with the nursing staff, primary PT, or MD?

_____

_____

_____

12. Are there any cultural, socioeconomic, or ethical issues presented in this case that might affect your interventions or communication with this patient? If so, how?

_____

_____

_____

_____

13. Re-review this case. Are there any coexisting medical diagnoses that might affect how this patient responds to physical therapy? If so, what are they, and how might they cause the patient to respond to physical therapy differently than you expected?

_____

_____

_____

14. After reviewing the other disciplines' notes regarding this patient, is there any other information that will help you to plan your treatment sessions?

_____

_____

_____

15. Compare your responses on this case with those of your classmates or instructors. What, if anything, would you change and why?

_____

_____

_____

Medical Update

01/05/2010

Upon discharge from the acute setting on 01/5/2010, the patient is S/P ORIF of right hip for intertrochanteric fracture. His laboratory results are as follows: CBC: hemoglobin 10.2, hematocrit 30.6, platelets 150,000; PT/INR 1.5. The following medications have been added: MS Contin 15 mg every 12 hours, hydrocodone 5 mg/325 mg three times daily for breakthrough pain, Coumadin 5 mg daily; and Tylenol arthritis 650 mg 1 to 2 tablets three times daily as needed for arthritic pain. The plan is to discharge the patient to ECF with physical therapy, occupational therapy, speech therapy, and social work consults and to follow up with orthopedic surgeon in 1 month. Weight-bearing, per the orthopedist, is as follows: TTWB until orthopedic follow-up. PT/INR is to be checked in 3 days.

BOX 12-2 | Parkinson Disease Treatment Principles

This summary was modified from lesson 6 of APTA's Self Study Course, Topics in Physical Therapy: Neurology, written by Margaret L. Schenkman, PT, PhD.[3]

The following scale helps define or classify where a patient with Parkinson disease is in the typical progression of the disease. The POC written by the PT will outline appropriate interventions and give guidance to the PTA; however, understanding the patient's stage of disease will help the PTA focus the treatment interventions appropriately.

Modified Hoehn and Yahr (H & Y) Staging

Stage 0	No signs of disease
Stage 1	Unilateral disease
Stage 2	Bilateral or midline involvement without impairment of balance
Stage 2.5	Mild bilateral disease; recovery on pull test
Stage 3	Mild to moderate bilateral disease; some postural instability; physically independent
Stage 4	Severe disability; still able to walk or stand unassisted
Stage 5	Wheelchair bound or bedridden unless aided

The following table describes the various direct effects of Parkinson disease and the secondary or indirect effects:

DIRECT EFFECTS OF PARKINSON DISEASE	INDIRECT EFFECTS (EXAMPLES)
Rigidity	Decreased muscle flexibility
Tremor	Decreased cardiorespiratory function
Postural instability	Increased thoracic kyphosis
Bradykinesia (akinesia, "freezing," motor planning problems with sequencing and simultaneous tasks)	Decreased lumbar lordosis
	Decreased spinal mobility

The following treatment principles can help the PTA focus interventions appropriately with patients who have Parkinson disease:

1. Treat direct effects (of the disease process) with compensatory and preventative techniques
2. Treat indirect effects with corrective and preventative techniques
3. Treat impairments first if needed to perform a functional task
4. Help patients optimize movement strategies by incorporating improved impairments into functional exercises
5. Use atypical strategies judiciously
6. Practice tasks in various environments and circumstances
7. Use sensory enhancement strategies such as auditory cues (external or internal) like music
8. As disease progresses, use more compensatory techniques:

   • Task or environment modification
   • Determine cost vs. benefit of assistive devices

9. Coordinate treatment sessions with medications
10. Encourage patient responsibility
11. General focus of interventions by H & Y stages:

    • H & Y 1 to 2: Improve impairments, prevent cardio and musculoskeletal impairments
    • H & Y 3: Use corrective and compensatory techniques to reduce fall risk and maximize functional ability
    • H & Y 4 to 5: Prevent further pathology, maximize comfort and quality of life, provide family and caregiver training

Skilled Nursing Facility Physical Therapy Evaluation

NAME	Alfred Jones
SOC DATE	01/06/2010
ONSET DATE	01/02/2010
PRIMARY DIAGNOSIS	Right hip fracture S/P ORIF
TREATMENT DIAGNOSIS	Difficulty in walking
PAYOR	Medicare A
SHORT-TERM GOALS	1. Bed mobility: Patient will transition from supine to sit with Min. A and 50% verbal cues for sequencing to increase level of independence. 2. Transfer: Patient will perform stand pivot transfer with Min. A and FWW and 50% verbal cues for sequencing to increase his level of independence. 3. Standing balance/Tinetti: Patient will increase his balance score to 12/16 and gait score to 8/12 for total of 20/28 on Tinetti balance test, placing him at moderate fall risk, to decrease his risk for falls and improve his ambulation in environment. 4. Gait: Patient will ambulate 50 feet with Min. A and 50% verbal cues and FWW for safety to increase level of independence. 5. Standing tolerance: Patient will tolerate standing for 5 minutes in parallel bars without a rest break to increase endurance for ambulation in environment.
OUTCOME (long-term, in 12 weeks)	Mod. I with ambulation to 300 feet indoors, 100 feet outdoors on varied surfaces and up/down one flight stairs with two rails in order to return to his home safely. Supervised for home exercise program.
PLAN	97001—Physical therapy evaluation 97110—Therapeutic exercise 97116—Gait training 97530—Therapeutic activities G0283—Electrical stimulation (unattended) to one or more areas, for indication(s) other than wound
The resident and/or responsible party understands the proposed treatment and	The rehabilitation potential is good. Prognostic indicator: The patient is able to follow multistep directions, is alert and oriented, and has good motivation and

the expected benefit and risks if any that are associated with the plan. The resident and/or responsible party agrees to the treatment as prescribed.

family support to return home at close to prior level of function.

FREQUENCY/DURATION	6 per week x 12 weeks
CERTIFICATION	N/A
PRIOR HOSPITALIZATION	From 01/02/2010 through 01/06/2010
PRECAUTIONS	TTWB RLE, fall risk, peripheral neuropathy
INITIAL ASSESSMENT (history, medical complications, level of function at start of care, reason for referral)	PLOF: The patient is Mod. I in his home, with two steps to enter and one rail, and with one flight of stairs with two rails inside the home to the upstairs bedrooms. He used a cane but also has an old walker that his wife used years ago. He has a tub-shower combo with grab bars installed and a raised toilet seat. He has been considering placing a ramp at the front of his home and remodeling a downstairs den into a bedroom. History: This 83-year-old patient fell at the bottom of the stairs while descending and fractured his right hip on 01/02/2010. He underwent ORIF and was admitted to a SNF setting 01/06/2010 for rehabilitation with a goal to return home. He also strained his right shoulder in the fall, with no fracture. He has a PMH including the following: Parkinson disease, DM II, HTN, peripheral neuropathy, osteoarthritis, left TKR, mild obesity, and aspiration pneumonia 1 year ago. He has a supportive wife at his bedside during assessment today. He states that his goal is to walk again and return to his exercise classes in the community designed for people with PD. He is also wondering whether an aquatic program would be good for him. He states he wants to lose weight. Although he wants to get home as soon as possible, he is willing to stay longer in order to be independent because he knows his wife cannot care for him.
DC PLANS	Return to home with wife to continue with cooking and cleaning but independent with self-care activities. Outpatient follow-up.

ASSESSMENT			

ASSESSMENT	Orientation: Alert and oriented x 4.		Left hip flexion 3+/5, quadriceps 4–/5,

ASSESSMENT

Orientation: Alert and oriented x 4.
Cognition: Follows one- or two-step directions; some STML.
Bed mobility: Mod. A
Sitting balance: Static: good, dynamic: fair
Sit to stand with FWW: Mod. A
Standing balance: Fair with FWW; Tinetti balance score 8/16, gait score 5/12, total score 13/28 placing him at high fall risk
Stand pivot transfer with FWW: Mod. A for sit to stand, then Min. A for pivot with verbal cues to maintain TTWB RLE
Posture: Stands with hips flexed, thoracic kyphosis, and forward head
Gait: Min. A x 10 feet with FWW and W/C follow; holds right hip in external rotation and flexion, needs verbal cues to maintain TTWB RLE
Endurance: Sits edge of bed x 15 minutes, in W/C x 60 minutes, stands x 1 minute
SpO_2 before activity: 98% on room air
SpO_2 during activity: 89% on room air; up to 92% after 3-minute seated rest break
Pain: Right anterior and lateral hip incisional pain and aching at 7/10 at rest, 9/10 with activity; right shoulder pain 5/10 at rest and 7/10 with use of FWW for standing and gait
MMT: Right hip flexion 2–/5, quadriceps 3–/5, ankle dorsiflexion and plantarflexion 4/5

Left hip flexion 3+/5, quadriceps 4–/5, ankle dorsiflexion and plantarflexion 4/5
AROM: Limited in right hip due to pain; others WFL, other than bilateral knee extension lacks 20 degrees and hips lack 5 degrees from neutral hip extension.
Tone: Rigidity throughout trunk and extremities
Sensation: Intact BLE for light touch
Protective sensation: Impaired bilateral feet
Proprioception: Impaired bilateral ankles and great toes

FUNCTIONAL STATUS AT SOC

1. Bed mobility: Patient transitions from supine to sit with Mod. A and verbal cues for sequencing.
2. Transfer: Patient is able to perform stand pivot transfer with Mod. A and FWW and verbal cues for sequencing.
3. Standing balance/Tinetti: Patient scores 8/16 on balance score and 5/12 on gait score for total of 15/28 on Tinetti balance test, placing him at high fall risk.
4. Gait: Patient ambulates 10 feet with Mod. A, W/C followed by second person and FWW for safety. Verbal cues 75% of time to maintain TTWB RLE.
5. Standing tolerance: Patient stands for 1 minute with FWW without a rest break.

Skilled Nursing Facility Nursing Note

01/06/2010   11:34 AM

This resident was admitted today S/P ORIF for right hip fracture. He transferred from a W/C onto a bed with two-person assist. He is able to make his needs known. An alarm has been placed for safety. Foley is draining light amber urine. He is continent of bowel. His vital signs are as follows: temperature 36.7°C, resting pulse 79 BPM, RR 18 respirations per minute, BP 120/72 mm Hg, SpO_2 95% on room air at rest. The resident complains of right hip pain at 8/10; he was given one Percocet tablet, with good relief 1 hour later. The resident will continue his medications from the hospital. He is on an ADA diet.

Skilled Nursing Facility Social Work Summary

01/09/2010   4:29 PM

The patient was admitted on 01/06/2010 S/P right hip fracture and ORIF. A care conference was held today with the patient, his wife, his daughter, PT, OT, SLP, LPN, and MSW present. The therapists are reporting a good start to rehabilitation in this setting, with the patient participating well but limited somewhat by pain. The nursing staff are to address improved pain control. The PT will also try electrical stimulation for enhanced pain control before therapy. The patient and his family express a desire to stay as long as possible to get as close to independent as he can. The current plan is to D/C home with outpatient physical therapy follow-up and an assistive device and other equipment to be determined. D/C tentatively planned for 8 to 12 weeks, depending on progress.

Skilled Nursing Facility Occupational Therapy Summary

01/07/2010   2:59 PM

The patient was evaluated today after admission yesterday from an acute setting S/P right hip fracture and ORIF. He is alert and oriented x 4, recalling TTWB precautions but having difficulty following them in standing. The patient has good potential to reach his goal of returning home, but progress will be slowed because of the combination of ongoing Parkinson symptoms and TTWB precautions. STG for the next 2 weeks are as follows:

1. Upper body dressing to Mod. I from seated position
2. Lower body dressing to SBA with reacher
3. Able to adjust clothing for toileting with SBA while the OT supports for balance and cues for weight-bearing precautions
4. Bathing of front of upper body to supervised in seated position; front of lower body with Mod. A using a long-handled sponge
5. Decrease right shoulder pain to 3/10 at rest and 5/10 with dressing activities through use of modalities to allow the patient to return to his prior level of function

---

Skilled Nursing Facility Speech Language Pathology Summary

01/07/2010   12:54 PM

The patient was evaluated today and found to have mild swallowing difficulties. He has been assigned to the supervised dining room for all meals and regular diet. He began exercises to promote improved vocal intensity, as well, and the PT, OT, and nursing staff will encourage the patient in speaking up during sessions. He will benefit from continued outpatient speech therapy to progress his exercise program after discharge.

SKILLED NURSING FACILITY CRITICAL THINKING QUESTIONS

After reviewing the skilled nursing facility physical therapy initial evaluation and other discipline notes, address the following:

1. What are the patient's impairments? Functional limitations? Is there a disability?

_____

_____

_____

_____

2. Find assessments of gait, strength, ROM, and balance if available from the initial evaluation and list.

   a. How could each potentially be used to assess function and demonstrate progress toward goals or show the patient's response to physical therapy interventions?

_____

_____

_____

b. What would be the most important items to document for this patient?

_____

_____

_____

3. After reviewing the POC and the treatment principles summarized in Box 12-2, describe a possible next treatment session.

   a. List the activities/exercises and your rationale for the order of treatment activities that you selected.

_____

_____

_____

4. What subjective information will you gather during your session to help in your treatment of this patient and why?

_____

_____

_____

5. What tests or measures will you use to assess the patient's progress and response to treatment?

_____

_____

6. What subjective or objective information that you gather during the treatment might cause you to alter your treatment for this patient and why?

_____

_____

7. How would you document your treatment in the SOAP or Patient/Client Management format?

_____

_____

_____

_____

8. If the treatment goes as expected, what will you do for the next treatment?

_____

_____

9. How would you expect this patient to progress over time?

_____

_____

10. If the patient does not progress as expected, what might be some reasons for a lack of progress?

_____

_____

11. What signs or symptoms, if observed or reported by the patient, would cause you to hold treatment and check with the nursing staff, primary PT, or MD?

_____

_____

12. Are there any cultural, socioeconomic, or ethical issues presented in this case that might affect your interventions or communication with this patient? If so, how?

_____

_____

13. Re-review this case. Are there any coexisting medical diagnoses that might affect how this patient responds to physical therapy? If so, what are they, and how might they cause the patient to respond to physical therapy differently than you expected?

_____

_____

14. After reviewing the other disciplines' notes regarding this patient, is there any other information that will help you to plan your treatment sessions?

_____

_____

15. Compare your responses on this case with those of your classmates or instructors. What, if anything, would you change and why?

_____

_____

Outpatient Physical Therapy Evaluation

NAME: Alfred Jones

DATE: April 22, 2010

DIAGNOSIS: Right hip fracture with ORIF, WBAT

SUBJECTIVE INFORMATION: The patient states that he has been home for a week from the SNF setting where he received physical and occupational therapy for his right hip and right shoulder. He is now independent with all self-care activities but has limited endurance and continues with pain, which is now rated at 4/10 in the right hip and minimal in the shoulder. His hip pain increases with walking and other weight-bearing activities and lessens with rest. He is still taking Tylenol for pain as well as one Percocet tablet about every other day. He can walk about two blocks with his FWW but is slow and feels he is walking "funny." He would like to return to a group exercise class and a regular walking program and is also interested in going to the pool. Overall, he has lost a few pounds during the past couple of months because of dieting but would like to continue with a weight loss program to alleviate some of the strain on his body along with the effects of the PD.

continued

Outpatient Physical Therapy Evaluation *continued*

OBJECTIVE INFORMATION		ASSESSMENT	The patient has limited PROM and limited strength and balance, leading to gait abnormalities. He also has postural dysfunction, likely related to PD, which contributes to his functional limitations. All of these contribute to and are a part of his pain presentation of the right hip S/P ORIF for fracture. The patient is unable to participate in an independent exercise program that will help him manage his long-term effects of PD and diabetes and will benefit from skilled therapy services to address the following goals:
POSTURE	Thoracic kyphosis and forward-head posture; right ilium appears higher than left		
GAIT	Mild **Trendelenburg** gait pattern bilaterally, right greater than left; ambulates with FWW with about equal step lengths, and inadequate ankle dorsiflexion for foot clearance		
BALANCE	BERG balance test total score 42/56		
STRENGTH	Right shoulder abduction 4–/5 with pain on contraction; otherwise BUE WNL Right hip flexion 4–/5, abduction 3–/5, quadriceps 4/5; left hip abduction 3/5; other BLE WNL Functional strength test: The patient is able to perform three step-ups on 6-inch step with good form on LLE and needs tactile cues to hip abductors to facilitate good form on RLE for one step up; unable to perform step-down with good form on either side	STG (2 weeks)	1. Increase PROM right hip to neutral extension bilaterally and ankle dorsiflexion with knees straight to 5 degrees bilaterally to allow more normal gait pattern and prevent further pain and dysfunction. 2. Decrease pain in RLE to 1/10 with activities that will allow him to return to a more independent home exercise program. 3. Increase BERG balance test score to 50/56 to increase safety and decrease risk for fall.
PROM	Right hip flexion 10 to 90 degrees; left hip flexion 5 to 110 degrees Right knee flexion 14 to 130 degrees, left knee flexion 10 to 125 degrees Bilateral ankle dorsiflexion with knees straight to neutral and knees bent to 5 degrees Right SLR 55 degrees; left SLR 65 degrees	LTG	The patient will be independent with a home exercise program of stretching, strengthening, and cardiovascular endurance activities on a daily basis with the use of a written home exercise program. He will be able to manage his pain through exercise and home use of heat and cold as needed.
PALPATION	Tenderness at right greater trochanter, proximal to distal iliotibial band and lateral knee, quadratus lumborum; right supraspinatus tendon insertion also tender to palpation	PLAN	Two to three times per week for 8 weeks, he will receive manual therapy and heat, cold, and electrical stimulation modalities to increase ROM and decrease pain, along with therapeutic exercise, including aquatic exercise and gait training. A progressive home exercise program will be developed.
SENSATION	Light-touch and hot-cold sensation intact on back, BUE, and BLE; impaired proprioception bilateral great toes and ankles		

BOX 12-3 | Physical Therapy Specialty: Aquatics

Aquatic therapy is a specialty within the practice of physical therapy and is used in many settings across the continuum of care but mostly in the outpatient setting because of limitations in the acute and subacute settings, such as open wounds, incontinence and greater difficulty with transfers and mobility, which can limit access. Many patients can benefit from the unique environment that water provides to help them reach their physical therapy and fitness goals. Some outpatient clinics have pools on site, and others use pools in the community to provide one-to-one aquatic interventions. Other patients can benefit from group exercise classes that can be taught by PTs, PTAs, or other trained exercise professionals. Some patients do not need sessions taught by physical therapy staff but are recommended to use community classes at the local YMCA, health club, or community pool. For more information on aquatic therapy, visit the following websites: http://www.aquaticpt.org for the APTA's Aquatic PT Section web page and http://www.aeawave.com for the Aquatic Exercise Association web page.

OUTPATIENT CRITICAL THINKING QUESTIONS

After reviewing the outpatient physical therapy evaluation, address the following:

1. What are the patient's impairments? Functional limitations? Is there a disability?

_____

_____

2. Find assessments of gait, strength, ROM, and balance if available from the initial evaluation and list.

   a. How could each potentially be used to assess function and demonstrate progress toward goals or show the patient's response to physical therapy interventions?

   _____

   _____

   _____

   b. What would be the most important items to document for this patient?

   _____

   _____

   _____

   _____

3. After reviewing the POC and the treatment principles summarized in Box 12-2, describe a possible next treatment session.

   a. List the activities/exercises and your rationale for the order of treatment activities that you selected.

   _____

   _____

   _____

   _____

4. What subjective information will you gather during your session to help in your treatment of this patient and why?

_____

_____

5. What tests or measures will you use to assess the patient's progress and response to treatment?

_____

_____

6. What subjective or objective information that you gather during the treatment might cause you to alter your treatment for this patient and why?

_____

_____

_____

7. How would you document your treatment in the SOAP or Patient/Client Management format?

_____

_____

_____

_____

8. If the treatment goes as expected, what will you do for the next treatment?

_____

_____

_____

9. How would you expect this patient to progress over time?

_____

_____

continued

OUTPATIENT CRITICAL THINKING QUESTIONS *continued*

10. If the patient does not progress as expected, what might be some reasons for a lack of progress?

_____

_____

11. What signs or symptoms, if observed or reported by the patient, would cause you to hold treatment and check with the nursing staff, primary PT, or MD?

_____

_____

_____

12. Are there any cultural, socioeconomic, or ethical issues presented in this case that might affect your interventions or communication with this patient? If so, how?

_____

_____

_____

13. Re-review this case. Are there any coexisting medical diagnoses that might affect how this patient responds to physical therapy? If so, what are they, and how might they cause the patient to respond to physical therapy differently than you expected?

_____

_____

14. After reviewing the other disciplines' notes regarding this patient, is there any other information that will help you to plan your treatment sessions?

_____

_____

15. Compare your responses on this case with those of your classmates or instructors. What, if anything, would you change and why?

_____

_____

CONTINUUM OF CARE CRITICAL THINKING QUESTIONS

After reviewing the continuum of care for this patient, consider the following:

1. How did the patient's problems change over the months after his fracture?

_____

_____

_____

_____

_____

2. How did this affect the goals and the interventions that the PT included in the POC?

_____

_____

_____

_____

3. How were the same interventions modified over time to progress the patient according to his changing needs?

_____

_____

_____

_____

4. What are some potential community resources that this patient might like to participate in and how would these help him to maintain and improve his physical fitness?

_____

_____

_____

IMPLICATIONS OF PATHOLOGY FOR THE PTA[2]

1. What are Mr. Jones' risk factors for falls and how might the PTA incorporate fall reduction education and techniques throughout the interventions in the different settings?

_____

_____

_____

_____

_____

2. What signs and symptoms should the PTA watch out for that might indicate the following kinds of complications, which are common with hip fracture: DVT, pulmonary complications, and infection? What would you do as the PTA if your patient exhibited any of these signs or symptoms?

_____

_____

_____

_____

_____

3. With patients who have had ORIF after a hip fracture, the physician will sometimes allow WBAT. Why is it important for the PTA to observe changes in the following areas when the patient is ambulating without weight-bearing restrictions, especially more independently: cognitive and decision-making capabilities, sensation including proprioception, upper body strength, vestibular function, and balance?

_____

_____

_____

_____

_____

4. How might the timing of Parkinson disease medications affect the physical therapy interventions?

_____

_____

_____

_____

_____

_____

_____

5. How would cognitive impairment, as is common with later stages of Parkinson disease, affect your approach during the physical therapy interventions?

_____

_____

_____

_____

_____

_____

6. What should the PTA be aware of when working with patients with the following:
   • Spinal fractures
   • Lower extremity fractures
   • Upper extremity fractures

_____

_____

_____

_____

_____

References

1. American Physical Therapy Association: Guide to Physical Therapist Practice, Second Edition. Alexandria, VA: Author, 2001.

2. Goodman CC, Boissonnault FG, Fuller KS: Pathology: Implications for the Physical Therapist, Second Edition. Philadelphia: Saunders, 2003.

3. Schenkman ML: Update on Clinical Features, Pathology/Pathophysiology, and Management, Lesson 6. Alexandria, VA: American Physical Therapy Association, 2002.

CHAPTER 13

Katie Wilson: A Patient With Cerebral Palsy

 Preferred Practice Pattern: Neuromuscular, Pattern C

CHAPTER OUTLINE

Introducing Katie Wilson

Katie is a 7-year-old girl with spastic diplegic cerebral palsy. According to the APTA's *Guide to Physical Therapist Practice* (the *Guide*), this patient could have a number of impairments, including the following:

- Impaired affect, arousal, attention, and cognition
- Impaired motor function
- Loss of balance
- Impaired communication

Functional limitations may include the following:

- Difficulty negotiating terrains
- Difficulty planning movements
- Difficulty with positioning
- Frequent falls[1]

Please refer to the *Guide*[1] for a complete list of possible impairments. As you work through this case, think about which of these the patient is experiencing. Also, keep in mind that a patient such as Katie will likely be receiving outpatient physical therapy services as well. Her physical therapy and other goals related to her special needs are linked with her education needs. Therapy is provided in the school setting if the team determines it is necessary for the student to benefit from their educational program. Providing the services the student needs to be as successful as possible is required by law. For information about the history of these laws in the United States, see the following website: http://www 2.ed.gov/policy/speced/leg/idea/history.html.

Vocabulary List

Hypertonicity	Anoxia
Neonatal	

BOX 13-1 | Physical Therapy Specialty: Pediatrics

Pediatrics is a large specialty within the field of physical therapy. Pediatric therapists and assistants work in a number of settings, including outpatient, acute care, and school settings with patients that range in age from premature babies to teens. They specialize in the treatment of common pediatric disorders, such as cerebral palsy and the effects of Down syndrome, but also work with children and adolescents who have sports or other injuries. It is important to remember that the disorders commonly seen in childhood, such as cerebral palsy, are often the cause of problems later in life and that these patients will often need ongoing or intermittent physical therapy to address their needs throughout the life span. When working with pediatric patients, the PT or PTA must also work closely with the parents to facilitate follow-through with the therapy program at home. Another feature of pediatric physical therapy is that often the therapy is designed to be "fun and games" in order to obtain the highest level of involvement possible with the child. Just as in therapy with the adult, PTs and PTAs are always looking at function and how the impairments affect function at home and in the work place; so with children, it is important to know how their impairments affect function in school, home, and other environments. For more information on the Pediatric Section of the APTA, see http://www.pediatricapta.org. In the following case, notice that the PT has used the School Function Assessment to provide objective data regarding this patient's functional status within the school setting. Because of the length of the assessment, the full document is not provided here, but only parts are summarized in Box 4-2. For more information on this particular assessment, please refer to the following website: www.pearsonassessments.com/HAIWEB/Cultures/en-us/Productdetail.htm?Pid=076-1615-709&Mode=summary.

Physical Therapy Initial Evaluation and Plan of Care

STUDENT	Katie Wilson	TONE	Increased in hamstrings, adductors, plantarflexors BLE
DATE	10/06/2010		
BIRTH DATE	06/19/2003	SENSATION	Impaired light touch below knees and proprioception of ankles, toes BLE
SCHOOL	Washington Elementary School		
PRECAUTIONS	Seizures, peanut allergy	STRENGTH	BLE able to move through partial range with gravity eliminated
MEDICAL HISTORY & MEDICATIONS	Cerebral palsy with **hypertonicity** affecting BLE; seizure disorder; peanut allergy Medications: Dilantin 50 mg PO three times daily; Baclofen 40 mg daily PO. Weight: 50 pounds	BALANCE/POSTURE	Sacral sits with legs adducted and needs Min. A to maintain position; needs Mod. A to maintain standing with BUE support.
		ENDURANCE	Fair, shortness of breath with stairs and ambulation
		TRANSFERS	Transfers from W/C to plinth using scoot-across technique with Min. A
PRIOR LEVEL OF FUNCTION	She has been needing assist with toileting, bathing, dressing, ambulation, and W/C mobility. She was working on ambulation in her prior school.	GAIT	She needs a posture-control walker, bilateral AFOs, and Mod. A with cues and tactile facilitation to decrease scissoring and increase step length for 50 feet on level surfaces. She needs Mod. A to ascend/descend four steps with two handrails. She is unable to run.
SOCIAL HISTORY	She lives with her single mother, her mother's boyfriend, and two siblings aged 3 and 9 years. She does not have contact with her father. She makes friends easily at school and is in the second grade with part-time special education classes.		
		WHEELCHAIR MOBILITY/SEATING	She propels herself in a manual W/C for 25 feet in 7 minutes. She is able to independently manipulate brakes and footrests but needs cues to remember brakes before transfers. An adductor wedge in the W/C promotes improved alignment and sitting balance.
LIVING SITUATION & EQUIPMENT	She lives in an upstairs apartment with a flight of stairs to enter. Her mother has been carrying her up and down stairs. She uses her posture-control walker to ambulate short distances with assistance. She uses a manual W/C inside the apartment and in school. She has bilateral AFOs and uses them all day.		
		TEST SCORES	School function assessment: See summary scores in Box 4-2.
		DIAGNOSIS	Neuromuscular pattern C
SYSTEMS REVIEW	Her cardiopulmonary and integumentary systems are clear. Her cognition and communication are mildly impaired. Her hearing and vision are adequate, and she wears glasses. She has behavioral problems at home and school with temper tantrums three or four times daily.	PROGNOSIS	The patient qualifies for and will benefit from skilled physical therapy intervention to address the following goals, with the ultimate outcome being improved ability to perform in school setting, promoting greater learning. She has good potential to meet the goals as stated. She has adequate family support, although her single mother who has two other children and works full-time needs additional resources to ensure best outcomes.
PROM	Bilateral ankle dorsiflexion 5 degrees from neutral Bilateral SLR 55 degrees Bilateral hip flexion 95 degrees, extension to neutral Bilateral hip abduction 10 degrees		

continued

Physical Therapy Initial Evaluation and Plan of Care *continued*

FREQUENCY OF THERAPY	45 minutes once per week
EXPECTED DURATION OF THERAPY SERVICES	One school calendar year to be re-evaluated annually for continued need
STRENGTHS	1. Katie can communicate problems or concerns related to her disability and participate in problem-solving solutions to address her needs. 2. Katie has shown progress in past therapy environments with ambulation and has a strong desire and motivation to improve in this area. 3. For her age, Katie has assumed a great deal of responsibility for her therapy program and works hard.
NEEDS	1. Katie needs to improve her speed and efficiency with W/C propulsion while negotiating the school premises. 2. Katie needs to improve her ability to transfer herself independently and safely to and from the wheelchair. 3. Katie needs to improve her strength, balance, endurance, and ROM for increased ease of movement and improved success with modified gross motor play activities at recess and during physical education classes.
PRIORITIES AMONG THERAPY INTERVENTION GOALS & OBJECTIVES	1. Katie will propel herself in the manual W/C 200 feet from her classroom to the cafeteria in 5 minutes by May 2011. 2. Katie will improve her strength, balance, endurance, and ROM to allow her to actively participate in physical education and recess activities for 20 minutes without a rest break in 2/3 opportunities by May 2011.

STUDENT IEP GOALS & OBJECTIVES	3. Katie will ambulate with a posture-control walker for 50 feet with supervision only to access classroom activities by May 2011. 4. Katie will be able to stand for 10 minutes at a table for appropriate classroom activities by May 2011.
STRATEGIES, METHODS, ACCOMMODATIONS, ENVIRONMENT USED TO ADDRESS NEEDS	Katie will receive specially designed instruction in the areas of reading, writing, and math. Physical therapy services will support her in these areas as well by improving her ability to achieve and maintain effective postures that will help her maximize attention and learning. Additionally, she will become more efficient with W/C propulsion and ambulation to allow her improved access to all school environments.
PLAN FOR RE-EVALUATION, METHOD OF DATA COLLECTION, DISCHARGE PLANNING	Strategies and methods: Direct physical therapy services, including therapeutic exercise and functional mobility training for transfer and W/C mobility skills; gait training and motor control activities as well as education for teaching staff and mother in the proper use of adaptive equipment and home exercise program. Environment: General and special education classrooms, playground or gym as appropriate. Katie will be re-evaluated at least every 3 years. Progress toward therapy goals will be documented in therapy notes. She will be discharged from therapy services when goals are met or she is unable to progress any further.

BOX 13-2 | Health-Care Team Member Role: Teacher

Teachers and their assistants are a vital part of the health-care team when working with children, especially within the school system. As indicated in the introduction to this chapter, therapy in the school setting must always be tied to the student's abilities and disabilities as related to his or her learning. Goals must always reflect the student's function in the school setting and be related to their academic level and activities. For preschool-aged children, appropriate therapies include fine and gross motor activities. As children age and move through the grade levels, therapy may focus more on using equipment and on teaching the student how best to function within his or her limitations. In all cases, the PTA must include the student's teachers and assistants. Often, the therapy staff will teach techniques or the best use of equipment. Other times, the teachers will provide therapy staff with much-needed information on the student's abilities within the classroom. Together with the rest of the team, therapists and teachers work toward the common goals of improving the ability of the child to learn. For more information on teaching and special education, see the National Association of Special Education Teachers website at http://www.naset.org.

Table 13-1 PARTS OF SCHOOL FUNCTION ASSESSMENT SUMMARY

	TOTAL RAW SCORE	CRITERION SCORE	STANDARD ERROR	CRITERION CUTOFF SCORE K-3
Part I Participation				
Regular Classroom	26	62	4	100
Part II Task Supports				
Physical Tasks—Assistance	25	54	5	100
Physical Tasks—Adaptations	24	53	5	100
Cognitive/Behavioral Tasks—Assistance	29	63	5	77
Cognitive/Behavioral Tasks—Adaptations	30	65	6	91
Part III Activity Performance				
Travel	55	62	2	100
Maintaining and Changing Positions	39	64	4	100
Recreational Movement	24	43	4	83
Manipulation With Movement	49	61	3	93
Using Materials	91	75	3	83
Setup and Cleanup	61	83	5	87
Eating and Drinking	56	100	15	100
Hygiene	58	83	8	92
Clothing Management	53	64	3	93
Up/Down Stairs	N/A			100
Written Work	37	66	4	73
Computer and Equipment Use	N/A			65

 Individualized Educational Program

DATE: October 12, 2010
STUDENT: Katie Wilson
STUDENT ID: 1234567
DATE OF BIRTH: June 19, 2003

Present Level of Educational Performance
MEDICAL-PHYSICAL: See Health Plan
ACADEMIC:
READING: She is reading at a mid-1st grade level. She uses strategies such as rereading and looking at picture cues. She needs continued instruction and practice to become more proficient in her decoding skills.

WRITING: She is able to write 24/26 upper case letters and 22/26 lower case letters with correct formation. She is beginning to work on capitalization, punctuation, and spacing. She needs to continue working on all of the above as well as begin working on the writing process.
MATH: She can count to 100 by 1s and 10s. She does not yet count by 2s or 5s. She uses the correct formation for all numbers except 4, 6, and 9. She can name and give values of coins with 90% accuracy. She can correctly answer addition problems using numbers 1 to 10 with 95% accuracy and subtraction problems using numbers 1 to 10 with 75% accuracy.

continued

Individualized Educational Program *continued*

FINE MOTOR:
Katie continues to work hard in therapy sessions. In occupational therapy, she is working on fine-motor skills to enhance her writing ability. Her mildly increased tone in both upper extremities reduces her success, but she is learning relaxation techniques to reduce tone and improve her writing. She is also working on manipulation skills to participate fully in classroom activities such as math manipulatives, games, and computer use.

GROSS MOTOR:
Katie receives physical therapy services as part of her IEP. She needs assistance to propel functional distances within the school setting in her manual W/C because of decreased strength and endurance. She needs assistance for transfers. She is beginning to work on ambulation skills using a posture-control walker and bilateral AFO braces. She has ROM, strength, balance, and endurance impairments that affect her ability to participate in physical education and recess activities with her peers.

Annual Goals and Objectives

READING: When given material at her instructional level, she will read the material with improved use of decoding strategies progressing to a mid-2nd grade level as measured by district assessment scores.

WRITING: When given a topic, she will follow the writing process to write 10 legible sentences using correct capitalization, ending punctuation, and spacing progressing to a mid-2nd grade level as measured by curriculum-based assessment and work samples.

MATH: When given math addition and subtraction problems using numbers 1 to 20, she will correctly solve problems with 90% accuracy as measured by curriculum-based scores.

FINE MOTOR: See Occupational Therapy Report
GROSS MOTOR: See Physical Therapy Report

Health Plan

HISTORY
Katie was born prematurely at 30 weeks to a mother who had uncontrolled maternal diabetes. Her **neonatal** period was complicated by low birthweight and **anoxia.** She has spastic diplegic cerebral palsy and uses a manual W/C for most mobility, although she is dependent on assistance.

PROBLEMS
• She has a seizure disorder related to the cerebral palsy and is on medication to prevent seizures.
• She has a peanut allergy.

NEED
School staff will recognize the signs and symptoms of potential impending seizure and allergic reactions to peanut exposure.

PLAN FOR RESOLUTION
Seizures
Symptoms and signs to observe:
• Headache
• Sudden mood change
• Lethargy
• Muscle jerking
• Stiffening; she may fall to the floor
Treatment:
• Lower her to the floor.
• Protect her from a fall or something falling on her during the seizure.
• Roll her onto her side if needed to maintain airway.
• If at any time she stops breathing, 9-1-1 should be called.
• Possible negative side effects of her medications include lethargy, nausea, irritability, and skin rashes. If these are observed, the nurse should be contacted or 9-1-1 called, if severe.

Peanut Exposure
Symptoms and signs to observe:
• Wheezing
• Low blood pressure
• Swelling
• Hives
• Clear, runny nose with or without sneezing
Treatment:
• Contact the school secretary immediately for epinephrine injection and call 9-1-1.

SEEING THE DIAGNOSIS IN ACTION 13-1

Children with cerebral palsy are often not diagnosed until they do not meet normal milestones for growth and development. There are different types of cerebral palsy, all affecting muscle tone and motor control. In general, there are types that cause lower-than-normal muscle tone and those that cause higher-than-normal muscle tone. PTs and PTAs who work with this patient population must understand the differences and learn facilitation and inhibition techniques typically used throughout functional activity training in order to promote more normalized motor control. However, depending on the severity of the disease, some patients with cerebral palsy may never achieve these normal movement patterns.

As an adult, persons with cerebral palsy may need physical therapy for ongoing or recurrent needs related to developmental progression and motor control. They may also require physical therapy for musculoskeletal dysfunction and pain related to abnormal muscle tone and function.

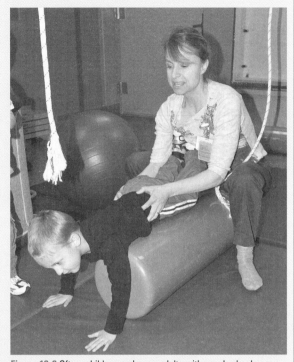

Figure 13-2 Often, children and even adults with cerebral palsy can learn more normal movement patterns by working in positions that are developmentally appropriate. In this photo, the patient performs a reaching activity while prone on a roll to improve balance reactions.

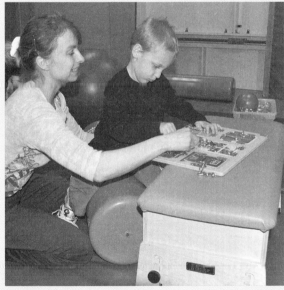

Figure 13-1 This patient with cerebral palsy performs a fine-motor activity while working on sitting balance. Often, these activities are addressed by both occupational and physical therapy, each discipline working toward the patient and family's goals in perhaps slightly different ways.

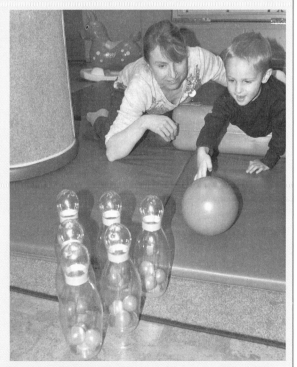

Figure 13-3 The prone position is one of the normal positions for development at certain stages in the infant. Using this position can help the child or adult to progress further in the developmental stages.

continued

SEEING THE DIAGNOSIS IN ACTION 13-1 *continued*

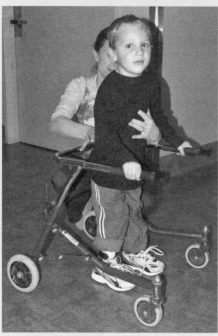

Figure 13-4 Once they have learned control in the earlier developmental positions of prone, supine, rolling, and sitting, patients can begin standing activities and then gait training. Here, the patient uses a posture-control walker to provide stability and facilitate more normal movement patterns. Adults with cerebral palsy may need physical therapy for ongoing or recurrent needs related to developmental progression and motor control. They may also require physical therapy for musculoskeletal dysfunction and pain related to abnormal muscle tone and function.

REVIEWING THE MEDICAL HISTORY

1. What do you already know about cerebral palsy?

_____

_____

_____

_____

_____

2. Review the vocabulary list, physical therapy evaluation, IEP, and health plan. Look up the meanings of any terms you do not understand in a medical dictionary or other text.

_____

_____

_____

_____

3. Review the diagnoses in the past medical history using a medical or pathology text, Internet resource, or other available resource.

_____

_____

_____

_____

_____

_____

_____

_____

_____

_____

_____

_____

4. Which diagnoses in the past medical history would be significant and potentially affect the patient's response to the physical therapy interventions?

_____

_____

_____

_____

_____

5. List the purpose and potential side effects for each of the medications the patient is taking.

_____

_____

_____

_____

_____

_____

CRITICAL THINKING QUESTIONS

After reviewing the physical therapy initial evaluation, IEP, and Health Plan, address the following:

1. What are the patient's impairments? Functional limitations? Is there a disability?

_____

_____

_____

2. Find assessments of gait, strength, ROM, and balance if available from the initial evaluation and list.

a. How could each potentially be used to assess function and demonstrate progress toward goals or show the patient's response to physical therapy interventions?

_____

_____

_____

b. What would be the most important items to document for this patient?

_____

_____

_____

3. After reviewing the POC, describe a possible next treatment session.

a. List the activities/exercises and your rationale for the order of treatment activities that you selected.

_____

_____

_____

_____

4. What subjective information will you gather during your session to help in your treatment of this patient and why?

_____

_____

5. What tests or measures will you use to assess the patient's progress and response to treatment?

_____

_____

6. What subjective or objective information that you gather during the treatment might cause you to alter your treatment for this patient and why?

_____

_____

_____

7. How would you document your treatment in the SOAP or Patient/Client Management format?

_____

_____

_____

_____

8. If the treatment went as expected, what would you do for the next treatment?

_____

_____

9. How would you expect this patient to progress over time?

_____

_____

continued

CRITICAL THINKING QUESTIONS *continued*

10. If the patient did not progress as expected, what could potentially be some reasons for a lack of progress?

_____

_____

11. What signs or symptoms, if observed or reported by the patient, would cause you to hold treatment and check with the educational staff, primary PT, or MD?

_____

_____

_____

12. Are there any cultural, socioeconomic, or ethical issues presented in this case that might affect your interventions or communication with this patient? If so, how?

_____

_____

13. Re-review this case. Are there any coexisting medical diagnoses that might affect how this patient responds to physical therapy? If so, what are they, and how might they cause the patient to respond to physical therapy differently than you expected?

_____

_____

14. Who are the health care team members in this case scenario and what are their individual roles and responsibilities?

_____

_____

15. Compare your responses on this case with those of your classmates or instructors. What, if anything, would you change and why?

_____

_____

SEEING THE DIAGNOSIS IN ACTION 13-2

Finally, as with other patients living with a disability from a disease, patients with cerebral palsy may need physical therapy off and on throughout their lives. Therapy interventions may be related to improving function related to the disease itself, or it may be concentrated on the treatment of a musculoskeletal or other injury related or unrelated to the disease. In either case, the PTA must be aware of the common problems associated with patients with cerebral palsy.

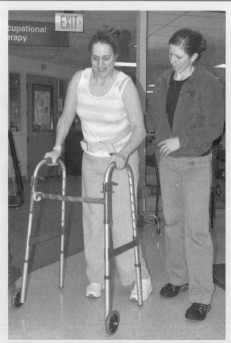

Figure 13-5 This patient with cerebral palsy performs gait training with a FWW.

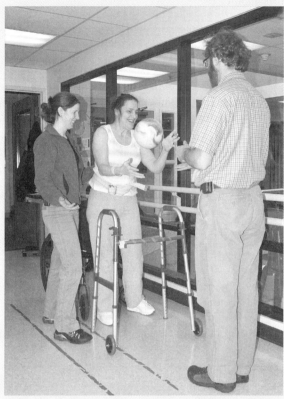

Figure 13-6 As with many patients, those with cerebral palsy often experience balance impairment. Here, the patient performs a balance activity using a ball-toss activity. The element of fun is useful for all patients but especially for those living with an ongoing disability.

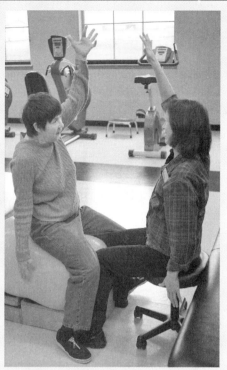

Figure 13-8 Therapy balls are a useful tool for patients with cerebral palsy. The ball provides an unstable surface on which to perform the balance activity.

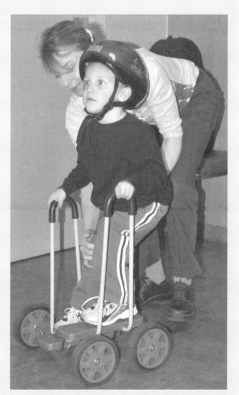

Figure 13-7 Here is another example of an activity to promote balance and improve gait in a patient with cerebral palsy.

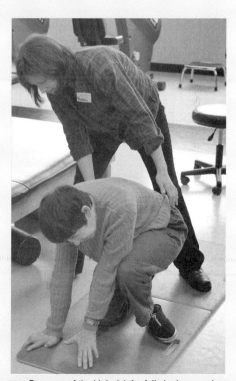

Figure 13-9 Because of the high risk for falls in these patients, training in floor transfer techniques is necessary. As patients age and begin to experience the effects of aging on joints and muscles, they may have more difficulty getting up after a fall. The PTA can instruct, assist, and train the patient in safe floor transfers for fall recovery as part of the overall POC.

IMPLICATIONS OF PATHOLOGY FOR THE PTA[2]

1. What should the PTA do in the event that the patient is exposed to peanuts?

_____
_____
_____
_____
_____
_____
_____

2. What should the PTA do if he or she observes signs of a seizure during the physical therapy session?

_____
_____
_____
_____
_____
_____
_____

3. What should the PTA be aware of when working with patients with the following conditions often seen in pediatric patients?
 • Spina bifida
 • Down syndrome
 • Hypotonia

_____
_____
_____
_____
_____

4. What precautions should the PTA take when providing modalities, especially ultrasound over or near a joint, for children?

_____
_____
_____
_____
_____

References

1. American Physical Therapy Association: Guide to Physical Therapist Practice, Second Edition. Alexandria, VA: Author, 2001.

2. Goodman CC, Boissonnault FG, Fuller KS: Pathology: Implications for the Physical Therapist, Second Edition. Philadelphia: Saunders, 2003.

Joshua Fletcher: A Patient With Down Syndrome

 Preferred Practice Pattern: Neuromuscular, Pattern B

CHAPTER OUTLINE

Introducing Joshua Fletcher

Vocabulary List

Physical Therapy Initial Evaluation and
   Plan of Care

Individualized Education Program

Health Plan

Reviewing the Medical History

Critical Thinking Questions

Implications of Pathology for the PTA

Introducing Joshua Fletcher

Joshua is a 3-year-old boy with Down syndrome. According to the APTA's *Guide to Physical Therapist Practice* (the *Guide*), he could have a number of impairments, including the following:

- Delayed motor skills and oral motor development
- Impaired locomotion
- Impaired sensory integration

Functional limitations may include clumsiness during play. Please refer to the *Guide*[1] for a complete list of possible impairments. As you work through this case, think about which of these the patient is experiencing. Also, keep in mind that a patient such as Joshua will likely be receiving outpatient physical therapy services as well. His physical therapy and other goals related to his special needs are linked with his education needs. Therapy is provided in the school setting if the team determines it is necessary for the student to benefit

from the educational program. Providing the services the student needs to be as successful as possible is required by law. For information about the history of these laws in the United States, see the following website: http://www2.ed.gov/policy/speced/leg/idea/history.html.

Vocabulary List

- Hypermobility
- Cruises
- Hyperreflexia
- Clonus
- Babinski
- Torticollis

BOX 14-1 | Peabody Developmental Motor Scales, Second Edition (PDMS-II)

Standard scores of 8 to 12 are considered average; quotient scores of 90 to 110 are considered average. For more information on the PDMS-II, please see the following website: www.proedinc.com/customer/productView. aspx?ID=1783.

Physical Therapy Initial Evaluation and Plan of Care

STUDENT	Joshua Fletcher	MEDICAL HISTORY & MEDICATIONS	Down syndrome with ventricular septal defect; moderately low tone throughout trunk and extremities; frequent ear infections; atlantoaxial instability (AAI)
DATE	10/14/2010		
BIRTH DATE	02/22/2007		
SCHOOL	Washington Elementary School		
PRECAUTIONS	Avoid activities that flex neck; cardiac		

continued

Physical Therapy Initial Evaluation and Plan of Care *continued*

PRIOR LEVEL OF FUNCTION	The patient's parents have been carrying him or using a stroller when going places; he commando crawls at home to reach toys and can push up to hands and knees to creep for short distances. He feeds himself finger foods and uses a spoon awkwardly, according to his mother. He plays with other children with minimal interaction. He is working in speech therapy on communication skills using sign language and speech vocalizations.
SOCIAL HISTORY	He lives with his parents and three older siblings. His father works in the accounting department of a local bank, and his mother is a homemaker. His grandparents live nearby. He is enrolled in a Head Start preschool.
LIVING SITUATION & EQUIPMENT	Two-story home; stroller for locomotion; sleeps in a crib
SYSTEMS REVIEW	Cardiopulmonary system is impaired due to a ventricular septal defect. Integumentary system is intact. Cognition and communication are impaired. Hearing and vision are intact. The patient has behavioral problems at home and school, with reported manipulating behaviors.
PROM	**Hypermobility** is present in all UE and LE joints.
TONE	Low throughout trunk and extremities
SENSATION	Sensation cannot be tested fully because of cognitive deficits, but the patient appears to have sensory integration impairment as noted during observation of movement patterns. Sensation will be tested more fully by the OT.
REFLEXES	Protective extension reactions, functional
STRENGTH	The patient is able to move his extremities through a full ROM and takes minimal resistance, but is unable to perform manual muscle testing because of his age and cognition.
BALANCE/POSTURE	He sits with rounded back and shoulders, posterior pelvic tilt, lumbar flexion, arms out to the side to stabilize, and hips abducted to increase base of support. In standing, he will bend at the waist to pick up toys. He is unable to squat to retrieve toys.
ENDURANCE	Impaired; the patient is able to scoot or crawl 30 feet toward a toy in 4 minutes with multiple self-imposed rest breaks because of shortness of breath.
TRANSFERS	The patient pulls himself to stand from sitting when furniture is available; he is unable to squat to pick a toy up off the floor but bends at the waist to retrieve a toy.
GAIT	The patient **cruises** along furniture for about five steps with Min. A for weight shifting and then sits; he scoots on his bottom in sitting, pulling himself forward with his legs. He commando crawls and occasionally creeps. He is just beginning to ambulate, with his two hands held and knees locked in hyperextension.
BALL SKILLS	The patient can fling a small foam ball from seated position 5 feet toward his mother with the ball landing about 4 feet to the side of mother; he can trap a ball rolled to him when seated. He is not yet successful with catching a large ball when tossed from about 2 feet in standing.
WHEELCHAIR MOBILITY/SEATING	His parents are using a standard stroller with added roll for neck support.
TEST SCORES	Peabody Developmental Motor Scales, Second Edition (PDMS-II): Stationary Standard Score = 6 Locomotion Standard Score = 1 Object Manipulation Standard Score = 2 Gross Motor Quotient (GMQ) = 55
DIAGNOSIS	Neuromuscular pattern B
PROGNOSIS	The patient qualifies for and will benefit from skilled physical therapy intervention to address the following goals, with the ultimate outcome being improved ability to perform in preschool setting, promoting greater learning. He has good potential to meet goals as stated and good family support, although the parents have three other children aged 6 to 14 years. His mother is a homemaker, and his father works full-time.
FREQUENCY OF THERAPY	30 minutes once per week
EXPECTED DURATION OF THERAPY SERVICES	One school calendar year

STRENGTHS	1. Joshua can communicate basic needs to therapy staff, teachers, and parents. 2. Joshua is a pleasant, gregarious child who engages with therapy staff easily; thus, he is ready to participate and learn new motor skills. 3. Joshua's family has participated in therapy services before this, which demonstrates good support, and Joshua has made progress toward therapy goals in the past.		3. Joshua's teachers will implement joint protection procedures during normal classroom and playground activities by May 2011. 4. Joshua will perform sit to stand without any assist or device in 2/3 trials by May, 2011 to participate fully in his classroom activities.
NEEDS	1. Joshua needs to progress his locomotion skills to independent ambulation to access his classroom and school environments. 2. Joshua needs to be able to stand up from sitting on the floor without any furniture or assistive device to participate more efficiently in classroom and playground activities. 3. Joshua needs to improve his strength, balance, and endurance for increased ease of movement and improved success with modified gross motor play activities at recess and during gross motor play time. 4. Joshua needs to have joint protection procedures in place to protect his lax joints from damage.	STUDENT IEP GOALS & OBJECTIVES	Joshua will receive specially designed instruction in the areas of prereading, writing, and math at the preschool level. Physical therapy services will support him in these areas as well by improving his ability to achieve and maintain effective postures that will help him maximize attention and learning. Additionally, he will become more efficient with ambulation to allow him improved access to all school environments.
PRIORITIES AMONG THERAPY INTERVENTION GOALS & OBJECTIVES	1. Joshua will independently ambulate 50 feet by May 2011. 2. Joshua will improve his strength, balance, and endurance to allow him to participate actively in group play activities for 20 to 30 minutes without a rest break in two thirds of opportunities by May 2011, including being able to independently squat to retrieve toys and return to standing again.	STRATEGIES, METHODS, ACCOMMODATIONS, ENVIRONMENT USED TO ADDRESS NEEDS	Strategies and methods include direct physical therapy services, including therapeutic exercise and functional mobility training for transfer skills. Gait training and motor control activities, as well as education for teaching staff and mother in the proper use of adaptive equipment and home exercise program, will also be provided. Environment: General and special education classrooms, playground, or gym, as appropriate.
		PLAN FOR RE-EVALUATION, METHOD OF DATA COLLECTION, DISCHARGE PLANNING	Joshua will be re-evaluated at least every 3 years. Progress toward therapy goals will be documented in therapy notes. He will be discharged from therapy services when goals are met, skills are functional for the school environment, and/or he is unable to progress any further.

BOX 14-2 | Health-Care Team Member Role: Family

The patient's family is always an important part of the health-care team but perhaps most of all in the area of pediatrics. Parents and siblings of the patient can often be a huge motivator and help to facilitate the follow-through of a home program designed by the physical therapy team. Because parents or guardians have responsibility for the child in all aspects, they must provide consent for all interventions. Effective communication between the therapy or health-care team and the family is crucial to ensure that therapy goals are met and interventions are effective.

Although ideally the family is a big part of the success of the patient, keep in mind that most families can experience a sense of being overwhelmed by the extraordinary amount and type of stress placed on the family because of a child's disability. If the patient has a chronic condition, the family members may experience various stages of grieving over the losses and will have a difficult time managing everyday life along with meeting the needs of the child. Parents and families will appreciate an understanding attitude and genuine caring and support from the PTA in these cases.

Individualized Educational Program

DATE: October 17, 2010
STUDENT: Joshua Fletcher
STUDENT ID: 1234567
DATE OF BIRTH: February 22, 2007

Present Level of Educational Performance

MEDICAL-PHYSICAL: See Health Plan
ACADEMIC:
PREREADING: Looks at books, turns pages, points to pictures correctly
PREWRITING: Scribbles with pencils and crayons, attempts to copy a circle but is unable to complete
PREMATH: Repeats numbers 1 to 10
FINE MOTOR:
Joshua participates well in therapy sessions. In occupational therapy, he is working on fine-motor skills to enhance feeding and prewriting skills. External support of trunk is needed to provide stability to allow him greater success with writing because of his low tone in both upper extremities and trunk. PDMS-II scores are as follows: Grasping Standard Score = 5, Visual Motor Integration Standard Score = 5; Fine Motor Quotient (FMQ) = 70.
GROSS MOTOR:
Joshua receives physical therapy services as part of his IEP. His primary means of mobility is scooting on his bottom or commando crawling. With Min. A, he is able to stand and cruise at furniture. He is able to ride a push toy but is not yet pedaling a tricycle. He is beginning to use a tricycle for LE and trunk strengthening and endurance during PE time. He has strength, balance, and endurance impairments that affect his ability to participate in classroom, PE, and recess activities with his peers.

Annual Goals and Objectives

PREREADING: Recognizes 10 letters
PREWRITING: Correctly copies a circle, triangle, and square
PREMATH: Counts 1 to 10
FINE MOTOR: See Occupational Therapy Report
GROSS MOTOR: See Physical Therapy Report

Health Plan

HISTORY
Joshua was born at term to a 45-year-old mother, the fourth child of the family. His neonatal period was complicated by feeding difficulties. His development has been delayed with sitting alone at 11 months and crawling at 21 months, and he is just now beginning to walk. He is beginning to speak in one-word sentences and says about 20 words.

PROBLEMS
He has atlantoaxial instability, affecting his ability to participate in activities that flex the neck.
He has ventricular septal defect, affecting his endurance for activities.
He has frequent ear infections.

NEED
School staff will recognize the signs and symptoms of cardiac distress, atlantoaxial instability, and ear infections.

PLAN FOR RESOLUTION

Cardiac Distress
Symptoms and signs to observe:
• Higher than normal heart rate with activity
• Greater than normal shortness of breath with activity
• Blue skin tone (cyanosis)
Treatment:
• Slow down activity.
• Monitor heart rate and respiratory rate until returns to normal levels.
• If Joshua stops breathing or becomes unconscious, call 9-1-1 and initiate CPR, then call parents.

AAI
Symptoms and signs to observe:
• **Hyperreflexia**
• **Clonus**
• Positive **Babinski**
• **Torticollis**
• Loss of strength
• Changes in sensation
• Loss of bladder or bowel control
• Decreased motor skills
Treatment:
• Stabilize neck immediately, call 9-1-1

Ear Infections
Symptoms and signs to observe:
• Redness around the ear
• Pain around the ear
• Pulling or tugging on the ear
• Fever
Treatment:
• Contact school secretary for Tylenol administration.
• Call parents to come take Joshua home.

SEEING THE DIAGNOSIS IN ACTION 14-1

When children are born with Down syndrome, as with other abnormalities, parents must cope with the emotional aspects of having a handicapped child while at the same time learning to provide for the specialized day-to-day needs of the child. Physical therapy can provide much education and support while teaching parents how to work effectively with their child and promote normal development as much as possible. As with children with other disease processes, therapy often is geared toward play for the child, making therapy a fun time that they will want to participate in.

Once the child has learned a level of control in sitting, therapy often progresses to the standing position and then to gait training. Many times, as the patient grows to adulthood, he or she is able to progress to using no device.

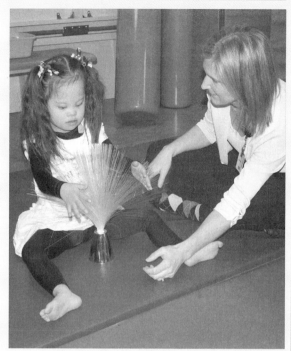

Figure 14-2 Once the child has developed some control in prone, he or she can progress to the sitting position. Here, the child has fun with a toy while learning to control sitting postures.

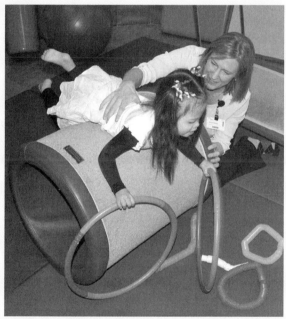

Figure 14-1 Patients with Down syndrome need help progressing through the normal developmental stages. Here, a child is engaged in a reaching activity while prone on a roll to improve balance reactions.

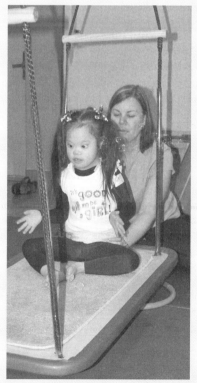

Figure 14-3 One dynamic surface used to promote sitting balance is the swing. Also, therapy balls can be useful to promote dynamic balance reactions.

continued

SEEING THE DIAGNOSIS IN ACTION 14-1 *continued*

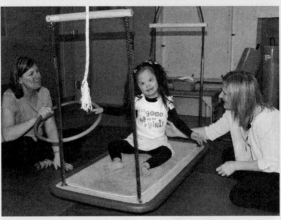

Figure 14-4 Although the equipment used with children is often specialized, it is often very similar to play equipment of normal children, and this can help children with a handicap feel more like they belong.

REVIEWING THE MEDICAL HISTORY

1. What do you already know about Down syndrome?

_____

_____

_____

_____

_____

2. Review the vocabulary list, physical therapy evaluation, IEP, and health plan. Look up the meanings of any terms you do not understand in a medical dictionary or other text.

_____

_____

_____

_____

_____

3. Review the diagnoses in the past medical history using a medical or pathology text, Internet resource, or other available resource.

_____

_____

_____

_____

_____

4. Which diagnoses in the past medical history would be significant and potentially affect the patient's response to the physical therapy interventions?

_____

_____

_____

_____

_____

_____

_____

_____

_____

5. List the purpose and potential side effects of each of the medications the patient is taking.

_____

_____

_____

_____

_____

_____

_____

CRITICAL THINKING QUESTIONS

After reviewing the physical therapy initial evaluation, IEP, and Health Plan, address the following:

1. What are the patient's impairments? Functional limitations? Is there a disability?

_____

_____

_____

_____

2. Find assessments of gait, strength, ROM, and balance if available from the initial evaluation and list.

   a. How could each potentially be used to assess function and demonstrate progress toward goals or show the patient's response to physical therapy interventions?

   _____

   _____

   _____

   b. What would be the most important items to document for this patient?

   _____

   _____

   _____

3. After reviewing the POC, describe a possible next treatment session.

   a. List the activities/exercises and your rationale for the order of treatment activities that you selected.

   _____

   _____

   _____

4. What subjective information will you gather during your session to help in your treatment of this patient and why?

   _____

   _____

   _____

5. What tests or measures will you use to assess the patient's progress and response to treatment?

   _____

   _____

   _____

6. What subjective or objective information that you gather during the treatment might cause you to alter your treatment for this patient and why?

   _____

   _____

   _____

7. How would you document your treatment in the SOAP or Patient/Client Management format?

   _____

   _____

   _____

   _____

8. If the treatment goes as expected, what will you do for the next treatment?

   _____

   _____

   _____

9. How would you expect this patient to progress over time?

   _____

   _____

10. If the patient does not progress as expected, what might be some reasons for a lack of progress?

    _____

    _____

11. What signs or symptoms, if observed or reported by the patient, would cause you to hold treatment and check with the educational staff, primary PT, or MD?

    _____

    _____

    _____

12. Are there any cultural, socioeconomic, or ethical issues presented in this case that might affect your interventions or communication with this patient? If so, how?

    _____

    _____

    _____

continued

CRITICAL THINKING QUESTIONS *continued*

13. Re-review this case. Are there any coexisting medical diagnoses that might affect how this patient responds to physical therapy? If so, what are they, and how might they cause the patient to respond to physical therapy differently than you expected?

_____

_____

_____

14. Who are the health-care team members in this case scenario and what are their individual roles and responsibilities?

_____

_____

_____

15. Compare your responses on this case with those of your classmates or instructors. What, if anything, would you change and why?

_____

_____

_____

_____

_____

_____

_____

_____

_____

_____

_____

_____

SEEING THE DIAGNOSIS IN ACTION 14-2

The adult with Down syndrome often has ongoing or recurring needs related to chronic problems associated with the disease process. These can be related to specific injuries because patients often have a higher risk for musculoskeletal injuries because of the low muscle tone and poor trunk stability typically associated with Down syndrome. Therapy may also be related to helping the adult patient learn skills to manage more independently at home or in the community.

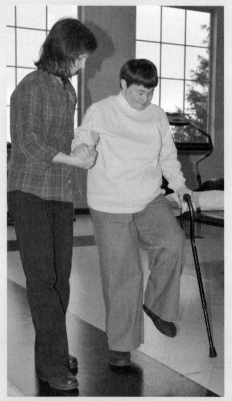

Figure 14-5 Here, the adult patient with Down syndrome performs gait training with a cane for needed stability.

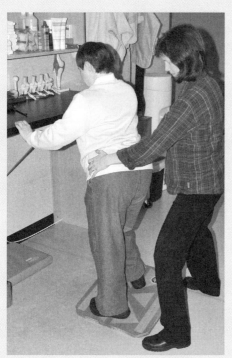

Figure 14-6 Higher-level balance activities help improve safety with ambulation for patients with Down syndrome. Here, the activity is performed on a rocker board for a dynamic surface.

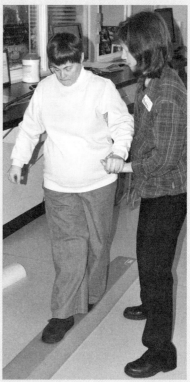

Figure 14-7 A balance beam can also be a fun way to incorporate a balance activity into the therapy session.

IMPLICATIONS OF PATHOLOGY FOR THE PTA[2]

1. What activities should be avoided with this patient and why?

_____
_____
_____
_____
_____
_____
_____
_____
_____
_____
_____

2. What are the possible implications of a ventricular septal defect on physical therapy?

_____
_____
_____
_____
_____
_____
_____
_____
_____
_____
_____

continued

IMPLICATIONS OF PATHOLOGY FOR THE PTA[2] *continued*

3. What are signs and symptoms of atlantoaxial instability or an acute ear infection?

_____

_____

_____

_____

_____

_____

_____

_____

_____

_____

_____

_____

4. What should the PTA be aware of when working with patients with the following conditions often seen in pediatric patients?

a. Spina bifida

b. Cerebral palsy

c. Hypertonia

_____

_____

_____

_____

_____

_____

_____

_____

_____

_____

References

1. American Physical Therapy Association: Guide to Physical Therapist Practice, Second Edition. Alexandria, VA: Author, 2001.

2. Goodman CC, Boissonnault FG, Fuller KS: Pathology: Implications for the Physical Therapist, Second Edition. Philadelphia: Saunders, 2003.

CHAPTER 2

Rebecca Graves, PT

Acute Care Setting

Mr. Anderson has not previously been diagnosed with cardiovascular disease but has risk factors of obesity, smoking, and a relatively sedentary lifestyle as well as a family history of cardiovascular disease. He does have a desire to reduce his risk for future heart attacks, specifically by exercising. In fact, he began an exercise program that apparently brought on his MI. In my experience as a PT for more than 20 years in a variety of settings, many patients present with lifestyle-related injuries or disease and do not wish to change their patterns of living to promote wellness and health. It can be difficult for the PTA to provide respectful care and communication in such a situation. However, happily in this case, Mr. Anderson is ready to begin an exercise program to help him live a longer and healthier life. PTAs can support this through respectful communication during treatment sessions and provide assistance by finding answers to the patient's questions.

Before seeing any patient in the acute setting, it is common practice to always check in with the nursing staff. Even though good practice dictates that clinicians read the nursing notes, sometimes significant changes can take place and are not yet documented. Also, it is helpful to know if the patient has been vomiting or having diarrhea; in such a case, the patient may need to stay close to his room rather than walking all around the nursing unit. Other possible scenarios include a change in neurological status that might mean the patient is having complications; in many cases, physical therapy needs to be put on hold until further testing is done and the patient is cleared for activity.

Assuming there are no complications from a nursing standpoint, the PTA can proceed with the planned interventions. His hospital stay should be relatively short, perhaps 1 to 3 days. Before he can be discharged, he will need to demonstrate that he can manage safely at home without assistance. The PTA must provide interventions related to the goals in the plan of care and work quickly to help the patient progress. As the patient works on the various activities, data should be collected that will support the evidence of progress toward those goals. For example, one goal is independence with bed mobility, transfers, and ambulation. He will likely progress quickly with these and primarily need help with learning to pace himself during these activities. While the PTA checks his vital signs and times his ambulation to monitor progress, Mr. Anderson should be instructed to check his own heart rate before, during, and after activity in order to ensure that he is not overworking himself. Some patients have a difficult time feeling their pulse so could also use the RPE (rate of perceived exertion scale). Additionally, he should be instructed in proper progression of his exercise program at home, which should be given to him in a written format.

Do you see a goal related to endurance in the physical therapy plan of care? Although there are many tests and measures available to assess cardiovascular endurance, time is limited in the acute setting, and often the patient's ambulation is timed to demonstrate progress. In this case, the PTA will need a stop watch or other watch or clock with a second hand to accurately time the patient during his gait training sessions. Often, patients will not have significant gait deviations, but if they do, these should be addressed during the treatment interventions. These may not be observed during the initial evaluation because the patient is walking more slowly and not as far as later on in the rehabilitation process. In addition to making sure the patient can safely increase his ambulation distance in less time, he needs to be able to do this without supplemental O_2. After the oxygen is removed in the hospital setting, the PTA must monitor his SpO_2 during therapy activities. This information is very helpful to the physician when planning discharge and in determining whether the patient will need supplemental O_2 at home. Typically, this is not the case. If the patient desaturates during activity, the PTA will need to check with the nurse or physician to see what orders are for supplemental O_2. Sometimes, orders will be to maintain SpO_2 above a certain level, with supplemental O_2 given as needed or up to a certain amount. Orders for supplemental O_2 must be followed closely to ensure the safety of the patient.

Lastly, an important goal to address before discharge is that of managing the stairs. Again, it is likely that Mr. Anderson will not have a problem actually going up and down the stairs but may need assistance in pacing himself with the activity.

At any time, if there is a question about the patient's safety upon discharge to the home setting, the PTA must discuss the concern with the primary PT. The PT can then set up a plan for communicating those concerns to the nursing and medical staff. In some facilities, the PTAs communicate their concerns directly with nursing staff, who can address the need for additional referrals if needed. At times, a referral to a medical social worker may be needed in order to assist the patient with obtaining any needed help at home so that he can be discharged safely.

In preparing the patient for discharge home, it is important to reinforce the need to continue with the exercise program. If he continues in an outpatient cardiac rehabilitation program, he can be monitored closely for any signs of problems along the way. Often, these programs are directed and run by exercise science professionals who are specially trained for providing care to these patients. Care can also be provided in an outpatient physical therapy clinic, where the PTA can assist the PT in providing the necessary follow-up. In that setting, it will be important to address any concerns regarding a return to work and leisure activities, including sexual activity. Although the doctor may discuss these with the patient, often questions arise during the physical therapy sessions, and the PTA will need to address the questions or refer the patient to the primary PT or other health-care professional.

Other patients who will likely have similar impairments and functional limitations include those who have progressed cardiovascular disease and have now had a CABG or other procedure such as angioplasty that may have certain precautions. In the case of a patient who has just had a CABG, there will be sternal precautions to avoid damage to the repair of the chest after open heart surgery. These generally include avoiding twisting or reaching back as well as pushing up, especially on only one side, and lifting—anything that would disrupt the healing of the chest wound. When

beginning gait training with these patients, some therapists use a cardiac walker, which helps to avoid any pushing down with the upper extremities through the use of platform for the forearms to rest on, as on a standard or front wheeled walker.

In general, patients with cardiovascular disease are typically quick to return to their prior level of function as far as safety goes but have a harder time returning to their prior activities because of endurance impairments. At all times, the PTA should watch for signs of cardiovascular distress or further progression such as blue skin, sweating, chest pain, numbness or tingling in the extremities or face, slurring of speech, difficulty with motor control, and the like. Remember that patients who have had a cardiac arrest are often also at risk for CVA.

Patients like Mr. Anderson are enjoyable to work with because they tend to progress quickly and can benefit greatly from physical therapy interventions. This gentleman may also consider other lifestyle changes to further decrease his risk, such as diet modifications, smoking cessation, and stress control. The PTA can support the patient with these endeavors through his or her encouragement but must remember that the role of the PTA does not include providing specific diet recommendations or other such information that is not in the scope of physical therapy practice.

1. What are the patient's impairments? Functional limitations? Is there a disability?
   Impairments include pain, decreased BLE ROM, decreased cardiovascular endurance. Functional limitations include difficulty with bed mobility, transfers, and ambulation. The patient is currently unable to participate in his normal work and leisure activities, which could be considered a disability, even if temporary.
2. Find assessments from the initial physical therapy evaluation and list. How can each be used to assess function and demonstrate progress toward goals or show the patient's response to physical therapy interventions? Which measurements are the most important to document for this patient in order to show progress?
   Assessments of pain, ROM, and endurance, as well as functional mobility and balance, are included and can all be used to show progress in those specific areas. The PT has listed several goals, both short- and long-term, that will be most important to address during each treatment session.
3. After reviewing the physical therapy POC and other pertinent information, describe a possible next treatment session. List the interventions and your

rationale for the order of activities as well as any equipment you will need.

If the patient is in his hospital bed, the next treatment session could begin with practice of bed mobility, teaching him ways to get in and out of bed more easily. The PTA should have the patient practice in an environment that simulates his home setting, such as with a bed that doesn't have a head that raises or bed rails, getting in and out of the side of the bed he generally uses at home. After a warmup of supine and/or seated AROM exercises, the patient could then participate in gait training with the appropriate gait device. It is important to note throughout your session why this is "skilled" therapy; this can include instruction for improving gait deviations, cues needed for pacing, the need for monitoring of vital signs, etc. Teaching the patient how to monitor his own vital signs is an important part of gait training.

4. What subjective information will you gather and document during your session and why?

Pain levels and complaints of shortness of breath, dizziness, or other symptoms might indicate an abnormal response to the activity. You will also want to find out how the patient is feeling in terms of improved ability to accomplish tasks, such as getting in and out of bed, going to the restroom, and sitting up in bed to eat. This information is helpful in showing progress.

5. What tests or measures will you use to assess the patient's progress or response to treatment?

HR and SpO_2 to monitor response to activities and timed ambulation as well as levels of assist needed for functional activities to demonstrate progress toward goals.

6. What subjective or objective information that you gather during the treatment might cause you to alter your treatment and why?

If the patient's heart rate was extremely elevated or the SpO_2 was below 92%, or the patient had complaints of chest pain, shortness of breath, or other symptoms, you would stop the activity, have the patient rest, and continue to monitor. If these did not return to normal, you would provide additional supplemental O_2 if the SpO_2 was low and if ordered by the physician. These are good opportunities to help the patient learn how it feels to overdo activity and also to learn to start pacing himself.

7. How would you document your treatment in the SOAP format?

Date

S: *Patient reports fatigue after physical therapy evaluation and some dizziness upon sitting up, but this is decreasing.*

O: *Resting HR 72, SpO_2 on 2 LPM O_2 99%*

   Supine to/from sit with bed flat and no handrails CGA with BLE onto bed

   Seated AROM BLE: hip flexion, long arc quads, ankle circles x 20 each

   Sit to stand and transfer: supervised with VCs to reach for chair before sitting down

   Gait training: 200 feet with FWW, CGA in 2 minutes, 20 seconds

   Activity HR 115, SpO_2 on 2 LPM O_2 98%

   After 5-minute rest HR 98, SpO_2 on 2 LPM O_2 98%

A: *Patient shows progress toward functional mobility goals with increased gait distance and decreased assist needed for bed mobility, transfers, gait. Vital signs stable throughout.*

P: *Provide written home exercise program, progress gait distance, try stairs next session.*

   Rebecca Graves, PT

8. If the treatment goes as expected, what will you do for the next treatment?

Provide a written home exercise program for seated AROM as warmups and a typical progression of walking for endurance over a 1- or 2-week period until the patient is able to start his outpatient cardiac rehabilitation program. Determine whether he could increase his gait distance and decrease his time and have him practice the stairs at the next session.

9. How would you expect this patient to progress over time?

He would show progress each session and would meet his goals quickly. You would expect that he would be able to manage safely and independently at home at discharge for ADLs. He might still need help with cooking meals and housekeeping and may not be able to return to work.

10. If the patient did not progress as expected, what might be some reasons for lack of progress?

The patient might have an underlying medical condition that has not yet been found. He might be depressed and not coping well with his condition and hospitalization. He might not have motivation to try and even participate in therapy sessions and may not be participating as much as needed. His body may not be responding well to the activity level because of prior deconditioning; he may need more time than originally thought to meet his goals.

11. What would cause you to hold treatment and check with the nursing staff, primary PT, or MD?

Abnormal symptoms (such as chest pain, shortness of breath, dizziness) or signs (heart rate too elevated, SpO_2 too low) that did not improve with rest or other modifications such as increased supplemental O_2; any nausea, vomiting, or diarrhea would be reported to the nursing staff. Any new or previously undocumented signs or symptoms that seem unusual (such as numbness into an arm or leg, new pain elsewhere) should be reported to the primary PT or another supervising PT. Depending on the severity of the symptoms and the potential for an unsafe situation for your patient, your interventions may or may not need to be held.

12. What is the discharge plan for this patient and how might you as the PTA help prepare the patient for discharge?

    The patient plans to go home and begin a cardiac rehabilitation program on an outpatient basis. Typically, these programs are located within a local hospital. Exercise physiologists and other personnel usually manage these programs.

    The PTA should help the patient prepare for discharge by providing high-quality services that enable the patient to meet his physical therapy goals by discharge. The PTA will also answer his questions about the cardiac rehabilitation program and as such should know about the program itself or be able to refer him to another source of information.

13. If the patient follows up with an outpatient cardiac rehabilitation program as recommended, describe how the patient would be expected to progress in his impairments and functional limitations. How can you prepare him while in the hospital for this type of program and what to expect long-term after such a program is completed?

    His endurance for activity should improve, and any symptoms of shortness of breath, chest pain, and so forth should diminish. He should be able to return to his job and other activities within a few weeks as recommended by his doctor.

14. Compare your responses to this case with those of other students or instructors.

    Remember, your ideas may differ from your classmates' and your instructors. We all have a different perspective and may think of different things. The important things are that you are considering closely the PT plan of care, goals, and how you can most effectively and efficiently meet those goals during your therapy sessions. You should also be able to give a rationale for why you are choosing each therapy intervention as well as the sequencing of interventions within each session.

CHAPTER 6

Mariisa Bonsen, PTA

Acute Care Setting

Reviewing the Medical History

After careful review of the patient's medical history, there are several issues that should be taken into consideration for physical therapy in the acute setting. First and foremost is that the patient has undergone a bilateral knee replacement, rather than the more common single knee replacement, after a long history of bilateral knee pain resulting from osteoarthritis,. Of concern with performing bilateral knee replacement are that the surgical procedure takes more time to complete and that it can be more physically demanding on a patient's body. Another disadvantage is that early rehabilitation can be more difficult because patients do not have a "good leg" to work with. Additionally, this patient is taking several medications, including venlafaxine used to treat anxiety and depression. It would be beneficial to monitor the patient's daily mood and to give continuous encouragement throughout rehabilitation to motivate and reassure her progress. The patient is also taking naproxen, which would be extremely beneficial in her recovery because it is a nonsteroidal anti-inflammatory drug that helps to relieve postoperative pain, tenderness, swelling, and stiffness. The patient's past medical history shows that she has borderline diabetes, which can lead to a poor rate of healing. She suffers from obesity, which may indicate poor endurance and limited activity tolerance. She has a history of chronic osteoarthritis not only in her knees but also in her hips and spine, which could affect her acute rehabilitation activity tolerance. Another medical issue that could limit the patient's activity tolerance is her history of a bladder cystocele with stress urinary incontinence, which can result in a sudden involuntary release of urine, causing rehabilitation treatment sessions to be concluded abruptly. Finally, the medical history indicates that the patient may live independently without family nearby but may have assistance from her boyfriend. It would be beneficial to make sure that when the time comes for the patient to discharge home, she will have full-time support and assistance of either close friends or family.

Critical Thinking Questions

Pretreatment: Initially, postoperative bilateral total knee replacement patients are limited by pain, stiffness, and decreased mobility. The physical therapy evaluation notes the following: the patient is hard of hearing, weight-bearing is as tolerated, she may be limited by urinary incontinence but currently is using a Foley catheter, she has limited bilateral knee weakness and range of motion, she benefits from being premedicated before physical therapy treatments, and she needs notable assistance with bed mobility, transfers, and ambulation. By reviewing the patient's baseline ability at the time of initial evaluation, you can easily document progression by looking at all areas in which the patient needs improvement and which the primary PT has listed as goals.

Treatment: After review of the plan of care, the next treatment after the initial evaluation could begin focusing on bed mobility, transfer training, gait training, and gentle supine lower extremity strengthening and mobility. Begin treatment by asking how the patient is "feeling," including sleeping at night and current pain level, and by checking current vital signs, such as blood pressure, heart rate, and oxygen saturation. This information gives a baseline that can be monitored as needed throughout the session. Primarily, pain level would typically be affected during the session, and you would want to know how much the pain increases or decreases during the treatment interventions. Next, begin working on bed mobility by getting the patient into a sitting position at the edge of her bed. Have the patient use the log roll technique by rolling onto her side at the edge of the bed and then pushing up with her elbow. This technique may be easier on the back, especially for someone who has arthritis and back pain. Because of limited mobility and strength, the patient would need maximum assistance with both lower extremities, gently maneuvering them over the side of the bed at the same time as she is pushing up into a sitting position. While the patient is sitting at the edge of the bed, make sure to ask her to report any dizziness or increased pain levels at any time throughout treatment, and then instruct the patient to stand using a front wheeled walker, pushing up from the bed using both upper extremities for safety. Next, have the patient use the walker to complete a stand pivot transfer (or take several small steps depending on pain level and mobility) to her wheelchair and sit down. Have her repeat this process several times, drilling her on safe hand placement and sequencing of the transition. Then begin gait training with her walker, bringing the wheelchair along or having a second person following closely behind patient with the wheelchair if needed for safety. Examples of VCs given for ambulation might include encouraging the patient to have a relaxed upright posture and instructing with heel-to-toe gait pattern and

breathing techniques. Then have the patient transfer back into bed and instruct the patient with bilateral ankle pumps, quadriceps sets, heel slides, and gluteal sets as tolerated. These exercises are typically used in the acute care phase of rehabilitation after a total knee replacement and are included in many protocols. If another protocol is used in your facility, follow that. Because of the patient's history of anxiety, provide ongoing reassurance and make sure the patient feels comfortable and confident as much as possible. At the end of treatment, ask the patient to report any increased or decreased bilateral knee pain and to ask any questions regarding surgery and treatment. Based on the patient's response, both verbally and physically, the primary PT may need to make modifications to the treatment plan. All pertinent information must be communicated to the primary physical therapist through the written notes, with verbal communication if necessary.

Post-treatment: Important items to document from the treatment session include the patient's current pain level or other valuable subjective information that demonstrates progress or lack of progress, current functional abilities, and interventions completed during the session with any verbal or tactile cues or assistance given. This is an example of what the SOAP note might look like following a treatment session:

Date

S: Patient states that she is not sleeping well at night because of "excruciating" bilateral knee pain. She rates her knee pain at 8/10 bilaterally. She notes taking pain medications half an hour before treatment.

O: BP 128/78 mm Hg, HR 88 BPM, O_2 @ 98% on room air. Instructed patient in bed mobility and transfer training, including supine to sit @ edge of bed using log roll technique with Min. A with bed flat. Patient requires Max. A with BLE in and out of bed and VCs for setup and pushing up using RUE. Sit to stand with Min. A with FWW, ambulated from bed to W/C using FWW with Min. A x 3 steps with VCs to lock W/C brakes and reach back for armrests. Gait training with FWW 5 feet x 2 with CGA to Min. A with postural cues and reminders for heel strike with W/C following by PTA. Instructed supine BLE therapeutic exercise, including ankle pumps, quadriceps sets, heel slides, and gluteal sets, 10 repetitions each. Right knee PROM flexion 12 to 72 degrees, left knee PROM flexion 10 to 74 degrees. Patient rates pain @ 5/10 post interventions. Observable fatigue at end of session and patient needing considerable encouragement to complete because of pain.

A: Patient has progressed with bed mobility from Max. A to Min. A. Is able to ambulate further with decreased assistance overall. Needs increased encouragement to complete exercises, especially with increased pain with heel slides. Fatigue at end of session about as would be expected.

P: Continue with bed mobility, transfer training, gait training, and strengthening, progressing as patient is able per plan of care.

Mariisa Bonsen, PTA

Things to Consider

Factors that may continue to affect treatment would include pain, which could easily limit activity tolerance, and bilateral knee ROM. It would be beneficial for nursing to continue medicating the patient before treatment and coordinating with the nursing staff on therapy times. Treatment may also be affected when and if the patient has her Foley catheter removed before leaving the hospital. Any signs of infection or increased reports of pain need to be immediately reported to nursing to help coordinate pain management. It also appears that the patient has a MRSA infection. Because of these precautions, the patient may be isolated in her room, and staff will be required to take precautions when entering and conducting treatment in the room to prevent contamination or contact. Because of the patient's history of anxiety and current living situation, it would be beneficial to work with social services, who will likely be included in treatment and discharge planning with this patient. Also, communication with occupational therapy will be important so that treatments don't occur simultaneously or back to back, causing the patient to become too fatigued or to decline treatment because she is overwhelmed.

Inpatient Rehabilitation Setting

Reviewing the Medical History

It appears that Ms. Harper continues to be treated for respiratory MRSA and is still in isolation after transitioning from the hospital to an inpatient rehabilitation facility. She is under continued monitoring from nursing with a new reported diagnosis of type 2 diabetes, which is being managed by insulin and diet. She also continues to be limited by poor pain management and anxiety but is participating well.

Pretreatment

After reviewing the current plan of care, it is clear that the patient needs continued work on bed mobility, transfer training, gait training, and strengthening. Additional instruction as she progresses would include balance activities, establishing a home exercise program, and using physical modalities to assist with pain management. It is also recommended to instruct in diabetic foot care training and pelvic floor strengthening because of the patient's diagnosis of DM II and urinary incontinence. Based on the patient's current diagnosis of respiratory MRSA, necessary precautions need to be taken during treatment interventions. Precautions typically include using a mask, gown, and gloves as well as using universal precautions when entering the patient's room. Often, patients are required to wear a mask, gown, and gloves when outside of their room.

Treatment

After reviewing the plan of care, it would be important to check with nursing before initiating treatment to make sure the patient has been premedicated and that there are no medical changes affecting therapies. Begin treatment in the patient's room after donning a mask, gloves, and gown. Next, obtain a current pain rating and assessment of vital signs. Then, reinforce prior education on bed mobility and transfer training with the patient. Once the patient is sitting on the edge of bed, have her use the FWW to ambulate short distances to and from the bathroom and in and around her room as she is able. Based on the patient's pain limitations and anxiety, she might benefit from having a split treatment session, once in the morning and once in the afternoon. In the inpatient rehabilitation setting, patients are also required to tolerate and receive at least 3 hours of combined therapies per day. Physical therapy will often include two 1-hour sessions, with occupational therapy providing another hour per day, depending on the patient's needs. Assuming two sessions per day for this patient, have her complete the most strenuous activities (possibly gait training and transfer training, but could be the exercise program for this patient) in the earlier session before the patient has become fatigued from daily activities. If allowed by nursing, have the patient leave her room to complete other activities in the hallway and rehabilitation gym. The patient in this situation should be wearing a mask at all times outside of her room. At most facilities, the hallways can be a great location for gait training. Using her FWW and having the W/C close behind, begin ambulating short distances. It appears the patient will need VCs addressing her gait pattern to increase foot stride length and postural awareness in her trunk and to avoid compensating by bilaterally circumducting. During a second treatment session later in the day, take the patient to the rehabilitation gym for instruction in seated lower extremity strengthening exercises, including: heel and toe raises, hip adduction ball squeezes, long arc quadriceps extensions, and seated knee flexion stretches. These are often a part of total knee protocols in the subacute phase, but as in the acute phase, follow the protocols established by the physician or primary PT. The patient can also continue supine exercises given in the hospital. Because the patient has stairs at home, instruct her in stair training while in the rehabilitation gym. At this time, ask her which of the two operative knees feels stronger or is less painful. This will help in determining which lower extremity the patient should lead with when going up and down stairs. Encourage the patient to use both handrails initially and go slowly when completing the activity, using a step-to pattern. If the patient has minimal complaints of fatigue or pain, encourage her to complete another short period of gait training before returning to her room. Allow for periodic rest breaks and frequently ask the patient how she is doing, including her current pain levels during each activity. Finally, it is typically important and one of the goals to increase PROM as much as possible during this phase, and depending on her progress with this, she may need joint or soft tissue mobilization or other modalities to help achieve this goal and may need to work on PROM at both morning and afternoon sessions. Because mobilization techniques are not mentioned specifically in the physical therapy plan of care, discuss these with the primary PT before using them. The patient will likely need instruction on how to encourage more ROM in her room during breaks between therapies. This patient may continue to require increased encouragement and reassurance to keep her motivated throughout treatment.

Post-treatment

Important things to document would be patient's pain levels and interventions completed during the session. Noting the patient's response to treatment as well as progression will help with planning for further treatment sessions. The SOAP note might appear like this:

Date

S: Patient reports 6/10 bilateral knee pain. Notes right greater than left knee stiffness, worse in AM. Per nursing, patient is ambulating to toilet with FWW

with Min. A. She is anxious to return home as soon as possible, stating, "I've got lots of things that I need to catch up on at home."

O: AM session: Training in bed mobility, scooting and rolling with SBA, supine to sit with head of bed flat SBA and Min. A with BLE with VCs for setup. Sit to stand transfers with FWW CGA to Min. A with VCs to push up off of bed and W/C. Gait training with FWW in and around room short distances 6 feet x 4 with CGA and verbal and tactile cues for upright posture to bring shoulders back and widening base of support. Ambulated 20 feet x 4 in hallway with W/C following by PTA and CGA with VCs to increase stride length and heel strike. Passive stretching bilateral knees into flexion followed by contract-relax stretching into flexion, then passive knee extension stretch with ice packs applied for 15 minutes to decrease pain and increase extension.

PM session: Instructed seated BLE exercises: long arc quadriceps extensions, heel/toe raises, hip adduction ball squeezes all x 15 repetitions. Seated bilateral knee flexion chair stretch x 3 with 15-second holds. Contract-relax knee flexion stretches bilaterally. Stair training up/down 4 steps with handrails x 2 with CGA and VCs for technique and sequencing. Right knee PROM flexion 8 to 80 degrees, left knee PROM flexion 8 to 82 degrees. Patient declined PM gait training due to increased right greater than left knee pain and stiffness. Reports right knee pain @ 8/10 and left knee pain @ 6/10 post interventions. Ice to bilateral knees in extension x 15 minutes at end of session. RN alerted and will remove at end of 15 minutes.

A: Patient demonstrated increased activity tolerance today with decreased knee pain with ambulation.

P: Continue to progress ROM, strengthening, transfer training, gait training, and stair training per POC. Discuss with primary PT whether soft tissue mobilization techniques could be added to POC to help increase ROM and decrease pain. Try ultrasound before stretching next session.

Mariisa Bonsen, PTA

Things to Consider

This patient may respond well to frequent encouragement and reminders of long-term goals such as returning home and to prior activities. As she progresses, it will be important to transition patient from a FWW to a single-point cane to increase her mobility. Also, adding balance activities and endurance/strengthening activities such as the NuStep machine or stationary bike will help increase ROM and her overall endurance. Because the patient is returning home and appears to have a limited amount of outside help from friends and her boyfriend, a home visit made by PT or OT would benefit her in that any potential hazards, fall risks, or home environment issues can be addressed before she is discharged. The patient has not yet had her Foley catheter removed, but she would benefit from pelvic floor strengthening and education before returning home. Finally, because this patient's pain levels may vary daily, it is essential to modify the interventions accordingly.

Outpatient Setting

Pretreatment

Upon recent discharge from the inpatient rehabilitation setting, Ms. Harper has made steady progress with ROM but continues with notable bilateral lower extremity weakness. It appears that she is still using the FWW for ambulation with notable gait deviations. The patient complains of poor prolonged standing tolerance and has difficulty ambulating on uneven surfaces and going up and down stairs. She would benefit from the use of manual therapy and modality interventions to increase ROM and decrease pain, progressive gait training to address gait deviations, and balance and endurance activities. She continues to have difficulty with urinary incontinence, and a pelvic floor retraining program will be implemented along with the other therapeutic exercise program.

Treatment

To begin treatment, have the patient start with a warmup on either the treadmill or recumbent bike to help loosen up and relax her lower extremity muscles. With the patient on the treadmill, address any gait deviations. Starting at a slow speed of 1.0 mph with no incline, have the patient concentrate on heel strike and a slow and steady gait pattern, making sure she has adequate stride length and good postural awareness. After warming up while addressing gait, perform manual therapy interventions with the patient lying supine on a treatment table. This would consist of gentle soft tissue mobilization to her quadriceps muscles and anterior knee joint, followed by some patellar mobilizations and scar massage to her incision sites. Next, use manual, passive knee flexion and extension stretching, incorporating breathing techniques to help the patient relax and

stretch further and more comfortably. This should be followed by instruction with supine and standing exercises, many of which she will continue to do at home for her home exercise program. Exercises that the patient may have progressed to by this point in her rehabilitation process might include supine hip abduction/adduction, flexion, and extension with resistance bands or cuff weights to add resistance if needed for strengthening; supine bridging; and any of the exercises from the inpatient settings that were still challenging, such as straight-leg raises, short arc quadriceps, and long arc quadriceps. Of course, to progress ROM, she will need to incorporate exercises to stretch, such as knee extension stretches with her foot on a pillow, allowing gravity to assist the knee into extension, as well as working on flexion. With some patients, it works well to increase flexion by sitting on a high barstool or other seat and letting gravity provide a small amount of distraction force at the knee while the patient actively bends the knee. At this point, she might also be ready to progress toward standing exercises to promote strength of BLE as well as balance, such as small squats, calf/toe raises, standing hip abduction and extension, and hamstring curls, all first without and then with weights for resistance as the patient progresses. While the patient is completing these exercises, begin incorporating pelvic floor education, teaching the patient how to complete a Kegel as well as engage her core and pelvic floor muscles during exercise. Conclude the session with application of ice and electrical stimulation for pain management. Interferential electrical stimulation can be tried first because this type of stimulation often is very comfortable and helps reduce pain and spasms.

Post-treatment

As Ms. Harper continues to progress, gait training with a single-point cane or without an assistive device should be completed. Incorporate higher-level balance activities and strengthening exercises as tolerated. Also, communicating with the primary therapist any changes or concerns is helpful in the patient's recovery in that if the patient is not progressing or is having continued pain management issues, the interventions can be modified accordingly. An example of a SOAP note might appear like this:

Date

S: Patient notes continued poor prolonged standing tolerance greater than 15 minutes. Notes difficulty with stairs and feels unsteady when ambulating outdoors in garden on uneven surface. Rates right knee pain @ 4/10 and left knee pain @ 5/10 today.

O: Patient completed 10 minutes on treadmill @ 1.0 mph, no incline with VCs for increasing stride length and heel strike. This was followed by 15 minutes of soft tissue mobilization to bilateral quadriceps and anterior knee with BLE elevated, including scar massage to incision sites. Then she performed gentle passive bilateral knee extension and flexion stretching with instruction for pursed-lip breathing. Instructed patient in pelvic floor and core trunk awareness. Supine BLE therapeutic exercise including hip abduction/extension/flexion/adduction with blue resistance band, short arc quadriceps extensions with 1# weights, bridging all x 10 repetitions. Heel slides x 20 repetitions with 15-second hold. Standing BLE therapeutic exercise including hip flexion/extension/abduction, hamstring curls, small squats, and heel raises x 15 repetitions each with cues to lighten BUE support on counter to achieve greater challenge to balance. Right knee PROM flexion 5 to 103 degrees, left knee PROM flexion 5 to 108 degrees. Applied interferential electrical stimulation with cold pack to anterior knees x 20 minutes at end of treatment session. Patient complained of mild increased soreness to 6/10 post treatment bilateral knees.

A: Patient is making steady improvements with decreasing gait deviations and decreased antalgic gait along with improved PROM and strength.

P: Begin gait training with single-point cane at next session and continue to progress strengthening exercise within pain tolerance.

Mariisa Bonsen, PTA

Continuum of Care Critical Thinking Questions

Since having bilateral knee replacement, Ms. Harper has faced several challenges. Anxiety, respiratory MRSA, DM II, urinary incontinence, and pain management are all factors that have affected her recovery. Although the patient is still using a FWW, she has been able to slowly progress from requiring minimal assistance in the hospital to being independent with the device. She has continuously been limited by pain, so she has had a slow progression with her ambulation, but she has continued to make steady gains with ROM. It is important to discuss with the patient throughout treatment in all settings the realistic outcome of having a bilateral total knee replacement. Modifications were made throughout the different treatment settings based on

the patient's multiple challenges. For example, her DM II was treated with diet and insulin, and her increased pain was addressed by premedication before therapy treatments. After discussing and clearing with the primary PT, encourage Ms. Harper to increase her physical activity outside the clinic by either joining a health club to use exercise equipment such as the treadmill and recumbent bike or to participate in an aquatic exercise class. It would be important for her to complete activities that would be nonimpact or low impact because she suffers from osteoarthritis in other joints.

CHAPTER 7

Jennifer Koivisto, PTA

Acute Care Setting

Reviewing the Medical History

After reviewing the patient's medical history, it is clear that several factors need to be taken into consideration for therapy in the acute setting. First, the patient will have hip precautions. These will depend on what type of surgical approach is used, either posterior or anterior, and are in place to prevent the hip from dislocating. Second, the patient is taking Coumadin, an anticoagulant, which may result in deeper bruising but will also reduce the risk for blood clots. The PTA must take care not to increase bruising during therapy interventions such as any hands-on techniques. The patient also has a history of atrial fibrillation, so monitoring the patient's vital signs before, during, and after activity will be imperative to ensure the patient is responding appropriately to therapeutic activities. The patient is also using 3 LPM of supplemental oxygen and has a history of smoking, which will affect his activity level, endurance, and rate of healing. It will be important to monitor and record his oxygen levels with activity. Also to be taken into consideration are his previous left TKA, back surgery, and early dementia. Prior surgeries may indicate residual muscle weakness, tightness, or pain that can affect his progress in therapy now. Because of the dementia, he may not be able to consistently remember his precautions and may need to have them posted in his room to help him.

Critical Thinking Questions

Pretreatment at this point, pain and keeping precautions will be the biggest limiting factors for this patient. From the evaluation, it appears he has weakness in bilateral lower extremities and needs considerable assistance for bed mobility and transfers. It appears that some of his cognitive deficits have improved, but he is still having trouble remembering his precautions consistently. By seeing the patient's ability at his evaluation, the PTA can easily document progress. For example, if he needs Mod. A for bed mobility at initial evaluation, the PTA can monitor the level of assist needed at each treatment to see how well he is progressing and which areas he will need more help in. This patient would benefit from being premedicated before therapy to reduce pain.

Treatment: After reviewing the plan of care, a possible next treatment session would include instruction in bed mobility, transfer training, and supine lower extremity strengthening exercises while providing verbal and tactile cues to help the patient maintain his hip precautions. Begin the session with this patient by asking how he's doing, determining his pain level, and checking pertinent vital signs such as blood pressure, heart rate, and oxygen saturation. Proceed with instruction in bed mobility, specifically how to sit up in bed and bring his legs over the edge while maintaining his precautions. While he is at the edge of the bed, instruct the patient to stand with his FWW, cuing him on keeping his 90-degree precaution because he had the posterior approach. Then, have the patient transfer over to an appropriate W/C by taking a couple of steps with his walker. The patient should then transfer back to the edge of the bed and go from sitting back to supine. It is a good idea to monitor the patient's oxygen levels and any shortness of breath and to allow appropriate rest breaks between tasks. While the patient is supine, instruct him in quadriceps sets, hamstring sets, active-assisted abduction, adduction with a pillow between knees, gluteal sets, short arc quadriceps knee extensions with pillow under his knee, and possible active-assisted straight-leg raises with focus on contracting his quadriceps if he is able. After exercises, check his oxygen levels and also ask his pain rating. This is a great way to see how the patient is responding to the treatment. Throughout the treatment, it is always beneficial to ask the patient how he's doing and instruct him to let you know if he needs to take a rest break. If the patient is complaining of increased fatigue and/or pain with activity, the PTA may need to decrease the duration of treatment, reduce the repetitions, or otherwise modify the activity to make the exercise easier to complete.

Post treatment: The most important things to document for this patient would be his pain level; functional abilities, including bed mobility, transfers, and gait; and any exercises or activities used to assist him towards stated goals. This is what the SOAP note for this patient might look like:

Date

S: Patient states he feels sore "all over," mostly focused on right hip region. He rates his current hip pain as 4/10. He received pain medication approximately 1 hour ago.

O: BP = 122/65 mm Hg, HR = 65 BPM, O_2 = 96% on 3 LPM. Patient is able to recall 1/3 hip precautions. Instructed patient on all hip precautions and placed sign in room to help patient remember. Treatment today consists of bed mobility supine to sit edge of bed with Min. A for BLE and VCs to maintain hip precautions. Transfer training, sit to stand with Min. A with FWW, two steps around to W/C with verbal and tactile cues to reach back before sitting and sit slowly. O_2 = 93% on 3 LPM. Sit to stand from W/C to FWW with Min. A, two steps to edge of bed with VCs to maintain precautions. Sit to supine with Mod. A for BLE onto bed. Patient able to position himself using trapeze for scooting, with VCs for technique. Instructed patient in supine RLE therapeutic exercises, including quadriceps sets, hamstring sets, AAROM hip abduction, hip adduction sets with pillow, and gluteal sets, all 10 repetitions each. Attempted active assisted SLR, but patient too tired and sore to complete. O_2 = 92% on 3 LPM, patient rates pain 6/10 post treatment. Instructed patient in deep breathing technique. After 1 minute rest, O_2 = 96% on 3 LPM.

A: Patient is progressing with bed mobility from Mod. A to Min. A. He tolerates most exercises well without substantial increase in pain or decrease in O_2 saturation and is able to complete 10 repetitions of each showing improved strength and muscular endurance. Patient complains of increased pain and fatigue with SLR but this toward end of session.

P: Progress bed mobility, transfer training, gait training, and strengthening per plan of care.

Jennifer Koivisto, PTA

Things to Consider

This patient should continue to progress well toward his therapy goals. Once his pain is managed, he will most likely tolerate more strengthening and gait training. With every postsurgical patient, infection is something to be watched for as well. Note any increase in pain, swelling, or redness. If observed, these need to be brought to the nurse's attention immediately as well as to the primary PT. Also, from reading the previous summary, the patient may be dealing with some depression. It sounds like he has some serious family issues to deal with and prefers to stay isolated in his room. This is a great time to collaborate with the social worker to get feedback on any tips for working with the patient. Other disciplines that may affect the physical therapy progress are occupational therapy and nursing. Scheduling around his occupational therapy visits will allow the patient adequate rest and improved performance with each therapy. Additionally, nursing staff are critical team members who help address pain control, nutrition, bladder/bowel issues, and his previous heart condition.

Inpatient Rehabilitation Setting

Reviewing the Medical History

Mr. Jenkins has made good progress since leaving the hospital and transitioning to the inpatient rehabilitation facility. He continues to be limited by some cognitive impairments that lead to impulsiveness and decreased safety awareness. He may also have difficulty cooperating with therapy because he doesn't feel he has any major deficits and is also having increased agitation related to his nicotine addiction. It appears he still has limited mobility and reduced strength. His oxygen saturation levels look stable, but it is always a good idea to monitor this and any shortness of breath.

Pretreatment

After reviewing the current plan of care, the PTA will need to continue to work on bed mobility, transfer training, gait training, and lower extremity strengthening. As the patient progresses, exercises will focus more on endurance activities and balance activities. He will likely continue to need cues to remember precautions. Also, because of his cognitive deficits, he may need more repetitions with transfers and gait training to help him to be more aware of safety. He may still need pain medication before treatment. The PTA should check the nurses' notes to stay updated on any changes in the patient.

Treatment

For this treatment session, begin by checking his oxygen levels and asking the patient how he is doing, getting a pain rating. Because it appears his other vital signs have been stable, check these from the nurses' notes. Also, ask the patient whether he remembers his three hip precautions. Because the patient is dealing with some depression, it may be very helpful to take the patient out of his room and to the therapy gym for treatment. It is often beneficial for patients to be around others who are going through similar experiences or to just have a change of scenery. Work on bed mobility with the patient first, focusing on rolling to his side, maintaining hip precautions, then sitting on the edge of the bed. From sitting, have the patient transfer with his FWW to his W/C, cuing him as needed for his precautions. Taking the patient out into the hall can provide an open, obstacle-free area for gait training. Next, instruct the patient in gait training, cuing him for any deviations such as lack of heel strike and decreased left leg swing-through. The PTA should watch the patient closely to look for signs of fatigue in the RLE, specifically his gluteus medius, which will exhibit as a Trendelenburg gait. He may only be able to ambulate short distances and may require multiple rest breaks. Performing multiple short ambulation distances will allow for more repetition to properly cue the patient for safety during transfers and gait. In the therapy gym, after the patient has had a good rest and his oxygen levels have returned to normal if they had decreased, instruct him in seated therapeutic exercises. Seated exercises for this patient might include ankle pumps, long arc quadriceps (knee extension), hip abduction with a light resistance band, and hip adduction with a ball or pillow. This is also a good time to work on transfer training to and from a chair or mat table that can be raised. The patient can also complete the supine exercises he did in the hospital setting. As the patient progresses with his strength and endurance, he may progress to standing exercises with his FWW or at a counter or parallel bars, including calf raises, short squats, right hip flexion (below 90 degrees per the precautions), right hip abduction, and extension. After giving the patient an appropriate rest break, encourage him to take part in some of the social activities or assist him back to his room, transferring him back to bed if that is what he desired. Again, throughout the treatment session, it is important to ask the patient how he's doing, determining his pain and fatigue levels.

Post-treatment

Some important things to note in documentation would be the patient's subjective pain rating; any treatment, such as bed mobility, gait training, and therapeutic exercise; and how the patient responded to these treatments. It is important to always be mindful of how the patients are progressing towards their goals. This is what an example SOAP note might look like:

Date

S: Patient states his hip continues to be painful, especially with movement. He rates his current pain 5/10, 1 hour post pain medication. He states he is ready to go home.

O: Treatment today consists of bed mobility supine to sit edge of bed with Mod. A and verbal and tactile cues for sequencing. Sit to stand with FWW with Min. A with VCs to push off from bed; transfer to W/C with cues to step around and not pivot on the RLE. Gait training with FWW in hall 20 feet x 3 with Min. A, VCs for equal step length bilaterally and posture. Patient also needed cues to reach back for chair before sitting. Instructed patient in seated therapeutic exercises: ankle pump, long arc quadriceps extension, hip abduction with yellow resistance band, hip adduction isometrics with ball. Sit to stand from W/C to FWW x 5 repetitions Min. A with VCs for hand placement. Patient states he has increased fatigue and soreness post exercise; rates hip pain 7/10. Patient declines offer to join social event and requests to transfer back to bed to rest. Transfer W/C to edge of bed with Mod. A secondary to increased fatigue, sit to supine with Mod. A for BLE, Mod. A for positioning in bed.

A: Patient progressing with ambulation distance and technique as well as endurance, although noted increased fatigue at end of this session requiring increased assistance for bed mobility; this is not typical for this patient and may be due to prior occupational therapy session today just before physical therapy session and patient more fatigued.

P: Progress strengthening, transfer training, gait training, and bed mobility. Coordinate next session after patient is able to have at least an hour rest in his room prior.

Jennifer Koivisto, PTA

Things to Consider

In planning treatment interventions for this patient, the PTA may want to start with the most fatiguing activity, in many cases, gait training. Seated exercises usually are not going to be nearly as taxing as ambulation with proper form and technique. As the patient fatigues, he will be less able to correct his gait pattern and thus be at a greater risk for falls as well as developing faulty movement patterns that may become habitual and difficult to correct later. Assuming the patient continues to progress well with seated exercises, plan to progress him to standing exercises and balance activities. Also, begin stair training with the patient even if he does not have stairs at home; he may go somewhere in the community where he needs to go up a couple of steps, and it would be beneficial if he already knew the safest, easiest way to ascend/descend stairs. Since this patient is returning to an assisted living facility, a home visit would not typically be required. It is fairly safe to assume he will have an appropriate living space and accessibility. Hold treatment at any time if the patient complains of much increased pain, swelling, or increased shortness of breath or generally is not feeling well. These would all be indications to consult with nursing and the primary PT before continuing to provide interventions for the patient. Communication with other disciplines will also help the patient progress. OTs will have great insight into any difficulties the patient may face with toileting, dressing, or showering. Nursing will have good ideas when it comes to the best time of the day to approach the patient and of course to coordinate medication. If the patient is not progressing well, it is very useful to have other disciplines' input to help figure out why, and this information should be communicated to the primary PT right away in case changes to the plan of care need to be made. There may be many reasons for lack of progress in this patient, including but not limited to pain, depression, history of smoking, slow healing of the bone, surgical complications, lack of motivation, and infection. It is a great idea to sit down as a team to discuss these factors and also plan for discharge.

Outpatient Setting

Pretreatment

Mr. Jenkins is continuing to make good progress but is limited by pain and muscle spasms. He is currently ambulating with a cane and has a Trendelenburg gait. His goal is to not use an assistive device for outdoors, uneven ground ambulation. This is important to note because he can begin working on high-level balance activities, which will help him reach this goal. Some of his gait deficits may be due to muscle spasms, pain, and weakness. These are the areas to begin working on.

Treatment

Begin with a warmup of walking on the treadmill or riding a recumbent bike to help loosen up his muscles.

Then perform soft tissue mobilization (STM) of his low back and piriformis region with the patient lying prone with pillows to support his back if he can tolerate it and can get into the position easily while maintaining his hip precautions. If not, help the patient to lie on his left side with a pillow between his legs to maintain precautions. Because of his hip precautions, it would be very difficult to actively stretch his piriformis muscle, so the STM may be helpful to allow him improved ROM and decreased pain with ambulation and other activities. Next, assist him to complete standing hip abduction, extension, and flexion bilaterally. By working bilaterally, the patient will be working the right stabilizing musculature while doing left hip exercises. Add standing short squats, focusing on contracting bilateral gluteal muscles. He could also do a standing hip flexor stretch bilaterally to help correct his standing posture. Then have the patient work on proper gait form with his single-point cane. If he is able to maintain correct form and proper technique, advance him to not using an assistive device. As the patient progresses, add high-level balance activities such as standing on a cushion, ball toss, and using a balance or rocker board. If possible, work with him outdoors negotiating curbs and uneven ground.

Post-treatment

Mr. Jenkins should continue to make good progress. His gait pattern and endurance should improve after his muscle spasms and pain decrease and his strength increases. Continue to progress his strengthening, endurance, and balance. If he is not progressing as expected or has significantly increased pain, consult with the primary PT to see what other changes can be made. Here is an example of a SOAP note from this treatment:

Date

S: Patient continues to complain of right hip pain 4/10 today. He also complains of tightness in his low back and muscle spasms.

O: Patient completed 10 minutes on recumbent bike at level 2 resistance to reduce muscle tightness, followed by 15 minutes of STM to the quadratus lumborum and piriformis on the right with the patient laying prone with pillows under his hips and ankles for comfort. Presents with increased tenderness/tightness palpated throughout right piriformis region. Instructed patient in standing BLE hip abduction/adduction/extension/flexion, all with green resistance band, short squats all

x 10 repetitions each with cues for proper technique and pacing. Gait training with single-point cane x 100 feet with VCs for sequencing and tactile cues to engage gluteus medius to correct Trendelenburg gait pattern. Patient able to correct with tactile cues.

A: Improving gait pattern, decreased Trendelenburg today. He is also progressing with exercise program, using increased resistance.

P: Begin dynamic balance activities at next visit; continue with gait training.

Jennifer Koivisto, PTA

Continuum of Care Critical Thinking Questions:

Over the weeks following Mr. Jenkins' hip replacement, he faced many challenges. He had to overcome pain, depression, and reduced mobility secondary to weakness and hip precautions. He continued to get stronger over time and was able to progress well to a cane and soon to ambulating without an assistive device. As the patient progressed, the level of difficulty with the exercises increased, and the level of assist and the need for assistive device decreased. Also, the patient needed to be continually observed for any new or changing behaviors or pain. For example, noticing in the inpatient setting that the patient was struggling with signs of depression allowed the medical staff to treat it with appropriate medication. The tight piriformis muscles and low back pain also needed to be monitored closely and addressed through STM or exercise modification. Because Mr. Jenkins lives in an assisted living facility, encourage him to participate in any group exercise programs if he can continually remember his precautions and encourage him to participate in any social events or gatherings to help with his depression. If the patient does not fully achieve good strength in his gluteus medius and reduce his piriformis tightness, he may exhibit more permanent gait deviations. This can be addressed in outpatient therapy and with a continued home exercise program as outlined by the primary PT in the plan of care.

CHAPTER 11

Susan Schofield, PTA

Acute Care Setting

The acute care physical therapy evaluation describes the patient as a 64-year-old female with a medical diagnosis S/P 1 day left CVA with right hemiparesis and a treatment diagnosis of decreased mobility. Patient presents with global aphasia (receptive and expressive), which prevents physical therapy assessments of pain, orientation, short-term memory, MMT, and sensation. The patient needs Max. A with bed mobility and transfers (using low pivot technique), has poor sitting/standing balance and right-sided neglect, and pushes and leans to the right. PLOF was active and independent. Interventions in the POC include bed mobility, transfers, balance training, home exercise program, therapeutic exercise, family education, and diabetic foot care education. PT to determine whether gait training is appropriate.

Precautions include poor balance and risk for falling, osteoporosis, dysphagia, NG tube, and elevated BP (per 2:00 PM nursing note).

Treatment based on the initial evaluation would include the following:

1. Stimulate patient orientation toward right side; PROM RUE/RLE
2. Family education regarding right unilateral neglect (if English-speaking family or other interpreter present or service available); enlist family's assistance with translating between English and Filipino for comprehension of treatment plan and verbal cueing
3. Assess BP/HR in supine
4. Bed mobility training: supine to sit with head of bed elevated for easier transition
5. Lower/flatten bed to place feet flat on floor; sitting balance drills on the edge of bed with tactile facilitation to trunk and extremities toward midline and to reduce pushing to the right
6. Assess BP/HR while sitting and if elevated or unstable alert nursing staff; if BP lowers drastically, especially with symptoms of lightheadedness, gently and slowly assist patient back to supine because of possible orthostatic hypotension.
7. Assess sitting balance and record level of assistance required, timed endurance for sitting, and ability to maintain with or without perturbations
8. Determine patient's tolerance for interventions and whether responses are appropriate (i.e., BP/HR stable, patient's level of alertness and participation, availability of second person for assistance if needed)
9. If patient has had a positive response thus far, attempt sit to stand, possibly with a second person to assist such as a CNA or nurse or physical therapy aide if available. Assess standing balance and BP/HR in standing, again, looking for possible orthostatic hypotension or BP or HR that is

elevated too much, demonstrating poor tolerance to standing.
10. Assist patient with transition from standing to sitting to right side lying to supine and position patient according to schedule; patients who are unable to reposition themselves are typically placed on a schedule to allow frequent position changes in order to prevent skin breakdown and pressure ulcers
11. Patient/family education focusing on any questions they may have

Skilled Nursing Facility Setting

The SNF physical therapy evaluation lists a medical diagnosis as "late effects of CVA" and a physical therapy treatment diagnosis as "general muscle weakness." Patient is now 6 days S/P left CVA with right hemiparesis upon admission to this facility. She has progressed from Max. A to Mod. A with bed mobility, sit to stand transfer with FWW, low pivot transfers with two-person assist, and standing balance. She is also able to follow one-step commands, verbalize "yes" and "no" consistently 75% of the time, and use the communication board. She requires verbal cueing 90% of the time to sequence movements for bed mobility, transfers, W/C mobility. She uses LUE and LLE to propel her W/C 25 feet with Min. A. Patient continues to have poor sitting balance, pushing strongly to her right side in both sitting and standing. She has been able to ambulate three steps in parallel bars with Max. A requiring facilitation to unweight RLE secondary to increased lateral shift/pushing toward right. She can tolerate sitting at edge of bed x 10 minutes and standing with FWW x 30 seconds to 1 minute. There is decreased tone in RUE and RLE but increased tone in the right plantarflexors. Plan of care includes therapeutic exercise, therapeutic activities, gait training, and electrical stimulation. To participate in therapy, the patient must be able to follow one-step commands and be alert and oriented x 3 (to person, place, and time). Precautions include aspiration and fall risk, osteoporosis, cardiac, PEG tube, and stage II decubitus ulcer on sacrum and stage I decubitus ulcer on left heel.

The preferred treatment based on the evaluation would begin with patient up and in her W/C and transported to the rehabilitation gym for the following:

1. Transfer training W/C to mat table toward her left side; typically, it is easier for a patient with hemiparesis to transfer toward his or her stronger side, and this is often a good place to start transfer

training. She will likely need Mod. A with VCs for sequencing

2. Mat activities:
   a. Sitting balance on edge of mat table with both feet on the floor using visual (mirror), tactile, and verbal feedback to improve midline orientation, BUE on stationary table in front of patient, PTA kneeling behind patient on mat table for RUE support, guarding and facilitation of neutral pelvis. Rest breaks as needed.
   b. Sitting balance on edge of mat table with both feet flat on floor using visual (mirror), tactile, and verbal feedback for midline orientation; BUE clasped together in lap (to decrease manifestation of "pusher syndrome" toward right side); PTA facilitating neutral pelvis and lateral weight shifts with emphasis on weight shift to left hip and LLE; assess required level of assistance.
   c. Transfer training for transition from sitting to right side lying (protecting right shoulder) and then to supine; assess required level of assistance.
   d. Supine bridging exercise with PTA stabilizing right knee and foot and facilitating weight-bearing through left foot (to combine hip extension with knee extension as pregait activity); assess required level of assistance and number of repetitions tolerated; repetitions and rest breaks as tolerated.
   e. Assist patient to bridge and scoot hips right and move to right side lying and to sitting on edge of mat; assess required level of assistance and monitor scooting to prevent skin shear secondary to skin breakdown on sacrum.
   f. After sitting a few minutes, practice partial sit to stand with patient's hands on PTA's forearms; progress to full sit to stand as patient is able; assess required level of assistance and number of repetitions tolerated and rest breaks needed.
3. Transfer training from mat table to W/C using low pivot technique toward right side this time; assess required level of assistance and need for verbal or tactile cues for sequencing.
4. W/C mobility training having patient use LUE and LLE as tolerated; assess distance and need for verbal or tactile cues; return to patient's room.
5. Instruct family and patient regarding pressure relief strategies when in W/C.

Outpatient Setting

The patient has been discharged to home from SNF with care from son, daughter-in-law, and AM/PM caregivers to assist with ADLs. She is now 3 months S/P left CVA with right hemiparesis. She can communicate with translation through her son and speaks a few Filipino words but primarily uses gestures and pictures on a communication board. She continues to have complications related to aphasia (i.e., can't comprehend pain scale). Pain continues in right shoulder requiring use of sling. The type of sling she is using allows use of her hand and elbow, supporting at the humerus to help hold the humeral head in the socket. She is still not able to manage the three steps to enter/exit her apartment. She is now able to ambulate 40 feet with modified FWW, right AFO, and Mod. A with decreased stance on RLE and unequal step length, with right greater than left. Her posture in sitting and standing has improved, although she continues to lean toward the right with head turned left owing to right-sided neglect. Her balance has improved to grade fair, and she can tolerate sitting at edge of mat table x 5 minutes with supervision and standing with left rail support x 8 minutes. Her total Tinetti score is 16/28, which indicates a high increased risk for falls. LUE and LLE MMT is WNL, and right extremities are not tested. She is to receive physical therapy three times per week x 4 weeks with the POC to include functional electrical stimulation/neuromuscular electrical stimulation to right shoulder for subluxation and pain control, motor control activities, therapeutic exercise, gait and balance training, cardiovascular exercise program, and home exercise program. Precautions include risk for falling and right shoulder pain due to slight subluxation.

The preferred treatment based on the evaluation is as follows (with family member or other translator attending):

1. Balance and posture training sitting on therapy ball:
   a. PTA facilitates gentle anterior-posterior pelvic tilts and lateral weight shifts, progressing to more dramatic movements to challenge balance and assess static and dynamic sitting balance; observe presence of normal righting responses
   b. Reaching with RUE in PNF pattern D2 flexion (flexion/abduction/external rotation) with head turning to follow hand movement to facilitate head/trunk rotation, PTA guarding and facilitating as needed from behind with aide or family member providing targets for reaching in front.
2. Standing balance and posture training with visual feedback (mirror):
   a. Instruct patient to stand in correct alignment while viewing self in mirror, PTA guarding from behind and to the right, assisting with RUE support; W/C close by if needed; provide tactile and

verbal cues to facilitate self-correction; time endurance for standing.

   b. RLE step-ups forward onto low, wide step, WBAT RLE, stepping up then down, high table nearby for LUE support; PTA behind and right for guarding and assisting with RUE support.

3. Gait training with body weight support system on treadmill, if available, or with FWW.

4. Family education regarding support and positioning of RUE and importance of increased use of RUE, decreased use of sling as tolerated to discourage learned nonuse.

5. Functional electrical stimulation of right shoulder seated at table with small cones for reaching/stacking using RUE.

Continuum of Care Overview

This patient made significant progress during approximately 3 months of skilled intervention by physical, occupational, and speech therapy. Her functional mobility progressed from inability to ambulate at all to ambulation x 40 feet with a modified FWW providing RUE support, Mod. A with tactile cues, and a right AFO to facilitate foot clearance during the swing phase of gait. Her sitting/standing balance progressed from poor to fair as she was able to sit/stand unsupported for 5/8 minutes, respectively. She learned to go up/down one step with a railing on the left with Max. A.

Her involved RLE changed from no motor control due to flaccid tone to fair motor control of the major muscle groups, and her RUE had beginning motor control of the elbow and wrist.

Her global aphasia progressed from no language skills to improved, although limited, use of words along with gestures and the use of a communication board in her native Filipino language. This enhanced her ability to communicate more directly with her therapists and caregivers because she doesn't speak English and has to rely on family members to translate. This language barrier does complicate her therapy because a translator ideally should be present for all sessions.

Her general medical condition improved with drug management of diagnosed HTN and DM II.

Uncontrolled blood pressure and blood sugar levels were present during the acute phase of her rehabilitation and could have limited her participation in therapies. She also started cholesterol-lowering drugs to help decrease the reoccurrence of MI or stroke.

Her family is able to take care of her at home with the assistance of part-time caregivers to help with bathing, dressing, and meals. This was what the patient and family had initially wanted as the discharge plan.

Continuing problems involve right shoulder subluxation, pain, and the need for a sling, which is often not the best long-term solution because further complications and problems related to the sling. She continues to require 24-hour care for assistance with ADLs and general mobility. She remains unable to enter/exit her home independently because of the three steps at the entrance. It is reasonable to assume she'll continue to progress if she participates in outpatient physical therapy, is compliant with prescribed home exercise programs, and leads a reasonably active lifestyle in a safe, modified, and supervised home environment.

CHAPTER 12

Susan Schofield, PTA

Acute Care Setting

The following is information from the initial physical therapy evaluation that should be considered:

Mr. Jones is an 83-year-old male; transported to the hospital by paramedics after sustaining a fall at the base of his stairs; he complains of right shoulder and right hip pain on admission; assessed with right intertrochanteric hip fracture and right shoulder and head contusions; ORIF right hip performed 1/2/10.

His PMH includes Parkinson disease, HTN, DM II, peripheral neuropathy, mild obesity, hyperlipidemia, osteoarthritis, aspiration pneumonia 1 year ago, left TKR 5 years ago.

PLOF: lives at home with 82-year-old wife; has a history of five or six falls last year; ambulates with a single-point cane independently.

Treating diagnosis: Decreased mobility S/P ORIF right hip

Current level of function: Bed mobility one-person Tot. A; transfers with FWW, TTWB RLE with two-person Tot. A, gait unable, stairs unable.

Sitting balance edge of bed good with BUE support x 10 minutes, standing balance poor, requiring Mod. A with FWW.

Precautions: TTWB RLE; fall risk; risk for skin breakdown secondary to decreased sensation plantar surfaces of feet; impaired proprioception bilateral great toes and ankles; short-term memory deficit, unable to remember weight-bearing precautions, aspiration risk. Monitor for any signs or symptoms of increased coughing, chest congestion, or difficulty breathing that could indicate aspiration pneumonia. Also, carefully observe his skin during intervention sessions to monitor for any signs of redness or other skin changes that might indicate developing pressure ulcers. Because of his short-term memory deficits, use concise directions when giving VCs and use repetition to enhance learning.

POC: Patient's goals are to return home after rehabilitation and to return to group exercise class for PD at YMCA.

Discharge goals: bed mobility and transfers, Mod. A; gait x 50 feet, Mod. A with FWW; home exercise program, Min. A.

Interventions included in the POC: bed mobility and transfer training, balance and gait training, therapeutic exercise, therapeutic activities, home exercise program, diabetic foot care education, family training PRN.

Intervention Strategies

Based on the initial evaluation and POC, consider the effects of his rigidity related to the clinical signs of PD, especially in neck/trunk, and also note limitations in BUE/LE ROM. Concentrate on isometric exercises, protected ROM, bed mobility, transfers, and gait as tolerated with TTWB RLE. Note that venous thrombosis is a common complication in elderly patients after hip fracture and be alert to signs and symptoms, such as aching, burning, tenderness, pain, and edema, especially in the affected leg. Before beginning, obtain the patient's perceived pain level of RLE and then proceed as follows:

1. Gentle, rhythmic PROM BLE supine in bed with goal of relaxation and decreased rigidity to allow improved function during following exercises.
2. Active bilateral ankle pumps with patient/family education to repeat this exercise frequently when in bed to increase circulation and decrease possibility of deep vein thrombosis.
3. Supine to sit at EOB with both feet on floor with RLE forward to decrease weight bearing.
4. Patient/family education regarding TTWB RLE in seated position.
5. Lateral, rhythmic weight shifts in sitting using BUE for support as needed.
6. Sit to stand to FWW, TTWB RLE with additional patient/family education regarding TTWB RLE in standing.

7. Stand to sit at edge of bed. Assess patient's response to treatment by asking pain level RLE, observing signs and symptoms of fatigue. Continue sit to stand drills if there is no significant increase in pain level and patient is willing.
8. Time standing tolerance, assess level of assistance required and standing balance with FWW.
9. Stand to sit to supine. Obtain pain level for RLE especially surgical site.
10. Patient/family education regarding weight-bearing precautions in supine, sitting, and standing positions, including possible complications of decreased mobility. Assess patient and family learning of precautions.

Document levels of assist for bed mobility and transfers; patient's ability to recall and adhere to weight-bearing precautions; pain level before, during, and after interventions; and sitting and standing balance levels. Note any difficulties following directions or initiating and sequencing movements, or motor planning deficits that could be related to PD. Document patient/family education related to complications of decreased mobility and importance of adhering to weight-bearing precautions.

At the next session, advance to gait with FWW and initiate BLE exercises in sitting.

Skilled Nursing Facility Setting

The SNF physical therapy evaluation lists a primary medical diagnosis as "right hip fracture S/P ORIF" and a treatment diagnosis of "difficulty in walking." Precautions continue to be TTWB for RLE, high fall risk, and peripheral neuropathy secondary to DM II. The patient has progressed to requiring Mod. A for bed mobility and transfers and Min. A for gait x 10 feet with FWW and TTWB RLE. Continues to require VCs for weight-bearing precautions. He reports 7-9/10 pain at surgical site and 5-7/10 pain in right shoulder. He has limited AROM right hip secondary to pain and −20 degrees bilateral knee extension. There is rigidity in the trunk and extremities. Patient demonstrates a flexed, stooped posture common in PD and often associated with weak trunk extensor muscles, although these are not included in the initial evaluation. This postural dysfunction may contribute to poor balance because body weight is forward to the base of support. He scores 15/28 on the Tinetti. The D/C plan continues to be a return to home with wife assisting with cooking and cleaning and patient independent with ADLs.

POC includes therapeutic exercise and activities, gait training, and electrical stimulation for pain.

The preferred treatment based on the evaluation would begin with patient up in W/C and transported to the rehabilitation gym. Check in with nursing before treatment time to ensure pain medication was administered in advance of physical therapy session. Proceed as follows:

1. Slow, repetitive, rhythmic, rotational movements before functional training to decrease rigidity of PD. Start with mat activities as follows:
   a. Deep breathing exercises: patient sitting on edge of mat table, feet on floor with RLE forward to lessen RLE weight-bearing, bilateral hands on mat and abducted as tolerated; therapist kneeling behind patient on table, facilitating anterior pelvic tilt and trunk extension during inspiration and posterior pelvic tilt and trunk flexion during expiration. Start with small trunk ROM and progress as indicated. Eyes closed if balance not affected to remove visual aspect of balance.
   b. Seated anterior/posterior pelvic tilting/rocking with BUE resting on thighs to challenge balance further.
   c. Sitting to left side lying to supine transition.
   d. Hook-lying position with BLE resting on therapy ball to facilitate slow, rhythmic side-to-side rotation (bilateral hip internal/external rotation) and anterior-posterior rotation (bilateral hip extension/flexion).
   e. Supine to left side lying to sitting transition.
2. Sit to stand to FWW, TTWB RLE with verbal and tactile cues for erect posture.
3. Gait training with FWW and W/C following with focus on posture, following weight-bearing precautions. Standing or seated rest breaks as needed.
4. Sitting in W/C, hip flexion and marching in place.
5. Sitting in W/C, knee extension and kicking a ball.
6. Gentle stretching in sitting for bilateral knee extension and ankle dorsiflexion.

This patient has postural impairments that contribute to instability and a high risk for falling.

He has significant pain in the affected hip that is exacerbated by exercise and functional activity. There is limited right hip and bilateral knee extension that contributes to an abnormal gait pattern, as does the weight-bearing precaution. Increased tone and rigidity in the trunk and extremities put the patient at risk for contracture formation, increased postural deformity, dysphagia, and dysarthria. Despite all this, the patient is improving

as he advances from acute to subacute rehabilitation. His level of assist has progressed from Max. A to Mod. A for bed mobility and transfers, and he can now tolerate standing and 10 feet of gait with a FWW while maintaining TTWB RLE. It is reasonable to expect continued progress for this patient as pain management measures effectively decrease right hip and right shoulder pain and overall strength and endurance increase. When the physician upgrades the patient to WBAT, he should be able to make even quicker progress toward functional goals. It will be important to begin each physical therapy session with relaxation exercises that temporarily inhibit rigidity caused by PD, allowing more extensive ROM throughout the trunk and extremities.

Document subjective data related to perceived pain of right hip and shoulder before and after interventions. Document level of assistance for functional mobility, including transfers, gait, and balance activities. Collect and report data on gait distance, need for VCs for safety, and patient's level of alertness and ability to follow multistep commands. Stay alert to signs and symptoms of deep vein thrombosis, pneumonia, skin integrity issues, orthostatic hypotension, cognitive dysfunction, and depression.

A change in any of these areas would be cause to notify the primary PT.

Outpatient Setting

Jennifer Koivisto, PTA

Mr. Jones is 4 months post right hip fracture with ORIF. He has spent 13 weeks in an inpatient rehabilitation facility and has progressed well with his strength and mobility. He currently is experiencing continued right hip pain, rating it 4/10. He is using Tylenol and occasional Percocet for pain. He complains of a "funny gait" pattern while ambulating approximately two blocks outside. Mr. Jones is independent with ADLs and is WBAT with the RLE using his FWW for stability. He would like to return to his local pool for exercises and continue losing weight. The patient will be seen two or three times per week for 8 weeks for manual therapy, heat/cold, electrical stimulation, modalities to increase ROM and decrease pain, therapeutic exercise including aquatic exercise and gait training, and development of progressive home exercise program.

Begin the first treatment session by asking Mr. Jones his current pain scale and observing his natural gait pattern upon arrival. Then have him warm up on either the recumbent bike or another type of lower extremity bicycle ergometer to improve strength, increase endurance, and improve ROM in the hip. Next, instruct the patient in standing hip exercises to strengthen the affected hip and gluteus musculature. Have the patient complete standing hip abduction, extension, and flexion bilaterally. By working bilaterally, the patient is working the right stabilizing musculature while doing left hip exercises. He could then complete standing short squats, focusing on contracting bilateral gluteus muscles, and standing hamstring curls to strengthen the hamstrings. In the pool, Mr. Jones could complete all his standing exercises and add kicking with a kickboard and walking in the water forward, backward, and sideways. As the patient progresses with his exercise program and endurance, add seated trunk rotation, side-lying clamshells, supine trunk rotation, step-up/down to increase quadriceps strength, balance activities such as static standing with eyes open/closed, single-leg standing, tandem stance, and backward walking. Include some passive hamstring/gastrocnemius stretching to decrease bilateral knee contractures to improve standing posture. Instruct the patient in outdoor gait training with his FWW focusing on correct posture, appropriate bilateral stride length, proper trunk rotation, and heel strike bilaterally. It is also important to observe the patient's use of his FWW and make sure it does not get too far ahead of him because many PD patients tend toward a forward flexed posture.

In documenting the patient's progress, it is important to note several key factors, including the patient's subjective pain rating; any other complaints the patient may have; what was done for treatment, durations, and frequency; the patient's level of assistance or assistive device; how the patient responded to treatment and any progress noted; and the plan for next treatment. It would also be important to make note of patient's gait and any deviation or corrections noted. Also note any significant changes or "red flags" that need to be brought to the attention of the primary PT, such as a fall, increased pain, poor response to previous treatment, or any other abnormal symptoms.

Continuum of Care Critical Thinking Questions

The patient has gone through many changes over the past few months. He has had to overcome pain, weight-bearing restrictions, decreased mobility, and transitions in care settings. It is important to note how the interventions of therapy and goals have evolved since he first had his fracture. In the beginning, the goals were primarily pain reduction, improving bed mobility, and transfer training, all very functional activities to help him move around his environment. Then, his care progressed to include strengthening and stretching as well as gait training with his weight-bearing restrictions to help him transition back to his home setting. Finally, in the outpatient setting, the goals become mostly focused on strengthening and gait training so that the patient can fully return to community participation, including going to his pool to work out. Therapy interventions must be constantly monitored and adjusted to increase the patient's mobility, without overdoing it. The exercises he began in the hospital setting eventually became too easy and were progressed from sitting to standing exercises and eventually dynamic balance training exercises. The patient has a great goal to return to his group exercise, which provides an important social outlet as well as an excellent environment for maintaining his mobility through the various stages of PD. He may be interested in some PD support groups.

Implications of Pathology for the PTA

1. Mr. Jones is at a higher fall risk because of PD. Some of the common symptoms of PD are shuffling gait, decreased stride length, and difficulty stopping and starting. With gait training focusing on stride length and initiation, some of these risks can be lessened. Mr. Jones would also benefit from high-level balance activities to challenge and maintain his balance.

2. Signs and symptoms of DVT include redness, swelling, increased warmth, and pain, usually in the calf. Symptoms of infection are fever, increased pain and redness at the incision site, swelling, and usually a general feeling of unwellness. For pulmonary complications, monitor the patient's shortness of breath and oxygen saturation with activity. If any changes are noted, first inform the primary therapist. In an inpatient setting, inform the nurse on duty. In any setting, it is important to document any changes as well.

3. Monitor cognitive and decision-making capabilities to make sure the patient understands what weight-bearing as tolerated means and how to avoid overdoing it. If the patient is having cognitive deficits and is impulsive, he may be putting himself at risk for further injury or reduced healing. Sensation, including proprioception, is important to monitor to make sure the patient has proper feeling and balance reaction to prevent falls or injury. If the

patient has impaired sensation, he may not be able to appropriately feel pain and may actually be injuring the affected lower extremity. If the patient is lacking proprioception, he may be at a greater risk for falls. Upper body strength is important to make sure the patient can take some of his body weight through his upper extremities to take some of the weight off his lower extremity. The patient's vestibular function and balance are important to note so that the patient does not accidentally try to "catch" himself with his affected lower extremity and thus increase his weight-bearing and injure the leg.

4. Properly timing the patient's PD medications is important because it will decrease the symptoms and allow for improved mobility. If the patient's medications are at their peak effectiveness, he will have reduced shuffling and be able to perform better with less fall risk.

5. Cognitive impairment may reduce the ability of the patient to follow VCs or multistep commands. The patient may need to be cued in easy one-step commands, with tactile cues for exercises. Cognitive impairment may also limit the effectiveness of the patient remembering commands. More repetition may be necessary to allow for implementation of gait cues.

6. With all these conditions, it is important to be aware of the patient's weight-bearing and mobility restrictions, pain, and overall health, which may limit the patient's ability to perform in therapy.

CHAPTER AND PRIMARY DIAGNOSIS	PAST MEDICAL HISTORY	OTHER FACTORS	AGE AND GENDER	PHYSICAL THERAPY SETTINGS
2: Myocardial Infarction	Obesity, HTN, appendectomy		51-year-old male	• Acute
3: Chronic Obstructive Pulmonary Disease	MS, anxiety, depression, emphysema, bronchitis, fibromyalgia syndrome, CAD, allergies	Socioeconomic	65-year-old female	• Acute
4: Rotator Cuff Repair	Hypothyroidism, high cholesterol, depression		38-year-old male	• Acute • Outpatient
5: Laminectomy	HTN, DM II, epilepsy	Cultural	45-year-old male	• Acute • Outpatient
6: Bilateral Total Knee Replacement	Bladder cystocele, urinary incontinence, anxiety, OA, DM II, obesity		57-year-old female	• Acutc • Inpatient Rehab • Outpatient
7: Total Hip Replacement	Prostate CA, atrial fibrillation, COPD, dementia	Ethical Socioeconomic	74-year-old male	• Acute • Inpatient Rehab • Outpatient
8: Below Knee Amputation	Obesity, HTN, elevated lipids, high cholesterol, DM II, neuropathy, retinopathy, GERD, DJD	Ethical Socio-economic	66-year-old female	• Acute • Inpatient Rehab • Home Health • Outpatient
9: Traumatic Brain Injury	Tonsillectomy	Social	13-year-old male	• Acute • Inpatient Rehab • Home Health • Outpatient
10: Spinal Cord Injury	ADHD, seizure disorder	Ethical Socioeconomic	17-year-old female	• Acute • Inpatient Rehab • Outpatient
11: Cerebrovascular Accident	Osteoporosis, MI, HTN, DM II, appendectomy, cesarean sections	Cultural	64-year-old female	• Acute • SNF • Outpatient
12: Hip Fracture and Parkinson Disease	HTN, elevated lipids, DM II, neuropathy, OA, obesity, aspiration pneumonia, prior TKR, PD		83-year-old male	• Acute • SNF • Outpatient

continued

CHAPTER AND PRIMARY DIAGNOSIS	PAST MEDICAL HISTORY	OTHER FACTORS	AGE AND GENDER	PHYSICAL THERAPY SETTINGS
13: Cerebral Palsy	Peanut allergy, seizure disorder	Ethical	7-year-old female	• School
14: Down Syndrome	Ventricular septal defect; frequent ear infections; atlantoaxial instability (AAI)		3-year-old male	• School

AAROM	active assisted range of motion
AROM	active range of motion
ABI	ankle brachial index
ADA	American Diabetes Association
ADHD	attention deficit hyperactivity disorder
ADL	activity of daily living
AFO	ankle foot orthosis
AKA	above knee amputation
ALF	assisted living facility
APTA	American Physical Therapy Association
ASIA	American Spinal Injury Association
BID	twice per day
BKA	below knee amputation
BLE	bilateral lower extremities
BM	bowel movement
BMI	body mass index
BP	blood pressure
BPM	beats per minute
BUE	bilateral upper extremities
BUN	blood urea nitrogen
C	celsius
CABG	coronary artery bypass graft
CAD	coronary artery disease
CBC	complete blood count
C-Diff	*Clostridium difficile*
CGA	contact guard assist
CM	centimeters
CMP	comprehensive metabolic panel
CNA	Certified Nursing Assistant
COPD	chronic obstructive pulmonary disease
COTA	Certified Occupational Therapy Assistant
CPS	Child Protective Services
CPR	cardiopulmonary resuscitation
CROM	cervical range of motion
CT	computed tomography
CVA	cerebrovascular accident
D/C	discharge or discontinue
DJD	degenerative joint disease
DME	durable medical equipment
DM II	type 2 diabetes mellitus
D.O.	doctor of osteopathy
DSHS	Department of Social and Human Services
DTR	deep tendon reflex
DVT	deep vein thrombosis
ECF	extended care facility
ECG	electrocardiogram

EMS	emergency medical service
FBG	fasting blood glucose
FWW	front wheeled walker
GERD	gastroesophageal reflux disease
H & P	history and physical
HEENT	head, extremities, ear, nose and throat
HDL	high-density lipoprotein
Hg A$_{1c}$	hemoglobin A$_{1c}$ or glycated hemoglobin A$_{1c}$
HOH	hard of hearing
HPI	history of present illness
HR	heart rate
HTN	hypertension
IADL	instrumental activity of daily living
ICU	intensive care unit
IEP	individualized educational program
IM	intramuscular
INR	International normalized ratio (pertains to prothrombin time)
IV	intravenous
KG	kilogram
LDL	low-density lipoprotein
LLD	leg-length discrepancy
LLE	left lower extremity
LPN	Licensed Practical Nurse
LTG	long-term goal
LUE	left upper extremity
LPM	liters per minute
LROM	lumbar range of motion
MD	Medical Doctor
Max. A	maximum assist
MI	myocardial infarction
Min. A	minimal assist
mcg	micrograms
mg	milligrams
mm Hg	millimeters of mercury
MMT	manual muscle testing
Mod. A	moderate assist
Mod. I	modified independent
MRA	magnetic resonance angiography
MRI	magnetic resonance imaging
MRSA	methicillin-resistant *Staphylococcus aureus*
MS	multiple sclerosis
MSW	Medical Social Worker
N/A	not applicable
NDT	neurodevelopmental technique

NKDA	no known drug allergies
NT	not tested
NWB	non-weight-bearing
O₂	oxygen
ORIF	open reduction internal fixation
OT	Occupational Therapist
PACU	postanesthesia care unit
PD	Parkinson disease
PEG	percutaneous endoscopic gastrostomy
PLOF	prior level of function
PMH	past medical history/pertinent medical history
PNF	proprioceptive neuromuscular facilitation
PROM	passive range of motion
PRN	as needed
PT	Physical Therapist
PT/INR	prothrombin time/International normalized ratio
PTA	Physical Therapist Assistant
PT/PTT	prothrombin time/partial thromboplastin time
PO	orally
POC	plan of care
PSA	prostate-specific antigen
PWB	partial weight-bearing
RCR	rotator cuff repair
RCT	randomized controlled trial
RLE	right lower extremity
RN	Registered Nurse
ROM	range of motion
RPE	rate of perceived exertion
RR	respiratory rate
RUE	right upper extremity
SBA	stand by assistance
SCI	spinal cord injury
SLP	Speech Language Pathologist

SLR	straight-leg raise
SNF	skilled nursing facility
SOAP	subjective, objective, assessment, plan (parts of a SOAP note)
SOB, SOBE	shortness of breath, shortness of breath on exertion
SOC	start of care
S/P	status post
SpO₂	oxygen saturation
ST elevation	refers to a type of MI with elevation of the ST segment on the ECG
STG	short-term goal
STML	short-term memory loss
TAH	total abdominal hysterectomy
TBD	to be determined
TBI	traumatic brain injury
THR, THA	total hip replacement, total hip arthroplasty
TFL	tensor fascia lata
TKR, TKA	total knee replacement, total knee arthroplasty
TLSO	thoracolumbosacral orthosis
TTWB	toe-touch weight-bearing
Tot. A	total assist
UTI	urinary tract infection
VC	verbal cue
VPS	Verbal Pain Scale
WBAT	weight-bearing as tolerated
WBC	white blood cell
W/C	wheelchair
WFL	within functional limits
WNL	within normal limits
X	for
#	number

Index